Biomedical Library

Queen's Un sity Be

Tel:

mail

BRAIN
DAMAGE
AND
RECOVERY

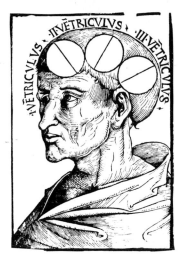

BRAIN DAMAGE AND RECOVERY

RESEARCH AND CLINICAL PERSPECTIVES

Stanley Finger

*Department of Psychology
and Neurobiology Program
Washington University
St. Louis, Missouri*

Donald G. Stein

*Department of Psychology
Clark University
Worcester, Massachusetts
and
Neurology Department
University of Massachusetts Medical Center
Worcester, Massachusetts*

ACADEMIC PRESS 1982
A Subsidiary of Harcourt Brace Jovanovich, Publishers

New York   London
Paris   San Diego   San Francisco   São Paulo   Sydney   Tokyo   Toronto

ACADEMIC PRESS, INC.
111 Fifth Avenue, New York, New York 10003

United Kingdom Edition published by
ACADEMIC PRESS, INC. (LONDON) LTD.
24/28 Oval Road, London NW1 7DX

Library of Congress Cataloging in Publication Data

Finger, Stanley.
  Brain damage and recovery.

  Includes index.
  1. Brain damage. 2. Nervous system--Regeneration.
I. Stein, Donald G. II. Title. [DNLM: 1. Brain injuries
--Rehabilitation. 2. Central nervous system--Physio-
pathology. 3. Brain damage, Chronic--Rehabilitation.
WL 354 F497]
RC387.5.F56   616.8   82-6846
ISBN 0-12-256780-3   AACR2

PRINTED IN THE UNITED STATES OF AMERICA

82 83 84 85   9 8 7 6 5 4 3 2 1

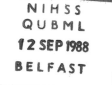

Contents

Preface

This book began as a review on recovery of function that was to be published with other essays on neuroplasticity and behavior. While writing, we soon became convinced that more had to be said about the whole question of recovery from brain damage and the relationship between the observed recovery, the underlying physiology, the theory of localization, and beliefs about how the nervous system may function in health and disease.

Almost everyone is aware of the tragedy that can occur when someone is afflicted with a brain injury or a disease of the central nervous system. In many cases, all that seems to be available are words of comfort for the family and hospitalization or pity for the victim. Why should the outcome of severe injury to the central nervous system be seen in such a pessimistic light? Is it really because there is no hope for treatment or recovery from brain damage? Or is it because theories and paradigms currently in vogue keep physicians and scientists from exploring new directions in therapy and considering alternative views about how the brain may work?

As we continued our exploration of the literature we realized that part of the problem was communicative. That is, the individuals who were studying recovery of function were not effectively conveying their findings to those who could make the most use of the new observations and information. There was no professional society devoted to the study of recovery from brain damage, no journal, and not even a monograph dealing with recovery from integrated anatomical, physiological, and behavioral perspectives.

For years, both of us worked on recovery from brain damage and in preparing our review we became convinced that a major attempt to piece the diverse findings together would be an exciting and worthwhile endeavor. We believed and wanted to demonstrate that the central nervous system could no longer be viewed as a static entity. The time had come to view the brain as an organ that is constantly in flux and as a structure capable of dramatic changes following injury or environmental challenges.

We began by returning to the historical literature. What were the early conceptions of brain function? When did scholars first begin to think of the brain as a collection of parts, each mediating a unique, specific behavioral function? What kinds of data were used to support various beliefs and claims? Our historical review showed us how current models of brain organization evolved and underscored the fact that some of the same concepts and issues that are debated today were proposed and argued decades, if not centuries, ago. Thus, we decided to make history one of the major themes in our book. In addition to devoting two chapters specifically to it, we also discuss the historical antecedents of the ideas that are examined in the other 16 chapters.

Another recurrent theme is the importance of casting recovery of function and neuroanatomical plasticity in a developmental perspective. This is because the ways that the central nervous system responds to injury are, in many cases, "age-linked" and because some of the best behavioral evidence for recovery can be found in articles on young children and animals that suffer brain injuries. Furthermore, there is reason to believe that some of the mechanisms thought to underlie recovery may not have evolved for this purpose at all. Indeed, survival and recovery from severe brain damage was and probably still is a very rare occurrence in nature in most circumstances. In this light, it may be worthwhile to consider those anatomical and physiological events that characterize early development and the idea that some anatomical and physiological effects of brain damage may represent a return to an earlier developmental state.

The third theme is that a multitude of factors can affect the outcome of a brain injury and consequently enhance or retard recovery of function. Many of these factors can be related to the condition of the remaining brain. Some of the variables that we consider are nutritional history, experiential background, the growth characteristics of the lesion, and the general health of the organism. One of the conclusions we reach is that recovery, when it is observed, cannot be attributed to only one type of event or series of happenings in the central nervous system. Recovery, in our estimation, has no monolithic explanation.

Although much of our book is devoted to the research findings on neural plasticity and recovery of function, the last two chapters were the most interesting and challenging for us. Here, we attempted a more complete integration of the data and asked the most perplexing of all questions: What does it all mean? We do not have all the answers, but many of the findings that we review do have relevance for brain-damaged patients, and physicians and scientists. Thus, in the final chapters we show how the principles discussed can be applied to patient care and treatment, and we also deal with the relationship between recovery of function and brain theory. We criticize blind adherence to the idea that brain lesions can reveal the functions of the damaged areas, and we propose that a greater effort should be made to use brain lesion techniques to understand why symptoms can vary so greatly across subjects and patients with similar lesions. We also argue for a more holistic view of brain function than is currently in vogue.

One of the most exciting things about brain research is that there is still room for many different approaches and many ways of thinking about how the nervous system works. Technical expertise and new tools are always needed, but so are new paradigms and conceptions of nervous organization, especially if they can show some of the limitations of looking at a problem in only one way. We hope that this book will lead to a greater appreciation of the problem and a sharper distinction between fact and theory. If the research literature on plasticity and recovery can achieve more recognition and more clarity as a result of our work, and if we can stimulate more thinking and new ideas about how the nervous system functions before and after brain damage, our efforts will have been worthwhile.

A brief statement must be made about the work we have done together. For the most part, writing this book as a joint venture was a pleasure. Both of us learned many new things, especially about the history of ideas in the brain sciences. We did not always share the same opinion and sometimes it seemed as if our differences might delay us in finishing our task. Yet, the differences in outlook turned out to be a blessing in disguise; we were often forced to reconsider and reevaluate our ideas and interpretations. Through this process, we both learned a great deal about neural ''plasticity'' and came to respect each other's way of viewing and interpreting the field to which we have devoted so much of our time and effort.

As the writing came to an end, we had to decide who would be first author. Both of us felt that the only reasonable way to decide was through the toss of a coin—the result appears on the cover and title page of this book.

BRAIN
DAMAGE
AND
RECOVERY

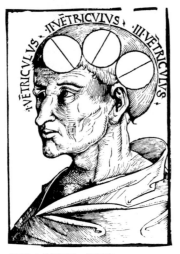

Problems and Paradigms

Pursuit of an anomaly is fruitful only if the anomaly is more than non-trivial. Having discovered it, the scientist's first efforts and those of his profession are to do what nuclear physicists are now doing. They strive to generalize the anomaly, to discover other and more revealing manifestations of the same effect, to give it structure by examining its complex interrelationships with phenomena they still feel they understand [Kuhn, 1977, p. 236].

This book is our attempt to examine a problem which some would consider to be an "anomaly" of brain function repeatedly observed. The anomaly derives from the observation that organisms, under certain conditions, are capable of dramatic recovery from traumatic and often extensive injury to the brain. When such recovery is seen, it is usually thought to represent an exception to the rules that cerebral functions are localizable and that damage to a specific area leads to an irreparable loss of function.

Contemporary neuroscience, with its emphasis on reductionistic philosophy and molecular techniques stressing unit recordings, ultrastructural analyses, biochemical assays, and the tracing of anatomical pathways, has reinforced the development of a "new phrenology" where each separate unit of the nervous system has its assigned role and specific function. In contrast, the alternate paradigm, which stresses an organismic–holistic approach to brain function, is thought of today as being essentially nonscientific or preparadigmatic. One reason for this is that the notions it proposes to account for brain–behavior relationships do not fall easily into the current reductionist paradigm. Although holists recognize that the reductionist model makes it easier to do research, they are quick to point out that currently accepted methodological approaches often avoid dealing with the complexity of cognitive behavior, or with the extensive variability in behavior among organisms of the same species or even those manifested by one subject at different times.

The reductionist view leads quite naturally to thinking of the brain as a collection of organs, each having a specified role in determining behavior. This, of course, is what we generally mean when we talk about *localization of function* in the central nervous system. In fact, we began our careers by attempting to confirm and follow the established views on localization by using the brain lesion method. As was being done by many other investigators, we created specific lesions in various parts of the brain in animals and then attempted to infer the functions of the damaged areas from the deficits and symptoms that we observed. However, as we began to look more carefully at our data and more critically at the journals, we started to note certain intriguing exceptions ("anomalies") to our accepted ways of thinking about lesion data and localization of function—exceptions that seemed to be largely ignored or treated as interesting curiosities by our colleagues working in research settings and by professionals treating patients in hospitals and clinics.

One such study that had tremendous impact on us was performed by John Adametz in 1959, while he was at the Washington University School of Medicine. Adametz decided to test the notion that the reticular formation of the brain was the "critical center" for the mediation and control of arousal and attention. In one group of cats, Adametz destroyed the reticular nuclei through the core of the formation. As expected, these animals fell into a deep coma and could not be induced into sustained arousal and consciousness by even the most intense stimulation. As would be predicted from the prevailing concept of *structure–function* (reticular formation–arousal) relationships, the animals soon died without ever manifesting normal sleep–wakefulness cycles or responses to peripheral stimulation like those seen in normal animals.

If Adametz had stopped his work with a comparison between the cats with lesions and those without central nervous system damage, his conclusion would have been simple—the reticular core of the brain is a necessary "center" for the control of arousal, a position strongly advocated by Lindsley (e.g., Lindsley, Schreiner, Knowles, and Magoun, 1949) and Magoun (1963) in their early studies on the "functions" of this brain-stem region of the central nervous system. Adametz, however, was not completely satisfied with this part of his experiment and so he went on to prepare another group of cats with the same extent of damage to the reticular formation of the brain, but this time inflicted in a number of discrete stages. Adametz spaced his multiple lesions 3 weeks apart so that the cats were allowed some recovery from each of the operations. Under these conditions, almost all of the cats survived massive destruction of the reticular core and eventually showed sleep–wakefulness cycles that closely resembled those of normal cats. Electrophysiological recordings from the cortex and a variety of behavioral indices also compared favorably with those taken from intact animals.

Thus, here was a clear anomaly. The data were difficult to interpret in the context of what was then being taught about localization of function because the findings did not support the idea that the reticular formation was in fact the critical center for sleep, wakefulness, and arousal. In short, the data presented by Adametz contradicted generally accepted ideas about how the brain was organized and how it ought to function. That is, according to formula, extensive damage to the reticular formation, no matter how inflicted, should have caused a severe disruption of consciousness. Yet, the animals not only survived, but even appeared to be alert and healthy!

To us, Adametz's experiment meant that it was time to reexamine some well-accepted views about how structure–function relationships could be derived for given brain areas, and the issue of just what was being localized in brain lesion experiments. Recalling Kuhn's statement at the beginning of this chapter, we thought that the findings were anomalous with respect to accepted reports and nontrivial with respect to the lesion-localization paradigm. Moreover, we were intrigued with these findings from a clinical perspective because they seemed to indicate that there might be ways to minimize the debilitating effects of brain injury. In any case, we attempted to see if the fast- versus slow-growing lesion effect would be found in our own experiments and, as Kuhn stated, tried to give it (the anomaly) structure by examining and relating the complex interrelationships with phenomena we thought we understood. As we will see (Chapter 9), our experiments did in fact show that staged brain lesions were less likely to be associated with symptoms and deficits than were similar lesions produced in a single operation, regardless of whether our target areas were classical sensory areas of the cortex (Finger, Marshak, Cohen, Scheff, Trace, and Neimand, 1971) or parts of the limbic system or association cortex (Stein, Rosen, Graziadei, Mishkin, and Brink, 1969).

In our enthusiasm to emphasize the recovery aspect of these staged lesion experiments and the contention that symptoms can vary in severity and perhaps not even appear at all after damage to supposedly "critical" structures in the brain, it might seem that we are trying to diminish the importance of studying the sometimes very severe consequences of acute brain damage. In our estimation, the clinical symptoms of acute brain damage are not trivial or unworthy of study. Quite to the contrary, the importance of systematically studying the severe effects of brain damage has long been recognized both by investigators working with animals in laboratory settings and medical personnel dealing with patients suffering from head wounds, strokes, and diseases of the central nervous system. The data collected in these investigations and more casual observations, bear directly on a number of practical issues in the health sciences. Such reports help physicians to judge whether symptoms might change with time, whether rehabilitation therapy might be helpful, and whether surgery should be attempted in certain cases.

In addition to these applied aspects of brain lesion research, such studies are important from a theoretical perspective. As we have already pointed out, the data allow us to speculate and hypothesize about the organization of the brain and how it might be functioning in both healthy and diseased states. Thus, for some people, the general premise is that by damaging cortical or subcortical struc-

tures and by assessing postoperative losses, structure–function relationships will
become apparent. Although the data obtained in these studies are subject to
multiple interpretations and hardly constitute "proofs" of such relationships,
brain lesion studies in the nineteenth and twentieth centuries have largely been
conducted and interpreted in this light.

The seemingly endless analyses of postoperative and posttraumatic behavioral
deficits, which began early in the nineteenth century, have contributed to the
development of functional maps of the brain (see Figures 1.1 and 1.2). These
maps depict the brain as a mosaic of identifiable parts, each of which is assumed to
play a role or a set of roles that, in at least some small way, distinguishes it from
other areas. The boundaries between the different areas are usually sharp and well
defined on these drawings, giving the impression that the dividing lines are
agreed upon by all investigators and that differences within a species are minimal,
if present at all.

As an example, let us take the drawings, figures, and verbal descriptions in
textbooks of neurology and biopsychology that tell us that the frontal lobes of the
brain play a very important role in higher intellectual functions. This idea stems
from animal research and some human case reports that have shown that after
these areas are damaged, subjects may be impaired on a number of cognitive
tasks, especially those utilizing spatial and temporal cues (e.g., French and

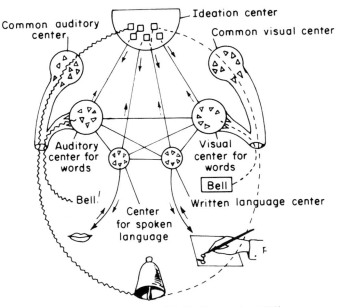

Figure 1.1. *Charcot's "Bell" diagram (ca. 1890).*

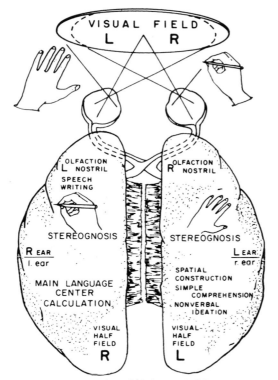

Figure 1.2. *Contemporary representation of higher cortical functions. (From Sperry, 1970.)*

Harlow, 1962; Settlage, Zable, and Harlow, 1948; Stamm, 1964). Nevertheless, even a quick review of this literature will show that cognitive deficits *do not* always emerge, even following massive frontal cortex lesions.

In like fashion, our textbooks tell us that the postcentral gyrus, or its homologue in mammals with nonconvoluted cerebral cortices, is the area of the brain that is responsible for tactile discriminative ability, especially on certain problems such as two-point discrimination (the subject must guess whether the skin is being touched by one or two points of a compass), and comparisons between surfaces differing in degree of roughness (e.g., Semmes and Mishkin, 1965). In fact, largely because of brain lesion experiments, the region just behind the Rolandic fissure in higher mammals, such as the monkey, is often called the "somatic" cortex or the "somatosensory" cortex. These are words that suggest that we know what the boundaries and precise functions of these areas really are. But if this were true, why are there differences of opinion over the boundaries of these zones (Woolsey, 1958)? Why would the deficits, following large lesions of somatosensory cortex, sometimes be transient (Norrsell, 1967; Schwartzman,

1972)? And why would the effects of these lesions be so variable among human patients that they might only be expressed as mathematical probabilities (Semmes, Weinstein, Ghent, and Teuber, 1960)?

Associations like these between structures and functions, of course, are not restricted to the cerebral cortex. A good example of a subcortical localization of function involves the hippocampus. Some lesion experiments on animals, and a few isolated human case reports, have led experimenters to conclude that this structure represents an important center for the formation of new memories. In the experimental literature, however, many new findings are confusing and contradictory, and the results most often cited have not always been easily replicated (Isaacson, 1974).

At the present time, there is not only a tendency to speak about the functions of general brain regions, such as the frontal association area or the hippocampus, but there is also a definite thrust to *subdivide* regions of the brain into even smaller units on the basis of morphological differences, cytoarchitecture and physiology, as well as on the basis of symptoms produced by subtotal lesions. In the case of the frontal cortex, for example, a sharp distinction has been made between the orbital and dorsolateral association zones (Goldman and Mendelson, 1977). Similarly, in subcortical zones, the amygdaloid complex is now being viewed as a number of nuclei, each of which may contribute something different to the symptoms that would be expected to appear if the entire structure were damaged. For instance, the basolateral part of the amygdala is perceived as having more to do with poor avoidance learning than the more corticomedial areas (Horvarth, 1963).

Correlative research in this tradition has advanced to the point where just about every area of the brain (and now even individual neurons) has been assigned a specific, behavioral function. Yet, despite the general acceptance of the paradigm employed to determine the functions of the various brain areas, the picture, as we have seen, is hardly one of agreement among investigators about what the precise and definitive functions might be in each case. After almost 200 years of making lesions to specify the "organs of the mind," one might ask why there is so much confusion, so little agreement, and why such limited progress has been made. Could this suggest that perhaps our interpretations extend well beyond our data, that our logic is faulty, and that possibly a "paradigm shift" might be helpful? We'll have more to say about these ideas later. Indeed, as we will see, attempting to understand the underlying nature of a deficit in a brain lesion study can be a very complex and challenging matter.

At the present time, with the help of modern technology in electrophysiology, biochemistry, and anatomy, there has emerged an implicit feeling that our beliefs about brain organization represent "truths," that is, that the paradigm need not be questioned. Indeed, some investigators have presented their data in a manner that would lead us to think that we have entered a stage in the history of the brain sciences where we finally understand, or at least are close to understanding, how the brain is organized and how it functions with respect to even highly complex cognitive behaviors.

Over the years, a number of principles and concepts have come to be associated with the notion that the brain is composed of a large number of distinct functional parts. From a developmental perspective, one of the more accepted concepts is that functions become associated with structures very early in life. Experiments performed on subjects of different ages, which may use anatomical, physiological, or behavioral measures, are interpreted as showing that by the end of the period of infancy, most structure–function relationships in the brain are firmly established or localized. It is further assumed that once a structure becomes "committed" to a function, it will lose its capacity for taking on new functions following damage to other parts of the brain. Thus, as the central nervous system develops and matures, it is viewed as progressing from a dynamic state to a more static or "fixed" state. With regard to brain damage, different rules are assumed to be operating in the two cases. This notion has played a major role in guiding the type of research that has been conducted on laboratory animals and has strongly influenced how we treat our patients in clinics and hospitals.

Two assumptions seem to follow from these "hard-wired" conceptions of brain organization and neuronal specificity. On a biological level, we have the idea that anatomical and single unit investigations will show the system to be lacking in dynamic, reorganizational capacity, especially after the period of infancy has passed. Failures to find evidence of regeneration of tissue or restoration of neuronal activity in the damaged, adult mammalian central nervous system are seen as consistent with the doctrine outlined earlier. Similarly, negative findings pertaining to regeneration have not only strengthened theoretical biases about how the nervous system is organized, but have had the effect of dissuading all but a handful of investigators from continuing to study these or related phenomena. As a result, the rush to look further or harder for evidence of morphological remodeling in the central nervous system has not been considered worthwhile by most investigators, at least not until a few years ago when some experimenters reported data that rearoused interest in these phenomena (e.g., Raisman, 1969). Historically, conceptions of brain organization and function emphasizing stability within the central nervous system have always held the dominant position; even today there is a tendency to compare the brain to a machine, or to make analogies between it and telephone lines or computers.[1] To many individuals,

---

[1] It is interesting to note that the tendency to use metaphors taken from other "more advanced" sciences to account for nervous function is not new. Earlier theorists, such as David Hartley, for example, applied Newtonian optics and physics (e.g., the movement of particles, pendulum motion) to explain how sensory "impulses" are conducted through nerve tissue. Apparently, each new technological development of the period finds its way into the jargon of disciplines attempting to establish their own scientific credibility. We might speculate that the less creative or emerging the discipline in

this approach is more consistent with what they believe localization theory demands than with ideas and models based on dynamic remodeling or neuroplasticity.

The second important assumption which stems from the tradition of viewing the brain as a mosaic of separate functional parts is that recovery of function probably does not occur. Here, the idea is that when a structure is damaged, the functions associated with it are lost and are not taken over by other brain areas. This, needless to say, would not prevent the organism from learning new "tricks" to deal with its problems in ways that might fool an investigator. The argument that is frequently heard in this context is that when recovery of function is reported it is only because the tests used to measure restitution are insensitive to the residual deficits. With better and more sophisticated testing procedures, we are told, recovery would not be seen after the period of infancy because each brain area and subarea is indeed unique in its functions and is closed to, or is incapable of, taking on new functions. The idea that some restitution could be due to neural "shock" wearing off tissue near to, or related to, the damaged region poses no threat to advocates of this position. Here the emphasis is strictly on the area permanently destroyed by the lesion—and the deficits that should remain when a structure is irreversibly damaged.

We should look at this bias in more detail. Clearly, one effect of this theoretical predisposition against the concept of recovery of function has been to diminish the attraction of doing research on recovery. The paradox is that the importance of understanding the effects of brain damage and the ability of an individual to resume seemingly normal or near-normal functioning has never been denied. Thus, on the one hand, recovery of function is sometimes treated as a threat or an embarrassment to established doctrines. Yet, on the other hand, there are certainly very practical reasons for increasing our understanding of recovery phenomena, regardless of our theoretical biases.

In some respects, it should be noted, evaluation of functional recovery falls victim to our strong reliance on group statistics. For example, it is not unusual to find studies in the literature in which lesions are comparable among the 20 or 25 subjects that comprise the group. If all but a single subject show a particular deficit, the presence of the deficit in the majority of cases is treated as if it were the only interesting finding in the investigation. Especially when the gross anatomy of the lesion appears to be the same in the "typical" and "deviant" cases, the one subject that does not show the effect is simply treated as an uninteresting or inexplicable exception. But how exceptional are the "exceptions"? How uncommon

---

developing original theories to account for its data, the more it will draw upon concepts and models borrowed from more technologically sophisticated domains whose measurement systems appear to be more precise. Whether a discussion of the measurement systems borrowed is relevant to the phenomena being measured by the borrower is often left for the philosophers of science.

is it to find individuals with massive brain damage that do not show any signs of it before they die of other causes, such as heart attacks and automobile accidents? Variability in response to brain damage, and a neurology of individual differences, represent a very important and legitimate area for research in our opinion. Moreover, findings of behavioral sparing after massive damage need not necessarily represent a complete and total *disproof* of current theories, although certain assumptions and interpretations associated with these theories may have to be modified (e.g., that all brains are comparable at birth, that environmental factors cannot affect the organization of the brain in a significant way). Moreover, as we will see, it may not be so much a question of whether there is any localization in the brain, but rather a question of what is being localized, especially in lesion experiments. Here it is important to remember that electrophysiological recordings or symptoms following acute brain lesions are not the same as, and should not necessarily be equated with, behavioral functions and that additional errors could be made in ascribing these psychological functions (e.g., aggressiveness, activity) to small parcels of tissue that are then thought of as being discrete, isolated entities in the brain.

In just the last few years, we have seen major advances in all areas of the brain sciences, with many previously held beliefs being challenged. Tying together some of these new findings represents one reason why we wrote this book. In addition, we felt the time had come to examine critically some of our general ideas about how the brain functions and what brain lesion data can really tell us about central nervous system organization. Are new findings consistent with time-honored views? Are present "laws" and "principles" still workable, or are we clinging unrealistically to outdated notions? Have we omitted looking at potentially important phenomena because they do not easily fit our theoretical frameworks? Do our experiments test what we think they are testing?

In the chapters that follow, we will concentrate on advances in two related subject areas dealing with brain damage, both mentioned previously. One is the capacity of the mammalian central nervous system to show structural and physiological changes in response to injury. The other is concerned with the nature and the extent of the behavioral recovery that may be seen after brain damage.

To put new developments into perspective, we will start by examining the development of the theory of cerebral localization of function from its roots in antiquity. The contributions of the Greeks and Romans will be mentioned, and the significance of the philosophical views of Gall and other phrenologists will be examined in detail. The roles of Pierre Flourens and Francois Magendie, in the early part of the nineteenth century, will also be reviewed. So will Broca's (1861) discovery of a faculty for articulate language, and Fritsch and Hitzig's (1870) classic experiments on the excitability of the motor cortex. The contributions of anatomists, neurologists, and surgeons at the beginning of this century will also be discussed.

Having done this, we will then look at our first broad subject area: the capacity of the central nervous system to "reorganize" itself after injury. We will examine new findings which we believe demonstrate that the central nervous system is not unmodifiable, hard-wired, nor directly comparable to a computer or some other man-made machine. The possibility that there is the potential for regeneration in the mature mammalian central nervous system will be examined very carefully. We will see, however, that other events, such as reactive synaptogenesis and the release of "latent" or blocked connections, may also play a role in the adaptation of the organism to its injuries.

After examining the evidence for anatomical and physiological plasticity in the injured nervous system, we will look at the behavioral literature on recovery of function itself. We will describe some conditions that might increase or decrease the probability of seeing impairments after brain damage. Here are a few questions that we will try to answer: How critical is developmental status at the time of injury? Are the symptoms solely dependent upon the locus of the damage, or do they also have something to do with how the damage is inflicted as was suggested by Adametz's "anomalous" finding after staged lesions of the reticular formation? Can stimulating environments affect the response to brain damage, either by acting as a therapy or in a pretraumatic "protective" role? In short, how can we begin to account for the behavioral variability that is found among patients and laboratory animals that suffer relatively comparable lesions?

In the next chapters we will look at the classical theories of recovery to see how they were formulated and how well they can explain the data that have been collected. These theories include the use of new strategies (behavioral compensation), the release of uninjured tissue from temporarily suppressed states (diaschisis), the possibility that one structure can take over another's functions (vicariation), and the use of existing but previously ineffective connections for guiding behavior (e.g., supersensitivity). Where possible, we will show how these theories can be related to anatomical and physiological events like sprouting and latent synapses. We will also devote considerable attention to the issue of whether these ideas are directly testable or only inferred from lesion data.

In the final chapters we will try to integrate the anatomical, physiological and behavioral data more fully and will attempt to show how the laboratory findings have clinical implications. We will talk about a number of issues that sorely need to be addressed by modern neuroscientists—issues that have received little attention in the rush to conduct a multitude of experiments with each and every new technique that comes along. One issue concerns the manner in which the functions of the brain can be defined. Another asks how we can be so sure that the psychological (behavioral) functions that we are now choosing are better than those mentioned by our predecessors and that they are indeed the functions of particular, discrete brain areas.

We also will offer another way of looking at brain lesion data; that is, we will offer an alternative to using the results of lesion studies only to try to localize functions in the brain. We will develop a conceptual framework for assessing lesion data that takes into account not only the locus of the lesion, but the natural history of the organism. This framework will deal with observable events and will concentrate on the individual at least as much as it does on the group. The applicability of this new approach to choosing a therapeutic setting, in determining how surgery should be performed, and for handling other aspects of patient care and treatment will be examined in detail.

Throughout all of the chapters we will try to make a number of distinctions that we think are important. One involves the tendency to confuse fact and theory—the proven and the assumed. Another concerns testable and nontestable ideas in the brain sciences. A third distinction was made about 100 years ago by John Hughlings Jackson, but has, for the most part, been forgotten. It is the difference between localizing psychological *functions* and localizing symptoms (or unit responses!).

By clarifying these issues and putting them into perspective, we hope that some "pseudoissues" can be identified and discarded, while truly important questions are singled out and properly addressed. In our view, it is only in such a context that valuable new directions and orientations can come forth and that theoretical "blind alleys" that may have limited progress in the past can be identified and avoided in the future.

In the final analysis, no one can deny the suffering that occurs after someone has been afflicted with traumatic, central nervous system injury. Until recently, there has been relatively little optimism concerning the victims of brain injury. We feel that the lack of hope and indeed the failure to ask the appropriate questions about central nervous system function and plasticity are derived from an uncritical acceptance of only one way of looking at the central nervous system—using one paradigm.

We certainly do not have all the answers because the problem and its solutions have only begun to be evaluated seriously. Much is still unknown, and there always is the risk of failing to ask the right questions of nature—but this is, in part, what makes the quest so interesting and demanding. Albert Szent-Györgi, who won a Nobel Prize in 1937 for his research on vitamins, once said

> Research means going out into the unknown with the hope of finding something
> new to bring home. If you know in advance what you are going to do, or even to find
> there, then it is not research at all: Then, it is only a kind of honorable occupation
> [1971, p. 1].

With this in mind, let us examine some of the challenges that lie ahead. Let us try to provide you with the opportunity to confront some of your own ideas and see if we can influence you to share in our enthusiasm and excitement about neuroplasticity and recovery of function.

References

Adametz, J. H. Rate of recovery of functioning in cats with rostral reticular lesions. *Journal of Neurosurgery*, 1959, *16*, 85–98.

Broca, P.-P. Remarques sur le siège de la faculté du language articulé: Suivies d'une observation d'aphémie (perte de la parole). *Bulletin de la Société Anatomique de Paris*, 1861, *36*, 330–357.

Finger, S., Marshak, R. A., Cohen, M., Scheff, S., Trace, R., and Neimand, D. Effects of successive and simultaneous lesions of somatosensory cortex on tactile discrimination in the rat. *Journal of Comparative and Physiological Psychology*, 1971, *77*, 221–227.

French, G. M., and Harlow, H. F. Variability of delayed reaction performance in normal and brain-damaged rhesus monkeys. *Journal of Neurophysiology*, 1962, *25*, 585–599.

Fritsch, G., and Hitzig, E. Über die elektrische Erregbarkeit des Grosshirns. *Archiv für Anatomie und Physiologie*, 1870, 300–332.

Goldman, P. S., and Mendelson, M. J. Salutary effects of early experience on deficits caused by lesions of frontal association cortex in developing rhesus monkeys. *Experimental Neurology*, 1977, *57*, 588–602.

Horvarth, F. E. Effects of basolateral amygdalectomy on three types of avoidance behavior in cats. *Journal of Comparative and Physiological Psychology*, 1963, *56*, 380–389.

Isaacson, R. L. *The limbic system*. New York: Plenum, 1974.

Kuhn, T. S. *The essential tension*. Chicago: University of Chicago Press, 1977.

Lindsley, D. B., Schreiner, L. H., Knowles, W. B., and Magoun, H. W. Behavioral and EEG changes following chronic brain stem lesions in the cat. *Electroencephalography and Clinical Neurology*, 1949, *1*, 455–473.

Magoun, H. W. *The waking brain*. Springfield, Ill.: Charles C Thomas, 1963.

Norrsell, U. A conditioned reflex study of sensory deficits caused by cortical somatosensory ablations. *Physiology and Behavior*, 1967, *2*, 73–81.

Raisman, G. Neuronal plasticity in the septal nuclei of the adult brain. *Brain Research*, 1969, *14*, 25–48.

Schwartzman, R. J. Somesthetic recovery following primary somatosensory projection cortex ablations. *Archives of Neurology*, 1972, *27*, 340–349.

Semmes, J., and Mishkin, M. Somatosensory loss in monkeys after ipsilateral cortical ablation. *Journal of Neurophysiology*, 1965, *28*, 473–486.

Semmes, J. S., Weinstein, S., Ghent, L., and Teuber, H. L. *Somatosensory changes after penetrating brain wounds in man*. Cambridge, Mass.: Harvard Press, 1960.

Settlage, P. H., Zable, M., and Harlow, H. F. Problem solution by monkeys following bilateral removal of the prefrontal areas. IV. Performance on tests requiring contradictory reactions to similar and to identical stimuli. *Journal of Experimental Psychology*, 1948, *38*, 50–65.

Sperry, R. W. Cerebral dominance in perception. In F. A. Young, and D. B. Lindsay (Eds.), *Early experience and visual information processing in perceptual and reading disorders*. Washington, D.C.: National Academy of Sciences, 1970.

Stamm, J. S. Retardation and facilitation in learning by stimulation of frontal cortex in monkeys. In J. M. Warren and K. Akert (Eds.), *The frontal granular cortex and behavior*. New York: McGraw-Hill, 1964, Pp. 102–135.

Stein, D. G., Rosen, J. J., Graziadei, J., Mishkin, D., and Brink, J. J. Central nervous system: Recovery of function. *Science*, 1969, *166*, 528–530.

Szent-Györgi, A. Looking back. *Perspectives in Biology and Medicine*, 1971, *15*, 1–5.

Woolsey, C. N. Organization of somatic sensory and motor areas of the cerebral cortex. In H. F. Harlow and C. N. Woolsey (Eds.), *Biological and biochemical bases of behavior*. Madison: University of Wisconsin Press, 1958, Pp. 63–81.

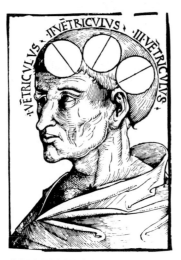

Localization in the Central Nervous System: Antiquity to Phrenology

As for me, arguing in accordance with the evidence revealed by dissection, it seems to be acceptable that the soul resides in the body of the brain where it produces reasoning, and the memory of sensible images is preserved there [Galen, 129–199 A.D.].

*God and the Brain;
nothing but God and the Brain* [Franz Gall, 1758–1828].

CHAPTER TWO

As we mentioned in the preceding chapter, many workers in the neurosciences have come to consider the brain as an organ that can be subdivided into a number of distinct parts, each of which may be subdivided further into smaller functional units, such as command neurons, hypercomplex cells, or cell assemblies. This viewpoint holds that each of these "units" is responsible for unique behavioral functions and is an extension of the general principle in biology that holds that structures with different shapes, such as the heart and eye, must have different functions (i.e., circulation and vision). In fact, since some parts of the brain can readily be distinguished anatomically from other parts, the concept of localization of function within the brain itself makes intuitive sense and has at least a face validity associated with it. Indeed, as we have already mentioned, morphological and functional "mapping" in the central nervous system have occupied anatomists for most of this century. Brodmann's maps of the cortex, from 1909, are still widely used and accepted today.

Even prior to written history, we have some evidence that neolithic tribes ranging from the Mediterranean bases to northern Europe had some idea that the head was important as the seat of behavioral functions. We can make this general statement because the practice of trepanning holes in the head was apparently a very widespread practice in Europe, Asia, and even South America. In various archeological sites, skulls with *healed* "rondelles" have been found dating back 30,000 years before the current era (B.C.E.). In some regions up to 25% or more of the skulls have been trepanned, and while it has been suggested that the practice may have had some religious rather than medical significance, no one is certain.

The first known written document describing brain functions and symptoms produced by brain injury was an Egyptian medical papyrus (3500 B.C.E.), translated by Edwin Smith. Apparently, the Egyptian physicians were aware of the fact that symptoms and signs of injury to the central nervous system could occur far-distant from the actual site of that injury. For example, the papyrus describes how focal damage to the head could result in impaired visuomotor coordination. It also mentioned the fact that the deficits usually occurred on the side of the body opposite that of the head injury. Remarkably, there is also a case description of a "contracoup" injury. Thus, we can see that over 5000 years ago there was a concern with the relationship between brain and behavior and that many of the observations made by that long-ago physician have sustained the test of time.

The idea that the brain was the site of the soul had been proposed by philosophers in Greece well before the current era. One of the first neuroscientists was Alcmaeon of Croton who performed the earliest recorded dissections of the human body (sixth century B.C.) and who is credited with the discovery of the optic nerves (McHenry, 1969). Based on his dissections and observations of nerve tissue, he argued that the brain was the central organ of sensation and thought. Other pre-Hippocratic writers, and many during the Golden Age of Greece, accepted and extended Alcmaeon's notions that the brain was important, but like him, most did not concern themselves with specific localizations of functions in the various parts of the cerebrum.

With Hippocrates (460–370 B.C.), diseases of the brain were recognized as being within the overall domain of medicine, although the physiology and pathology of the day were based upon the four humors (blood, phlegm, black and yellow bile). As far as we can determine, Plato (ca. 380 B.C.) was one of the first of the ancient philosophers to argue for relatively specific localization of function in brain tissue. He thought that the part of the "soul" subserving sensation, reason, and movement was found in the cerebrum (cortex), although appetite and drives were located in the brain stem (a position not unlike that of many contemporary thinkers!).

The idea that the brain was the locus of "mind," however, was a matter of contention and debate for centuries. The controversy was stimulated in part by the writings of Aristotle who forcefully argued that the *heart* was the seat of all cognitive and emotional functions. Aristotle thought that the bone marrow and blood were more important because they were warm to the touch, whereas the brain was cool. It should be remembered that the Greeks felt that fire (warmth) was one of the four basic elements of which all matter consisted, and that warmth distinguished living (animate) from nonliving (inanimate) things.

According to Aristotle, the brain served to temper the heat and passions of the heart. One might thus consider the brain as a "cooling organ" devoid of any complex, cognitive functions. Aristotle felt that the soul (and therefore rational thought) was located in the heart because he had observed that the beating heart is the first organ found in the embryonic chick.

The cardiocentric versus encephalic arguments over where to locate the soul continued until almost the end of the sixteenth century. Shakespeare indicated the confusion in several of his plays (see Rosner, 1974). For example, in the *Merchant of Venice* (Act III, Scene II) Shakespeare has Portia say "Tell me where is fancy bred, Or in the heart, or in the head?"

Even those who thought that the head was more important than the heart could not agree on where to locate the functions of the mind. Thus, while Plato thought the cerebral tissue critical for thought and feeling, Herophilus (ca. 300 B.C.), who dissected hundreds of bodies, argued for the importance of the ventricles and specifically pointed to the lower end of the fourth ventricle as the part of the sensory-motor "soul" (Clarke and O'Malley, 1968; McHenry, 1969).

Herophilus proposed that "animal spirits" (the liquid substance that gave movement to limbs) were generated by the tissue of the cerebrum, but these spirits were controlled by the soul, which interacted with the spirits in the "rete mirabile." This structure, found in ungulates, but never seen in man, is a sort of vascular plexus at the base of the brain surrounding the pituitary gland. The rete mirabile was destined to be given an important role in subsequent theories of brain function until finally its importance was questioned by Descartes and others in the seventeenth century.

Perhaps the most influential of all the early medical writers was Galen, physician to the Roman gladiators in the second century C.E. (current era). Galen was an authoritative figure who was completely opposed to the cardiocentric theory of Aristotle. In fact, he stressed an important role for the liver in mediating "psychic functions." Galen proposed what today might be termed an *organismic theory* of psychic functions in which he stressed the importance of nutrition in influencing physiological and behavioral functions (Singer and Rabin, 1946). In Galen's view, food is converted to "chylo" in the intestines and is then conveyed to the liver where it is changed into blood and mixed with "natural spirits." The blood then travels to the heart where it mixes with "vital spirits" coming from the ventricles of the brain. Galen carefully described the rete mirabile where the vital spirits were transformed into animal spirits, which were stored in the ventricles or "pneuma" until needed by the body. The pneuma, when called upon by psychic influences, would then enter the brain through pores in the walls of the ventricles and directly influence the nerves and muscles into action.

Galen thus attempted to provide a structural basis for most behaviors based upon the interaction of various body organs. The ventricles "stored" the necessary animal spirits, but it was the material substance of the brain that executed sensory and motor functions. As a natural observer, Galen dissected animals and traced the paths of the motor and sensory nerves, distinguished dura from pia mater, and defined structures, such as the corpus callosum, four ventricles, fornix, pineal and pituitary glands, and infundibulum. He claimed that the sensory regions of the brain were anterior to the tentorium, whereas motor functions were posterior to it. Shortly after his death in 201 A.D., many of his 400 treatises were lost although some 180 have been recovered. Galen's ideas, however, were the dominant guiding force in Western and Arabic thinking about brain function for almost 1500 years! As a specific example, most diagrams of the human brain, into the eighteenth century, showed the rete mirabile at its base, even though Galen could only have visualized it in oxen. In addition, although Erastistratus had earlier intimated that the complexity of the cerebral convolutions was directly related to intelligence, Galen's position that the cerebral convolutions played no role in mental functions was widely accepted until a few hundred years ago, in spite of attempts by investigators, such as Willis, to show that this was probably not the case at all.

As Edwin Clarke and Kenneth Dewhurst (1972) have noted, the principal concepts handed down from antiquity to the sixteenth century were to describe the seat of the soul, to distinguish between motor and sensory activities somewhat, and to define the role of the rete mirabile in the integration of the psyche with basic bodily functions. A fourth concept, to localize mental functions in the ventricles of the brain, was anticipated in Greek thinking and to some extent in the writings of Galen, although it remained to be developed by the Syrian bishop, Nemesius, in the fourth century C.E., who claimed to be a follower of Galen.

> The lateral ventricles were considered one cavity, the first cell; our third ventricle was the second cell, and our fourth, the third. The first cell received sensation from the special senses and from the rest of the body and thus accommodated the "sensus communis" or "common sense." Images were created from this sensation and so "imaginativa" (imagination) and "fantasia" . . . were either in the posterior part of the first cell or in the second. The latter part, however, was also the seat of reasoning. . . . Memorativa (memory) was contained within the third cell [Nemesius, cited by Clarke and Dewhurst, 1972, p. 10].

In a way, the ventricular theory of localization can be viewed as a "compartmentalization" and extension of Galen's thinking since he proposed that imagination, reasoning, and memory could be affected separately by injury, although he did not attempt to localize each function in a different part of the brain.

The ventricular theory, which is illustrated in Figures 2.1–2.3, was subject to various modifications over the years (e.g., additional cells or functions being added) and was accepted in both Islamic and Christian countries before it began to decline at about the time of the Renaissance. The theory was ultimately rejected for a number of reasons. First, by the sixteenth century, anatomists and scientists were examining their material more carefully. Leonardo da Vinci, for example, injected wax into the ventricles around 1490 to reveal their true shape—a shape which failed to correspond to earlier descriptions and diagrams

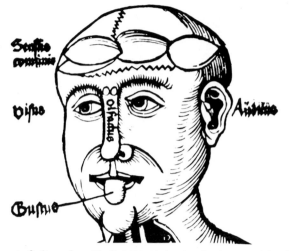

Figure 2.1. *Segment of a figure from Pleyligk (1518) showing the three ventricles of the brain. (From* Philosophiae Naturalis Compendium, *Leipzig: M. Lother, 1499.)*

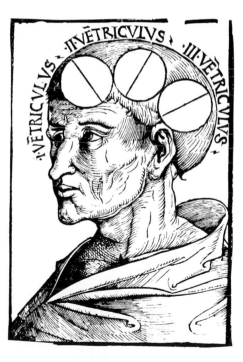

Figure 2.2. *Ventricular organization as depicted in* Philosophia Naturalis. *Basle: M. Furter, 1506. (See Clarke and Dewhurst, 1972.)*

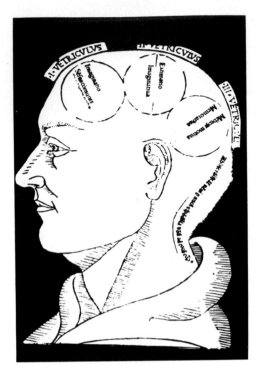

Figure 2.3. *Ventricular organization as depicted by Albertus Magnus in the thirteenth century. (From* Philosophia Pauper um sive Philosophia Naturalis, *Brescia: Farfengus, 1490.)*

that were widely accepted. His drawings, such as the ones shown in Figure 2.4, are now well known. Second, it was only a matter of time before it became clear that the ventricles were filled with a watery fluid (the cerebrospinal fluid), and it was deemed unlikely that mental processes, such as reasoning and memory, could reside in such a medium. A third consideration came from the work of Andreas Vesalius (1514–1564). This investigator examined human ventricles during anatomical dissections and was forced to conclude that they were virtually identical to those of animals that did not have the reasoning powers or other faculties of human beings. How then could the ventricles govern higher mental processes? Vesalius stated

> All our contemporaries, so far as I can understand them, deny to apes, dogs, horses, sheep, cattle, and other animals, the main powers of the Reigning Soul—not to speak of other (powers)—and attribute to man alone the faculty of reasoning; and ascribe this faculty in equal degree to all men. And yet we clearly see in dissecting that men do not excel those animals by (possessing) any special cavity (in the brain). Not only is the number (of ventricles) the same, but also all other things (in the brain) are similar, except only in size and in the complete consonance (of the parts) for virtue [Rosner, 1974, p. 8].

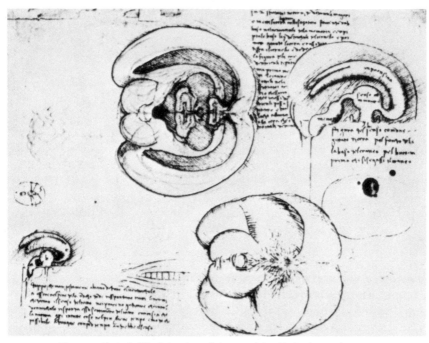

Figure 2.4. *A da Vinci drawing of the ventricles. Early sixteenth century.*

A drawing made by Vesalius in 1543 appears in Figure 2.5. At about the same time, Volcher Criter (McHenry, 1969) cut open the ventricles in living animals without finding very noticeable changes in their behaviors.

Slowly but surely, the hallowed ventricular theory began to lose ground; the brain substance itself, and even the cerebral cortex, began to attract attention. As we have seen, this represented a rejection of Galenic thinking since Galen had been firm in his conviction that the cortex played no role in mental activity. In fact, from the time of the ancient Greeks to the nineteenth century, the cortex has been likened to either the small intestine (Erasistratus of Alexandria) or to a plate of macaroni! In brief, as shown in Figure 2.6, no anatomical divisions of the cortex were really recognized at this time, and it thus followed that there should be no functional subdivisions either. This can be seen by the fact that careful anatomical descriptions or even faithful artists' renderings of the brain did not begin to appear in textbooks with any regularity until the eighteenth and nineteenth centuries (see Clarke and Dewhurst, 1972).

The first real break with tradition occurred when Descartes (1596–1650) selected the pineal body, a small gland near the back of the brain, as the seat of the soul. Although Descartes's contributions were generally philosophical, his con-

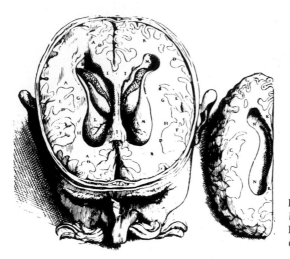

Figure 2.5. *Ventricles as depicted by Vesalius.* [*From* De Humani Corporis Fabrica, *Basle: Oporinus, 1543. (See Clarke and Dewhurst, 1972.)*]

tribution to science was very important. Descartes was one of the first "modern" philosophers to stress the materialist basis of behavior and argued that behavior resulted from the activation of a specific neuronal subsystem of the brain (Rosner, 1974). Thus, as illustrated in Figure 2.7, we see the introduction of the concept of a brain center as well as the notion that many complex responses could be explained in terms of simple movements (reflexes) controlled by a region of nervous tissue.

At about the same time as Descartes, others were drawing conclusions based upon anatomical observations. Thus, Sylvius (Franciscus de la Boë, 1614–1672)

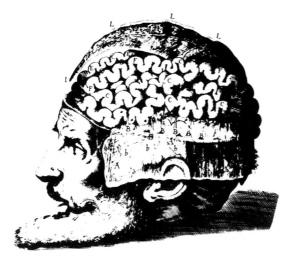

Figure 2.6. *Copperplate by Casserio (1561–1616). (In* Tabulae Anatomicae LXXIIX, *edited by D. Bucretius, Venice: Deuchinum, 1627.) This Renaissance drawing of the cerebral convolutions shows no clear notion of their organization.*

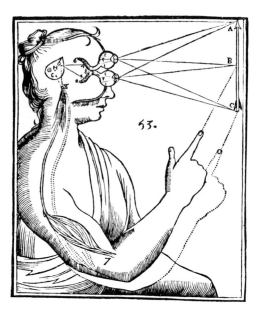

Figure 2.7. *Descartes' drawing illustrating how light enters the eyes and how the images go by hollow nerves to the ventricles and from there to the pineal gland (H) to initiate movement. (From* L'homme, *Paris: Le Gras, 1664.)*

and Thomas Willis (1621–1675) suggested that mental activity could be traced to the cerebral or cerebellar cortices, and they argued against the ventricles being the seat of higher functions. In particular, the system proposed by Willis is intriguing. He suggested that the corpus striatum was the center for "sensus communis," that the cerebral white matter (then called corpus callosum) was responsible for imagination, and that the grey matter that made up the cerebral cortex was involved in memory!

Niels Stensen (Steno) (1638–1686), a contemporary of Willis, also argued that there is a fundamental organization to the brain that should be examined more closely:

We need only view a Dissection of that large Mass, the Brain, to have ground to bewail our ignorance. On the very Surface you see varieties which deserve your admiration; but when you look into its inner Substance you are utterly in the dark, being able to say nothing more than that there are two Substances, one greyish and the other white, which last is continuous with the Nerve distributed all over the body. . . . If this substance is everywhere Fibrous, as it appears in many places to be, you must own that these Fibres are disposed in the most artful manner; since all the diversity of our Sensations and Motion depend upon them. We admire the contrivance of the Fibres of every Muscle, and ought still more to admire their disposition in the Brain, where an infinite number of them contained in a very small Space, do each execute their particular Offices without confusion or disorder [Steno, 1665/1950; see Gibson, 1962, p. 944].

Despite an analysis of the cortical grey matter by Van Leeuwenhoek in 1719, the concept of localization of function within the brain tissue itself still was not completely accepted. Yet, the notion of a functional organization was in the air (see Gibson, 1962; Rosner, 1974), as evidenced by an increasing number of clinical reports, such as the following, which appeared in 1691:

> A very Tall and well Set Gentleman, Aged about 24 years, by a Fall from his Horse, had his Skull broken in several places, and being a Person of good Estate, had several Chirugeons to attend him in the course of his Sickness, during which he was divers times Trephan'd, and had several pieces of his Skull taken off, which left great Chasms . . . between the remaining parts. Within about three days after his Fall, this Knight . . . was taken with a Dead Palsy on his Right side, which did not equally affect his Arm and his Leg: The use of the latter being sometimes suddenly Restor'd to him in some measure . . . But his Arm and Head were constantly Paralytical, being wholly depriv'd of Motion; and having so little Sense, that it would sometimes lye under his Body without his Feeling it. . . . And when the Chirugeons were going to close up his Head, as having no more to do; one of them . . . (alleged) that, if they did no more, the Gentleman would lead a Useless and very Melancholy Life; and that he was confident, the Palsey was in some way or other occasion'd by the Fall, which had left something in the Head that they had not yet discover'd. And the Knight himself agreeing to this Man's notion, his Head was further laid open; and at length, under a piece of proud Flesh, they found, with much ado, a Splinter, or rather Flake of a Bone, that bore hard upon the dura matter, and was not pull'd out without great Hemorrhage, and such a stretch of the Parts, as made the Patient think his Brain itself was tearing out. But this Mischief was soon Remedy'd, and his Hurts securely Heal'd up; and he is now a Strong Healthy Man [Boyle, 1691, see Gibson, 1962, p. 945].

Before turning to the revolution in Brain function in the nineteenth century, brief mention should be made of one remarkable investigator whose name is often overlooked by historians in the brain and behavioral sciences. Emanuel Swedenborg (1688–1772), who founded the New Jerusalem Church (The Swedenborgian Church), devoted much time and energy to the physical and natural sciences prior to his full-time commitment to theology in 1749. In surprisingly modern terms, he proposed that the cerebral cortex was responsible for sensation and movement and stated

> From the anatomy of the brain it follows that the brain is the *sensorium commune* with respect to its cortical substance, which is the brain proper, since to it are referred the impressions of the external sense organs as if to their one and only internal centre. The cortical substance is also the *motorium commune voluntarium,* for whatever actions are mediated by the nerves and muscles are determined beforehand by the will; i.e. initiated by the cortex [Swedenborg, 1847, pp. 194–194].

In addition, Emanual Swedenborg argued that the sensory cortex could be subdivided into specific parts:

The cerebellula are thus wisely arranged in order that they might correspond exactly to the various external sensations. For these cerebellula are compacted into a certain number of units, and those are united into new and still larger groups, until they make up the largest unit, which is the cortex itself. Individual areas are separated by fissures and sulci, to which correspond meningeal compartments and vascular patterns. The number of areas so formed is analogous to the various forms of sensation. In this way, every type of external sensation—vision, hearing, taste and olfaction— can be received distinctly, together forming the *sensorium commune* [1740–1741, p. 153].

Swedenborg even seems to have inferred the somatotopic organization of the motor cortex as it is known today. Yet his work was little circulated in his lifetime, and it seemed to have had virtually no impact on his contemporaries (Akert and Hammond, 1962). Even when his works were republished 140 years after they were written, these remarkable insights were treated as a series of strange premonitions that did not affect the evolution of scientific thought. It remained for nineteenth- and twentieth-century investigators to come to these same conclusions before the scientific community and the public at large would be willing to accept them.

Most historians of medicine trace the theory of localization of function in its modern form to Franz Joseph Gall (1758–1828) and to the theory of phrenology which he developed. With his pupil, Johann Caspar Spurzheim (1776–1832), Gall proposed that the surface of the brain (i.e., the cortex) could be subdivided into a mosaic of functional units, that each was responsible for a different faculty (music, speech, mathematical ability, etc.), and that the contribution of each organ to the total personality could be ascertained by examining the cranium overlying the cortex for size differences, protuberances, and depressions. This theory, which achieved considerable popularity at the beginning of the nineteenth century, might be viewed as an outgrowth of "physiognomy," the idea that personality and temperament can be judged by physical characteristics such as facial features, stature, and stance.

Phrenology was the first theory to attract specific attention to the cerebral cortex and to its convolutions. It not only suggested a finer localization than had previously been considered, but turned to "precise" measurement and naturalistic observation for its support. The method of measuring the features of the cranium with calipers and related instruments was called "cranioscopy" or "craniometry," and in itself it represented a marked departure from metaphysical and introspective approaches to brain function (Critchley, 1965).

Oddly, while stressing empiricism, Gall seems to have had little use for data derived from brain-damaged people or from animals subjected to brain lesions. He argued that the same exact lesion could not be replicated from case to case, that it was inconceivable to think that a lesion in one part of the brain would not affect surrounding tissue and other parts as well, and that animals rarely survived long enough to permit adequate observation. In addition to technical objections such as these, he raised a number of theoretical points, such as whether studies on animals in the absence of adequate data on humans really could convey any information of value.

It is often forgotten that Gall was an established physician, an accomplished anatomist, and a man of great stature at the time that he was presenting his ideas about the functions of the brain and their cortical localization. For example, after studying medicine in Strasbourg and Vienna, he contributed significantly to the study of the origin of cranial nerves II, III, V, and VI, the decussation of the corticospinal tract in the pyramids, and the central anatomy of the visual system. He also made major contributions in the field of spinal cord anatomy (the first descriptions of the cervical and lumbar spinal enlargements) and drew attention to the commissural pathways in the brain, including the corpus callosum. Yet, from even his earliest notes and letters, it is clear that the functions of the brain dominated his thinking to the point that he is even critical of his medical school training for having nothing to say about this matter (see Young, 1970, p. 13).

Gall's principles of localization were derived from observations that he had made of friends and acquaintances, and later, to a much greater extent, of men of genius, criminals, lunatics, prominent citizens, and other ''extremes'' of society. He noted different cranial features in these cases and went on to reason if nature had constructed a particular apparatus for each function: why would nature have made an exception of the brain? Why would nature not have destined the different parts of the brain for particular functions (Gall, 1835)? Gall then made the erroneous assumption that the skull itself reflected the development of the underlying brain and published his ideas in a massive series of volumes entitled, *Anatomie et Physiologie du Systeme Nerveaux en General, du Cerveau en Particulier* (1810–1819). Spurzheim collaborated with him on the first two works of this series, but then left for Scotland and America to establish the discipline and win new adherents to the phrenological movement.

To understand the relationship between the skull and the faculties of the mind better, Gall collected and measured skull casts of individuals with remarkable faculties and personality characteristics. By 1802, Gall presumably had over 300 crania of people for whom he knew the mental characteristics. He also had over 120 casts of distinguished living persons. These collections continued to grow in subsequent years (Bentley, 1916).

One of the things that is clear from Gall's writings is that his first chore was to define the functions of the brain; only after the functions were known could a detailed anatomy be accomplished. As a result, he devoted the majority of his time to examining behavior and crania:

> When he met or heard of a man or animal endowed with a striking talent or propensity, he set out to determine if this remarkable behaviour was the work of nature: a

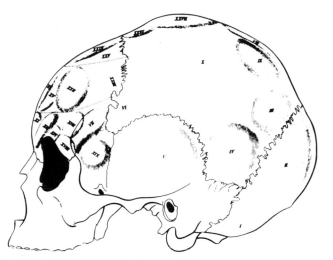

Figure 2.8. *Depiction of the skull showing the general placements of Gall's basic faculties. (From an anonymous manuscript,* Exposition de La Doctrine Physiognomique du Docteur Gall, ou Nouvelle Théorie du Cerveau, Considéré Comme le Siège des Facultés Intellectuales et Morales. *Paris: Henrichs, 1803.)*

truly fundamental faculty. The main criterion was that it be manifested *independent* of the other characteristics of the individual or species. When he found men or animals with an eminent talent or propensity he examined the form of the head for a cranial prominence. He collected and compared as many such correlations as he could find [Young, 1970, p. 33].

In all, Gall believed that there were 27 independent faculties that could be localized in distinct cortical centers ("organs"). This is shown in Figure 2.8. Nineteen of them were common to man and animals and included such things as reproductive instinct, courage, sense of color, and sense of space. The remainder were viewed as unique to man: wisdom, sense of metaphysics, satire, poetic ability, mimicry, compassion, religion, and firmness of purpose. Gall did not attempt to circumscribe the extent of each organ exactly, and they did not follow the convolutional patterns of the cortex. As Young (1970) has stated, "Gall was content to specify the areas and to admit freely that he neither knew the functions of all the cerebral parts nor the precise limits of those parts whose functions he had specified [p. 28]." He felt that in discovering the functions of the brain he had made a significant contribution and that future investigators would now find it easier to precisely delineate each of the cerebral organs.

Gall's followers showed a great propensity for adding functions and for filling in the "gaps" in his cortical diagrams. Spurzheim, for example, spoke of 35 faculties (see Figure 2.9) and the Fowler brothers, in the United States, delineated 43. Although these investigators felt confident that they understood the dorsal

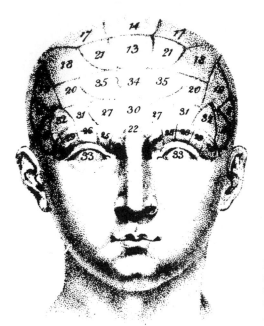

Figure 2.9. *Spurzheim's organs of the mind. (From his* Phrenology, or, the Doctrine of the Mind; and of the Relations between its Manifestations and the Body. *London: Knight, 1825, 3rd edition.)*

aspect of the cortex, they had less to say about the organs at the base of the brain, which were not readily available for cranial measurements or inspection. Gall himself suspected that these areas played a role in hunger and thirst and in the perception of heat and cold.

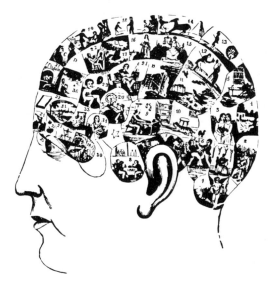

Figure 2.10. *Diagrammatic representation of the faculties of the mind. Such drawings were common in late nineteenth century and early twentieth century phrenological publications. (See Clarke and Dewhurst, 1972.)*

As we know, phrenology (Spurzheim's term) as a science was eventually discredited. Nevertheless, Gall's conviction that the cortex could not be viewed as an equipotential organ (see Figure 2.10) represented a major step in the development of localization theory. Although cranioscopy proved to be an invalid way of approaching the problem of cortical localization, the logical outcome of the work of the phrenologists was to have the cortex examined with more care. Only 30 years after George Combe (1836), a devoted follower of Spurzheim, described the cortex as a "curiously convoluted" structure, modern, impressively labeled maps of the cortex began to appear. A new era in brain research had begun.

References

Akert, K., and Hammond, M. P. Emanuel Swedenborg (1688–1772) and his contribution to neurology. *Medical History*, 1962, *6*, 255–266.

Bentley, M. The psychological antecedents of phrenology. *Psychological Monographs*, 1916, *21*, 102–115.

Boyle, R. *Experimenta et observationes physicae*, 1691.

Clarke, E., and Dewhurst, K. *An illustrated history of brain function*. Berkeley: University of California Press, 1972.

Clarke, E., and O'Malley, C. D. *The human brain and spinal cord*. Berkeley: University of California Press, 1968.

Combe, G. *A system of phrenology* (4th ed., 2 vols.). Edinburgh: Maclachan, Stewart and Anderson, 1836.

Critchley, M. Neurology's debt to F. J. Gall (1758–1828). *British Medical Journal*, 1965, *2*, 775–781.

Gall, F. J., and Spurzheim, J. C. *Anatomie et physiologie du système nerveux en général, et du cerveau en particulier*. Paris: Schoell, 1810–1819.

Gibson, W. C. Pioneers in localization of function in the brain. *Journal of the American Medical Association*, 1962, *180*, 944–951.

McHenry, L. C. *Garrison's history of neurology*. Springfield, Ill.: Charles C Thomas, 1969.

Rosner, B. Recovery of function and localization of function in historical perspective. In D. G. Stein, J. J. Rosen, and N. Butters (Eds.), *Plasticity and recovery of function in the central nervous system*. New York: Academic Press, 1974, Pp. 1–29.

Singer, C., and Rabin, C. *A prelude to modern science*. Cambridge: Cambridge University Press, 1946.

Steno, N. [*Dissertation on the anatomy of the brain, by Nicholas Steno*] (E. Gotfredsen, Ed. and trans.) Copenhagen: Nyt Nordisk Forlag Arnold Busck, 1950. (Originally published, 1665.)

Swedenborg, E. *Oeconomia regni animalis. I. De sanguine, ejus arteriis, venis et corde. II. De cerebri motu et cortice et de anima humana*. Amsterdam: Changuion, 1740–1741.

Swedenborg, E. *Oeconomia regni animalis. III. De fibra, de tunica arachnoidea, et de morbis fibrarum*. Posthumus edition by J. J. G. Wilkinson. London: W. Newbery, 1847.

Young, R. M. *Mind, brain and adaptation in the nineteenth century*. Oxford: Clarendon Press, 1970.

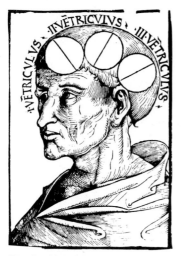

Localization in the Central Nervous System: Flourens to Present

It was a memorable day when Broca demonstrated before the Société d'Anthropologie in Paris—with his old father looking on in silent admiration—the brain lesion of his first patient who had suffered from aphémie (renamed aphasia by Trousseau). From this and subsequent observations he concluded that the integrity of the posterior part of the left third frontal convolution was indispensible to articulate speech, and therefore he termed this region the "circonvolution du language" [Goldstein, 1953, p. 14].

CHAPTER THREE

Although the significance of Gall's concept of cortical localization cannot be overestimated, the inadequacy of his method (cranioscopy) for localizing functions at the cortical level was quickly recognized by a number of scientists. Jean-Pierre-Marie Flourens (1794–1867), a man whose philosophy and approach to brain function was in direct opposition to that of Franz Gall, was probably Gall's sharpest and most influential critic. Flourens' first experimental paper, in fact, appeared in 1822, the very year that the first part of Gall's last book began to appear. Unlike Gall, who was a "society favorite," but who was not taken seriously by the scientific establishment of the day, Flourens, who is shown in Figure 3.1, received a seat in the French Academy of Sciences and numerous prizes (e.g., the Legion of Honor in 1832) for his work. His contributions were not only in experimental neurology, but in comparative anatomy, anesthesiology, embryology, and physiology.

David Krech (1962), writing on the history of cortical localization of function, states that Flourens regarded Gall and Spurzheim as fair game for sarcasm, verbal abuse, and all kinds of practical jokes. One example of this can be seen in Flourens' small book, *Psychologie Compareè* (1864), in which the following story is included about Magendie and Spurzheim:

> The famous physiologist, Magendie, preserved with veneration the brain of Laplace. Spurzheim had the very natural wish to see the brain of a great man. To test the science of phrenology, Mr. Magendie showed him, instead of the brain of Laplace, that of an imbecile. Spurzheim, who had already worked up his enthusiasm, admired the brain of the imbecile as he would have admired that of Laplace [p. 234; Krech, 1962, p. 44].

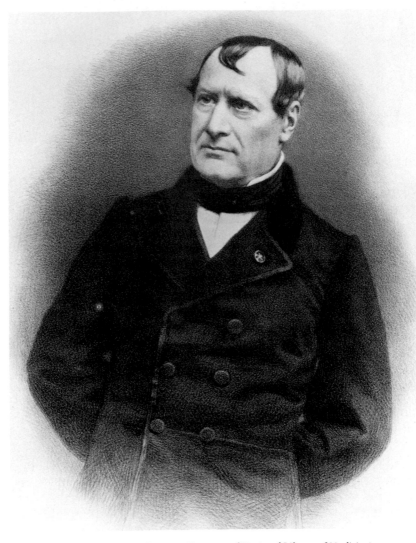

Figure 3.1. *Jean-Pierre-Marie Flourens. (Courtesy of National Library of Medicine)*

Flourens was committed to the "experimental method," that is, to understanding the brain by examining it with ablation and stimulation techniques.
Gall, as we pointed out, objected strongly to experimental ablations and studying
the accidents of nature, and Flourens attempted to take at least some of Gall's
criticisms into account when doing his own work. His philosophy and approach to
studying brain function were stated very clearly in his 1842 book:

Everything, in experimental researches, depends on the method; because it is the method which gives results. A new method leads to new results; a vague method can only lead to confused results. . . . Thus, the method which I have employed: 1st isolate the parts; 2nd remove, when necessary, the entire parts; and 3rd always prevent the complication of the effects on the lesions due to the effects of effusions [pp. 502, 510].

Historians in the brain sciences are quick to point out that Flourens did not originate the ablation method. DuVerney supposedly excised the cerebrum and cerebellum in 1697 (see Walker, 1957), and in 1809, Luigi Rolando (1773–1831) employed it to study the role of the cerebral hemispheres in birds. Other attempted uses of the ablation method prior to Flourens have been documented, but Flourens clearly popularized the use of this technique and was more rigorous and influential than any of his predecessors.

Flourens published his experiments in a book entitled *Recherches Expérimentales sur les Propriétés et les Fonctions du Système Nerveaux dans les Animaux Vertébrés*. The work first appeared in 1824, but was revised and expanded considerably in 1842, the year of the second edition. In these volumes, Flourens carefully described his ablation method, which was combined with naturalistic observations. The latter were, by present standards, crude and somewhat unsystematic. After ablating both cerebral hemispheres of a hen, he stated

I brought nourishment under her nose, I put her beak into grain, I put grain into her beak, I plunged her beak into water, I placed her on a shock of corn. She did not smell, she did not eat anything, she did not drink anything, she remained immobile on the shock of corn, and she certainly would have died of hunger if I had not returned to the old process of making her eat myself. Twenty times, in lieu of grain, I put sand into her beak; and she ate this as she would have eaten grain [p. 57].

The conclusions drawn from experiments like these often represented sweeping generalizations that seemed unjustified by the observations that were made. Thus, whereas Flourens concluded that the cerebellum was responsible for coordinated movements and that the medulla was necessary for the ''vital'' functions of the body, notions that are generally accepted today, he also asserted that the cerebral hemispheres had no direct role in the movement of muscle groups and argued vociferously that if one cortical faculty is destroyed, all are destroyed.

Flourens held that the cortex functioned as a whole in mediating intelligence, will, and perception (giving meaning to sensory stimuli). Thus, his position with regard to the cortex was decidedly antilocalizationist. As he stated in the 1824 edition of his book:

All sensations, all perceptions, and all volition occupy concurrently the same seat in these organs. The faculty of sensation, perception, and volition is then essentially one faculty [see Tizard, 1959, p. 133].

In part, Flourens' failure to find specific perceptual deficits after lesions limited to one part of the cortex and not to another part may have been due to his choice of experimental animals. He worked primarily with hens, pigeons, ducks, and frogs, all of whom have little cortex to speak of relative to mammalian forms. The use of birds and amphibia would also explain his failure to find any part of the cortex playing a convincing role in motor functioning. Still, Robert Young (1970) reminds us that Flourens occasionally worked on mice, and even cats and dogs.

Flourens was probably the first experimentalist to draw attention to the phenomenon of recovery of function. In the second edition of his book (1842) he devoted considerable space to this subject:

> We have just seen that it is possible to remove a certain portion of the cerebral lobes without these lobes losing their functions completely; there is more: they can recover them in their entirety after having lost them completely. I uncovered a pigeon's central node by stripping off gradually successive layers of the two lobes; I stopped as soon as, by the effect of this removal, the animal had lost the use of all its senses and all its intellectual faculties.

> From the very first day, the two mutilated cerebral lobes became enormous; their tumefaction diminished on the second day; it had almost disappeared on the third. Beginning then, the pigeon gradually reacquired sight, hearing, judgment, volition, and the rest; after six days it had recovered all; and what must be especially noticed is that as soon as it recovered one of its faculties, it had recovered them all [pp. 85–110, Krech, 1962, p. 45].

It is generally stated that the enduring contribution of Flourens to localization theory lies not in his findings, nor in his theoretical notions of brain function, but rather in the fact that he drew attention to a method for assessing the functions of the parts of the brain which was better than that of his predecessors or contemporaries. His contribution, however, really should be viewed as more than a technical one. Flourens did in fact provide the first "experimental" demonstration that suggested that the cerebrum, cerebellum, and medulla have different functions, and his discussions of recovery of function after cortical lesions represent a major contribution themselves. In addition, it was Flourens' work that stimulated the growth of more sophisticated experimentation in the brain sciences and that cooled much of the enthusiasm for phrenological theory.

The acceptance of the experimental method was, in part, due to the success that Francois Magendie (1783–1855) had with it (see Figure 3.2). Magendie, who is often cited as a founder of the French school of experimental physiology, called attention to the value of inquiring by experimentation in his text, *Précis Élémentaire de Physiologie* (1816–1817) and in a journal that he founded, which presented animal experiments and cited human case reports (*Journal de Physiologie Éxpérimentale*). Magendie, like Flourens, was a member of the French

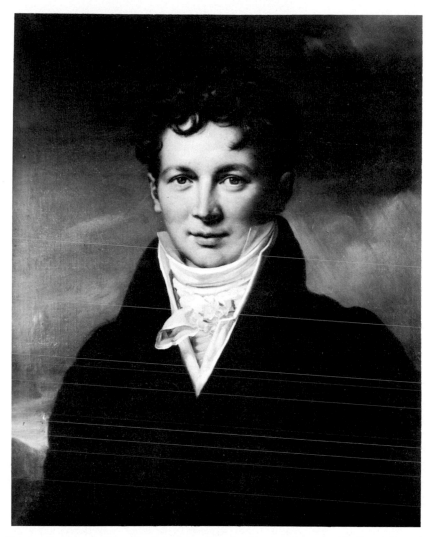

Figure 3.2. *François Magendie. Portrait attributed to Guerin. (Courtesy of Collège de France)*

Academy of Sciences, where he assumed a position of leadership and also was very influential.

Although Magendie contributed to the fields of pharmacology, circulation, digestion, respiration, and infectious diseases (cowpox, cholera), he is best known for his discovery of the functions of the spinal roots in 1822. In his landmark paper, he reported that after cutting the posterior roots of the spinal cord in some puppies, the animals retained the ability to move their limbs, whereas movement was lost and sensation remained when only the anterior roots were severed. After repeating his experiment, he wrote, "It is enough for me to announce today as positive, that the anterior and posterior roots of the nerves that arise from the spinal cord have different functions; that the posterior roots appear more particularly related to sensation, and the anterior to movement [cited in Clark and O'Malley, 1968, p. 301]."

Since a roughly similar conclusion had been alluded to by Charles Bell in 1810,[1] the credit for the distinction between the spinal roots became a matter of debate (Clarke and O'Malley, 1968; Olmstead, 1944). At any rate, the "Bell–Magendie Law," as it is now known, represented one of the most important single discoveries in the history of localization theory. It was reasoned that if a sensory–motor functional division could be found at the spinal root level, why should one not be able to make such a distinction among parts at even higher levels? As a result of such thinking, distinct sensory and motor areas of the brain were sought even more fervently than before. Flourens's conclusion that the cortex functions as a unit and does not play a direct role in initiating motor activity would now be challenged on both clinical and experimental fronts, despite his strong opinions and influence on the brain scientists in the first half of the nineteenth century.

The first localization at the cortical level that was widely accepted was presented in 1861. This was when Pierre-Paul Broca (1824–1880; Figure 3.3) described a "faculty for articulate language" in the left cerebral cortex. Prior to Broca, it seems that oral and written reports supportive of language localization were presented, but not broadly accepted. We know that Jean-Baptiste Bouillaud argued for a language center on the basis of clinical evidence as early as 1825: "The movement of the organs of speech, in particular, are controlled by a special, distinct, and independent cerebral center [p. 44]." Ernest Auburtin (1861) supported this position, and even Franz Gall discussed a case of a young man, with a sword wound of the left hemisphere, who could not remember names, yet had adequate faculties for recognition and comprehension. All of these men, moreover, believed that speech was represented somewhere in the frontal lobes. In addition, in a remarkable report dated 1836, Marc Dax described a large number of cases of speech disturbances (and right-side paralyses) and pointed out that in every instance the left hemisphere was affected (Benton and Joynt, 1960). Questions have been raised, however, as to whether Dax actually presented the

---

[1] Even when Bell replicated his findings and published them in 1811, he did not come out and directly state that the posterior roots were sensory. His conclusion, which has led to considerable controversy over who should get credit for the law of the spinal roots, was that the posterior roots represented the cerebrum, while the anterior roots projected to the cerebellum. The cerebrum, at the time, was viewed as the center for sensation and motion, and the cerebellum was believed to be the center for involuntary or reflexive action (see discussion by Clarke and O'Malley, 1968).

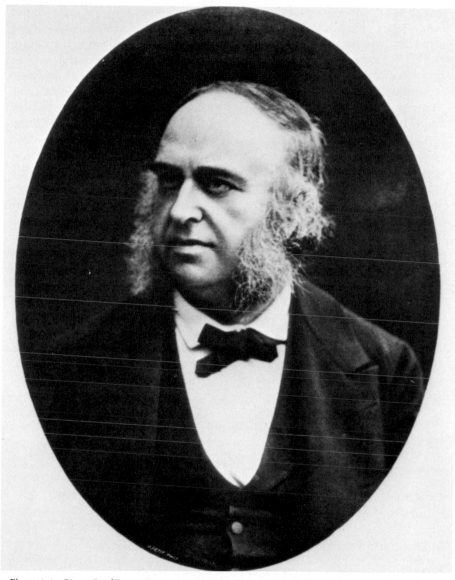

Figure 3.3. *Pierre-Paul Broca. From an engraving of a portrait by Lafosse. (Courtesy of the Wellcome Trustees)*

report at a regional medical congress at Montpelier, as intended. Gustav Dax, his son, came forth with the paper supposedly presented by his father only after Broca's key findings had been published (Joynt and Benton, 1964).

Broca's findings were presented shortly after Bouillaud offered a sum of money to anyone who could show a case of speech loss *without* a lesion of the frontal lobes. His patient, "Tan" (one of the only sounds that M. Leborgne could utter), had lost his speech 21 years earlier and had been confined to the Bicêtre ever since. One week before the patient died, Broca carefully examined him. The brain of M. Leborgne was removed immediately after his death and, 1 day later, presented to the Société d'Anthropologie as a confirmation of Bouillaud's and Aubertin's views of frontal localization of speech functions. The reaction that day (April 18, 1861) was somewhat muted, but this changed in August of the same year when Broca was able to present a more complete report of his case in which he attempted to determine more precisely the critical site of damage at the time of speech loss through a combination of anatomy, symptom history, and knowledge of lesion growth characteristics. This was necessary because the autopsy revealed a massive softening of much of the brain and because the patient showed a progressive increase in the number of symptoms that he displayed over the period of his hospitalization. That is, not only was there a loss of speech, but there was also a paralysis of the right limbs, weakened vision of the left eye, facial weaknesses, and the like. Broca deduced that the lesion originated in the third frontal convolution on the left side of the brain and, since speech was the first overt symptom, he singled out this area as the critical center for this function.

Broca came forth with a second case (M. Lelong, age 84) later the same year in which there was aphasia ("aphemie") for 1 ½ years, without a host of other symptoms, and a lesion better confined to this frontal area. By 1863 he had collected over 20 cases of aphasia. All had left hemisphere damage, and in only one of them was the "critical" frontal region spared. After considering some of these cases, Broca remarked

> Here are eight instances in which the lesion was in the posterior third of the third frontal convolution. This number seems to me to be sufficient to give strong presumptions. And the most remarkable thing is that in all the patients the lesion was on the left side [1863, p. 202].

Henry Head, the outstanding twentieth century British neurologist, summarized the impact of Broca's reports when he wrote

> These communications produced the greatest excitement in the medical world of Paris. They were specially selected for comment by the Secretary of the Societe Anatomique, in his Annual report for the year 1861. Bouillaud and his son-in-law, Auburtin, greeted Broca as a convert to their doctrines. Localisation of speech became a political question; the older Conservative school, haunted by the bogey of phrenology, clung to the conception that the brain "acted as a whole;" whilst the younger Liberals and Republicans passionately favored the view that different functions were exercised by the various portions of the cerebral hemispheres. During the next few years every medical authority took one side or the other in the discussions [1926, vol. 1, p. 25].

In the face of formidable opposition, Broca's position was successful in winning many adherents and converts to the localizationist position. Moreover, many of the skeptics in the experimental camp seemed to accept these findings of a cortical localization more readily after becoming aware of an experiment on dogs that was conducted in Prussia in 1870.

Eduard Hitzig (1838–1907; Figure 3.4) and Gustav Fritsch (1838–1927) were young physicians at the time that they conducted their study on a dressing table in the bedroom of the former's Berlin house. Following some initial experiments in which Hitzig passed current through the "central organ" in man to elicit eye movements, and some preliminary work on the rabbit, they undertook a detailed experiment to see if the cortex of the dog would be electrically excitable, and if so, to ascertain whether the sensitive area would be limited to only one part of the cortex.

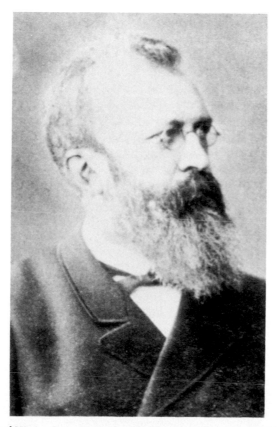

Figure 3.4. *Eduard Hitzig. (From Haymaker:* The Founders of Neurology, *1953. Courtesy of W. Haymaker and with permission of Charles C Thomas, Publisher, Springfield, Illinois.)*

The Fritsch and Hitzig (1870) experiment followed a number of early reports claiming that movements could be elicited by cortical stimulation. In general, these results were treated as artifacts due to the spread of intense current to lower centers, for not only did Flourens and Magendie deny that the cortex played a direct role in the initiation of movement, but the third great experimentalist of the time, Johann Müller (1801–1858), shared this view with them.

Clinical findings suggestive of a motor cortex were treated equally poorly despite the fact that monoplegias of an arm or a leg were beginning to be correlated with specific cortical lesions. Such reports, nevertheless, suggested a "seat" for motor functions at the cortical level, a conclusion reached by John Hughlings Jackson, among others. Nevertheless, only those findings that were indicative of no cortical localization of motor function were generally accepted prior to 1870, a point made very clear in the opening section of Fritsch and Hitzig's famous paper.

Using minimal intensity electric stimulation (enough to cause a distinct sensation when applied to the tip of the tongue), the young Germans were able to define five sites within reasonable proximity to each other that responded with specific musculature reactions. These areas represented the neck, the muscles of the front and hind leg on the opposite side of the body, and the face. This is shown in Figure 3.5.

Fritsch and Hitzig confirmed the location of the dog's motor zone by ablating

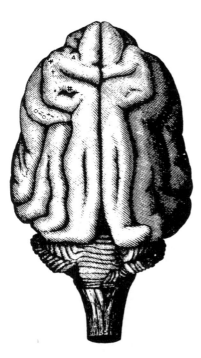

Figure 3.5. *Fritsch and Hitzig's (1870) depiction of the motor cortex of the dog (△ = neck; + = forelimb; # = hindlimb; ∞ = facial area).*

the area from which they were able to elicit bodily movements. Their ablations did not cause complete paralyses, but they clearly led to impairments in the motor performances of the dogs. Although the ablation findings were confined to a few brief sentences, the investigators were very certain about the meaning of their stimulation and ablation work. There was no question in their minds about there being a motor zone in the cortex.

Why then had this not been found by all other investigators who had attempted such experiments in the past? Fritsch and Hitzig postulated that because the motor cortex is very difficult to expose, previous experimenters probably trephined above the more posterior parts of the cortex where there are no motor fibers. When they did not find movements resulting from electrical and mechanical stimulation, they did not feel compelled to continue their explorations of the cortical surface since Flourens, Magendie, and other leading scientists stated unequivocally that the cortical surface was equipotential–that which would be found in one area would also be observed in other areas as well.

In retrospect, the isolation of the motor cortex by Fritsch and Hitzig represented the first *experimental* demonstration of localization of function at the cortical level that was widely accepted. These workers not only challenged the theory of equipotential in a controlled experiment, but raised the suggestion that more than a motor zone would be found at the cortical level (the 1870 paper does not cite Broca). In the last paragraph of their famous report, they made a statement that then attracted, and still is attracting, many adherents. They concluded that "certainly some psychological functions and perhaps all of them . . . *need* circumscribed centers of the cortex [p. 332]."

The period immediately following Fritsch and Hitzig's (1870) report can be characterized as one dominated by researchers trying to identify motor centers in other organisms, as well as attempts to define still other centers at the level of the cortex. These endeavors were aided by new and more precise stimulation and ablation techniques. To some extent the efforts were led by Sir David Ferrier (1873, 1874, 1876, 1878, 1886), a British investigator (Figure 3.6).

Intrigued with the idea that the cortex was electrically excitable, Ferrier was the first to confirm the findings of the German investigators and to extend them to the monkey. Not only did he define the motor cortex in the primate, but he also described 15 different subareas of it based on his stimulation techniques. Ferrier claimed that his experiments owed much to the thinking of John Hughlings Jackson and to his descriptions of patients with epilepsy. The seizures resulting from these "rude experiments of disease" led Jackson to state that a well organized motor cortex would be found in higher forms.

Ferrier continued to work on this problem and eventually was able to produce convulsions experimentally. He also was able to map the motor cortex in rabbits, cats, guinea pigs, and dogs, thus showing that localization of the motor zone represented a general principle of the mammalian cortex. Ferrier also performed

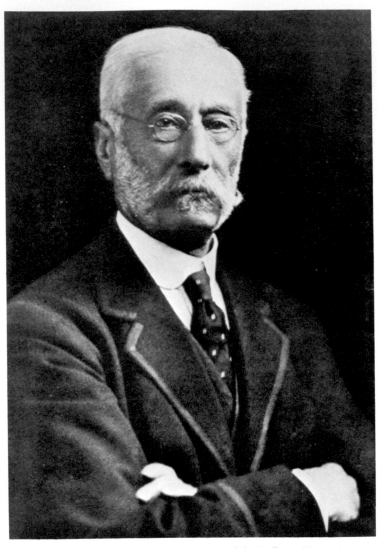

Figure 3.6. *Sir David Ferrier. (Courtesy of the Wellcome Trustees)*

ablations of the motor zone, some of which had rather dramatic impact. In 1881, when one of his monkeys with a unilateral motor cortex lesion was brought before a medical congress in London, Charcot, upon seeing the contralateral hemiplegia, reportedly remarked, ''It's a patient! [Thornwald, 1960].''

Confirmation of a motor cortex in a human being came in 1874 when Dr. Robert Bartholow (1831–1904), an American, was shown a patient with a malignant ulcer of the scalp which produced a large cranial opening that allowed him to see and stimulate the patient's brain electrically. He found that Mary Rafferty, his feeble-minded patient, showed well-defined muscular contractions on the right side of the body when the left hemisphere was stimulated. These revealing experiments had to be terminated when his patient went into seizure. She died soon afterward from complications due to her disease.[2]

While these experiments were being conducted on the motor areas, the search for restricted sensory cortical areas continued. Johann Müller's "doctrine of specific nerve energies" was generally accepted by the end of the 1800s, and his theory implied that each sensory system had its own receptors and pathways for transmitting information to the central nervous system, regardless of the mode of stimulation (e.g., pressure on the retina would still result in visual sensations, typically referred to as phosphenes). It seemed logical that an equivalent condition existed within the nervous system itself, with different cortical areas receiving information from each of the senses.

In the case of the visual system, there was good, early evidence that the occipital cortex was the center for visual perception, at least in birds (Walker, 1957). This assertion was confirmed in 1874 by Hitzig, in an experimental study of the effects of posterior cortical lesions on the behavior of dogs. Hitzig noted that such lesions produced blindness and paralytic dilation of the pupils. The work of David Ferrier on monkeys, dogs, and cats led to a more precise localization of the visual cortex at the back of the brain, and in 1911, Minkowski showed that the visual cortex had an anatomical correlate in the striated part of the occipital lobe. From that point on, the concept of a visual cortex seems to have been treated more as a fact than as a theory, although differences of opinion centered on the extent of the critical zone and the deficits which follow its destruction.

The association between hearing and the temporal lobes is usually attributed to Ferrier (1876). He believed that auditory functions were localized in the first temporal convolution since electrical stimulation of this area caused monkeys to perk up the opposite ear. Ferrier, in 1881, claimed that deafness resulted when this area was bilaterally ablated. He cauterized the superior temporal cortex bilaterally in a monkey and 6 weeks later took that monkey and the one with hemiplegia to a medical congress in London. When he fired a percussion cap, only the hemiplegic animal reacted to it. His conclusion was treated skeptically al-

---

[2] Most early descriptions of the motor cortex did not confine its boundaries to the precentral gyrus, as is frequently done today. Ferrier himself believed that the excitable region included parts of the parietal lobe and the superior temporal gyrus. Horsley and Schäfer (1888), in their investigations of monkeys and apes, agreed that the motor zone included at least some of the postcentral gyrus. This position was abandoned, however, when Grünbaum and Sherrington presented their ablation and stimulation studies of the cortices of primates, including chimpanzees and gorillas. Their findings, which began to appear in 1892, restricted the motor cortex to the precentral gyrus and soon represented the generally accepted position.

most from the beginning. Munk, for example, conducted a series of ablation experiments in which deafness per se was not found, although the animals had trouble recognizing sounds ("psychical deafness"). It is now clear that lesions like those made by Ferrier have little effect on intensity or frequency discrimination, although the area is "auditory" in the sense that lesions here tend to impair the localization of sound in space and auditory pattern perception.[3]

In addition to contributing to our knowledge of the motor and sensory areas of the cortex, David Ferrier (1874, 1878) was among the first of the experimentalists to try to localize higher functions in discrete zones of the cerebral cortex. He found that there was little change when he electrically stimulated the region anterior to the motor zones, but that when he ablated it, his animals behaved as if they were suffering from dementia. His conclusion (1886) was that the frontal lobes were likely to be the "substrata of those psychical processes that lie at the foundation of higher intellectual operations [p. 467]." This conclusion was not entirely original. Hitzig (1874) believed that animals with these lesions had weak memories, whereas Goltz stated that such subjects could be characterized by stupid facial expressions and lack of normal fear.

Another individual who contributed to this line of thought was the Italian neurologist, Leonardo Bianchi (1848–1927). Bianchi's important papers on the intellectual functions of the frontal lobes date from 1895 and are summarized in a book that appeared in 1920. The following sentence can be found in the latter publication:

> The first experiments that I undertook on dogs permitted me to express myself in an initial communication in the sense that, for the time being, it was possible to conclude that the *unilateral* mutilations of the prefrontal lobe of the experimental animals were not followed by any noteworthy symptoms; and that the bilateral mutilations in the dogs had produced a distinct change in character, especially prominent in all the psychic manifestations; defective perceptive judgment, exaggerated fear through defective critical power and through inability to avail themselves of their physical powers, actually preserved; amnesia and a psychically blind

---

[3] The localization of the somatosensory cortex proved to be especially troublesome to the early investigators, and there were marked differences of opinion on this subject. This is brought out very clearly in a review of this subject dating from 1890 (Mills). The review shows that some investigators localized the somatic cortex anterior to the Rolandic fissure, some placed it posterior, and some claimed that it crossed the fissure. C. E. Beevor and Victor Horsley (1890), for example, argued that the precentral cortex was primarily motor, the postcentral cortex was primarily sensory, and that a "zone of confusion" existed between the maximal motor and maximal sensory zones. Such a position is consistent with the findings of more modern investigators, like Clinton Woolsey, who tend to speak of motor-sensory and sensorymotor cortices because they feel that the sensory and motor areas do in fact overlap each other (Woolsey, 1958). Sherrington and his coworkers, however, restricted the somatic cortex to the anterior part of the parietal lobe, and their position has been the dominant one for the last 80 years, in spite of ablation, stimulation, and electrical recording data showing that the sensory zone is probably much broader than this.

behavior, defective initiative and resourcefulness, lack of finality in complex movements, revealed by incoherent conduct and lessened vivacity (lowering of the
psychic tone), so that any ordinary person would have judged the animals to be im-
becile [pp. 89–90; translated by Clarke and O'Malley, 1968].

The new localizations soon found practical application in the hands of the
neurosurgeons who could now use the symptoms displayed by their patients to
make better judgments about the nature and locus of the insult and the need for
surgery. In 1879, William Macewen, A Glasgow physician, performed a series of
operations in which the damage was localized with the aid of Ferrier's publications on localization. On November 25, 1884, a tumor, whose size and locus were
predicted on the basis of Ferrier's experimental studies, was removed from a patient by Rickman Godlee at the National Hospital, Queens Square. Godlee's patient was a 25-year-old man with evidence of a lesion near the central part of the
cortex of the right hemisphere. He displayed Jacksonian epilepsy (attacks beginning in the face, then spreading to the tongue and arm), left arm weakness, and
headache. Both David Ferrier and John Hughlings Jackson supposedly were present in the operating room when their predictions were confirmed (Trotter, 1934).

The efforts of physicians like Bartholow, Macewen, and Godlee soon led to the
use of electrical stimulation of the brain in human subjects undergoing surgery
for removal of epileptic foci and related disorders. Harvey Cushing (e.g., 1909)
was a pioneer in this area. He found that somatic "sensations without movements" were possible. In addition, he noticed that stimulation of the postcentral
cortex often resulted in sensations of tingling, pressure, and touch, but not
temperature or pain. This was confirmed many years later in the studies of Wilder
Penfield and Theodore Rasmussen (1950), at the Montreal Neurological Institute. Cushing's division among the skin senses had a tremendous impact on the
thinking of Henry Head. Head later postulated that pain and temperature were
subcortical functions, while the sensory cortex was responsible for tactual shape
recognition, two-point discrimination, and related higher tactile functions. Such
conclusions opened the door for others to try to correlate various subcortical nuclei
and tracts with functions, much as was being done at the cortical level.

At the same time that these clinical and experimental investigations were
being conducted, anatomists were hard at work attempting to determine if each
of the newly delineated cortical areas had unique cellular characteristics that
would distinguish them from other areas. Oscar and Cecile Vogt were the leading early figures in this endeavor and are often credited for founding the science
of "functional neuroanatomy." One of their students, Korbinian Brodmann
(1868–1918) claimed that there were 52 cytoarchitectural areas of the human cortex and devised a number code that is still being used today. (Figure 3.7 shows two
of his drawings.) Nevertheless, disagreement existed about the exact number of
areas and their boundaries. Grafton Eliot Smith, an Australian working in Cairo
at the time claimed the number was 56 after examining numerous specimens with

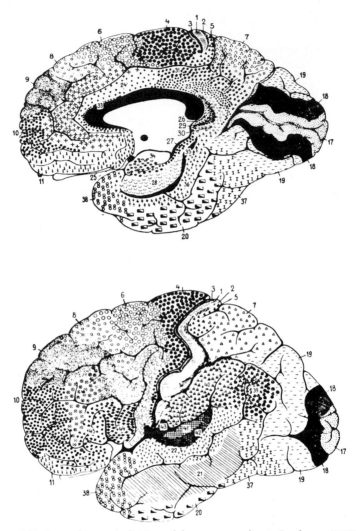

Figure 3.7. *Cytoarchitectonic divisions of the cortex according to Brodmann (1909).*

a hand lens. In fact, the Vogts at one point spoke of over 200 anatomical fields, each with distinguishing cytoarchitectonic and/or myelination patterns.

Brodmann (1909) summarized the views of this school when he wrote the following:

> The specific histological differentiation of the cortical areas proves irrefutably their *specific functional differentiation*—for it is based as we have seen on a division of labor. The great number of specifically prepared structural areas suggests *a special*

separation of individual functions. Moreover, the outlines of the fields in which all cases are sharp, finally allows us to conclude that a *strictly circumscribed localization* of the physiological activities which correspond to the area is necessary [cited in von Bonin, 1960, p. 304].

Physiologists were contributing to localization as well. Richard Caton, of Liverpool, was probably the first to record the spontaneous electrical activity of the brain, although his research is rarely cited today. Not only did he precede Hans Berger (1929) by many years, but he even noticed that light falling on the retina increased the electrical activity of the occipital region more than other regions (see Gibson, 1962).

From these anatomical, neurological, and physiological roots, twentieth-century investigators have gone on to localize literally hundreds of "functions" in cortical and subcortical areas of the brain and are now subdividing these areas even further. In fact, the tendency to localize functions is currently so well accepted by individuals in the neural sciences that even indirect or suggestive associations along these lines have ceased to be viewed as theoretical. This, in turn, has led to a very rigid conception of neuronal organization that has dominated thinking about such issues as recovery of function.

As we stated in Chapter 1, we will now raise a number of questions about this type of thinking. The first to be addressed is whether the central nervous system is capable of any sort of reorganization after injury, or whether the capacity of central nervous system neurons to make new connections and undergo "remodeling" is lost very early in development. We will then ask about the possibility of recovery after brain damage. If the circuitry is in fact unmodifiable, especially after the neonatal period, and if each structure has its own unique functions, one might expect little recovery following strokes, trauma, or other types of brain insult. On the other hand, if recovery is more pervasive than is usually thought, even after damage to supposedly "critical" centers in the brain, a number of possibilities would have to be addressed more seriously. One possibility, for example, is that neuronal plasticity and remodeling could underlie some of the observed recovery. Another is based on the notion that some psychological (behavioral) functions that have been assigned to particular structures are simply incorrect and represent ideas that extend well beyond the data at hand. In the last chapter we will emphasize the point that localization of a unit response or even a symptom following acute, focal brain injury has a certain heuristic and clinical relevance. However, equating such events and observations with psychological functions and centers for such activities as aggressiveness, memory, and forethought may require more in the way of inferences, suppositions, assumptions, and theories than immediately meets the eye.

With this in mind, let us begin to look at the data. The first issue to be addressed is whether the central nervous system of mammals is fixed and incapable of regeneration or reorganization following damage, or whether the synaptic organization of the brain is in flux and capable of regenerative and/or other dramatic anatomical and physiological changes after injury and disease.

References

Auburtin, S. A. E. Reprise de la discussion sur la forme et le volume du cerveau. *Bulletin de la Société Anthropologie le Paris*, 1861, *2*, 209–220.

Bartholow, R. Experimental investigations into the functions of the human brain. *American Journal of Medical Science* (New Series), 1874, *67*, 305–313.

Beevor, C. E., and Horsley, V. A record of the results obtained by electrical stimulation of the so-called motor cortex and internal capsule in the orangutang. *Philosophical Transactions*, 1890, *181*, 129–258.

Bell, C. *Idea of a new anatomy of the brain submitted for the observations of his friends.* London: Strahan and Preston, 1811. (Reprinted in *Journal of Anatomy and Physiology*, 1869, *3*, 147–182.)

Benton, A. L., and Joynt, R. J. Early descriptions of aphasia. *Archives of Neurology*, 1960, *3*, 205–222.

Bianchi, L. [The functions of the frontal lobes] (A. Watteville, trans.) *Brain*, 1895, *18*, 497–522.

Bianchi, L. *La meccanica del cervello e la funzione dei lobi frontali* Turin: Fratelli Bocca, 1920.

Bouillaud, J.-B. Recherches cliniques propres à démontrer que la perte de la parole correspond à la lésion des lobules antérieurs du cerveau, et à confirmer l'opinion de M. Gall, sur le siège de l'organe du language articulé. *Archives de Médicine Géneral*, 1825, *8*, 25–45.

Broca, P.-P. Perte de la parole, ramollissement chronique et destruction partielle du lobe anterior gauche du cerveau. *Bulletin de la Société Anthropologié de Paris*, 1861, *2*, 235–238. (a)

Broca, P.-P. Remarques sur le siège de la faculté du language articulé: Suivies d'une observation d'aphémie (perte de la parole). *Bulletin de la Société Anatomique de Paris*, 1861, *36*, 330–357. (b)

Broca, P.-P. Localisation des fonctions cérébrales—Siège du language articulé. *Bulletin de la Société Anthropologié de Paris*, 1863, *4*, 200–202.

Brodmann, K. *Vergleichende lokalisationslehre der grosshirnrinde in ihren prinzipien dargestellt auf grund des zellenbaues.* Leipzig: J. A. Barth, 1909.

Clarke, E., and O'Malley, C. D. *The human brain and spinal cord.* Berkeley: University of California Press, 1968.

Ferrier, D. Experimental researches in cerebral physiology and pathology. *West Riding Lunatic Asylum Medical Reports*, 1873, *3*, 30–96.

Ferrier, D. The localisation of function in the brain. *Proceedings of the Royal Society*, 1874, *22*, 229–232.

Ferrier, D. *The functions of the brain.* London: Smith and Elder, 1876.

Ferrier, D. *The localisation of cerebral disease.* London: Smith and Elder, 1878.

Ferrier, D. *The functions of the brain* (2nd ed.). London: Smith and Elder, 1886.

Flourens, J.-P.-M. *Recherches expérimentales sur les propriétés et les fonctions du système nerveux dans les animaux vertébrés* (2nd ed.). Paris: Ballière, 1842. (Originally published, 1824.)

Flourens, P. *Psychologie compareé* (2nd ed.). Paris: Garnier Freres, 1864.

Fritsch, G., and Hitzig, E. Über die elektrische erregbarkeit des grosshirns. *Archiv für Anatomie und Physiologie*, 1870, 300–332.

Gibson, W. C. Pioneers in localization of function in the brain. *Journal of the American Medical Association*, 1962, *180*, 944–951.

Goldstein, K. Paul Broca (1824–1880). In W. Haymaker and F. Schiller (eds.), *The founders of neurology.* Springfield, Ill.: Charles C Thomas, 1953, Pp. 12–16.

Head, H. *Aphasia and kindred disorders of speech* (2 vols.). Cambridge: Cambridge University Press, 1926.

Hitzig, E. *Untersuchungen über das gehirn*. Berlin: Hirschwald, 1874.

Horsley, V., and Schäfer, E. A. A record of experiments upon the functions of the cerebral cortex. *Philosophical Transactions of the Royal Society of London*, 1888, *179B*, 1–45.

Joynt, R. J., and Benton, A. L. The memoire of Marc Dax on aphasia. *Neurology*, 1964, *14*, 851–854.

Krech, D. Cortical localization of function. In L. Postman (Ed.), *Phychology in the making*. New York: Alfred A. Knopf, 1962, Pp. 31–72.

Magendie, F. *Précis élémentaire de physiologie*. Paris, 1816–1817.

Magendie, F. Expériences sur les fonctions des racines des nerfs rachidiens. *Journal de Physiologie Éxpérimentale et Pathologie*, 1822, *2*, 276–279.

Mills, C. K. Cerebral localization in its practical relations. *Brain*, 1890, *12*, 233–288; 358–406.

Olmstead, J. M. D. *François Magendie*. New York: Schuman, 1944.

Penfield, W., and Rasmussen, T. *The cerebral cortex of man*. New York: Macmillan, 1950.

Thornwald, J. [*The triumph of surgery*] (R. Winston and C. Winston, trans.) London: Thames and Hudson, 1960.

Tizard, B. Theories of brain localization from Flourens to Lashley. *Medical History*, 1959, *3*, 132–145.

Trotter, W. A landmark in modern neurology. *Lancet*, 1934, *2*, 1207–1210.

von Bonin, G. *Some papers on the cerebral cortex*. Springfield, Ill.: Charles C Thomas, 1960.

Walker, A. E. Stimulation and ablation: Their role in the history of cerebral physiology. *Journal of Neurophysiology*, 1957, *20*, 435–449.

Woolsey, C. N. Organization of somatic sensory and motor areas of the cerebral cortex. In H. F. Harlow and C. N. Woolsey (Eds.), *Biological and biochemical bases of behavior*. Madison: University of Wisconsin Press, 1958, Pp. 63–81.

Young, R. M. *Mind, brain and adaptation in the nineteenth century*. Oxford: Clarendon Press, 1970.

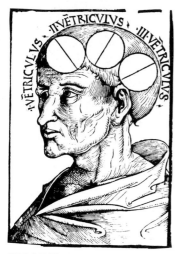

Regeneration in the Central Nervous System

CHAPTER FOUR

Once development was ended, the founts of growth and regeneration of the axons and dendrites dried up irrevocably. In adult centers, the nerve paths are something fixed, and immutable; everything may die, nothing may be regenerated [Santiago Ramón y Cajal, 1928, p. 750].

The phenomena of neural growth and regeneration and the possibility that they might serve as a basis for functional restitution after damage to the mammalian central nervous system have prompted a new and exciting area of research in neurobiology. Even before the turn of this century some theorists had suggested that some axonal regrowth after spinal cord injury in mammals was possible, but the regenerative process was thought to be very limited at best and therefore of questionable functional significance (Guth, 1975; Guth and Windle, 1970).

In reviewing the early literature, Carmine D. Clemente (1964) noted that early experimenters

> were especially responsible for the thesis that the regenerative efforts in the central nervous system of adult mammals resulted in abortive growth. In their opinions, central nerve fibers commenced to regenerate, but for some reason, the newly formed sprouts would not continue across the transection site and make functional connections in the opposite stump [p. 283].

Quite clearly, the best anatomical evidence for regeneration of tracts in the central nervous system comes from work on nonmammalian organisms, such as amphibia and fish. In this context, the retinal projections of frogs, newts, and goldfish have been carefully studied by Roger Sperry and his colleagues (Attardi and Sperry, 1963; Meyer and Sperry, 1974; Sperry, 1943, 1944, 1945). Sperry's group has shown that regenerating retinal fibers grow along specific pathways to reach "target points" in the tectum. In the goldfish, even after the fibers are divided and scrambled, Meyer and Sperry (1974) found that, "they somehow unsort themselves and regrow the appropriate topographic projections required for optokinetic orienting and visual discriminative behavior [p. 47]."

In some experiments, these investigators surgically rotated the eyes 180°. Afterward they found that the nerve fibers grew back into their normal locations and that the animals behaved as if their visual fields were upside down. The fact that the regenerating axons always terminated in an extremely orderly manner led Sperry (1963) to develop his "chemoaffinity" hypothesis, which basically holds that sites have specific chemical markers that guide growing and regenerating axons to their appropriate destinations.

How critical is it for damaged nerve fibers to grow back to their original points of innervation? This is an important question that must be addressed if neuronal regeneration is to be related to the behavior of the organism. For example, if visual fibers grow into an auditory region of the brain, they would not be expected to provide any information that would be helpful in recovering lost auditory abilities, and such "abnormal" growth could even interfere with normal auditory processing. In the visual system, appropriate topographical (point-to-point) representation is assumed to be essential for normal functioning, and the expectation is that regenerating fibers will follow the same general course as the original axons that were injured.

Myong G. Yoon (1973) examined the assumption of point-to-point topography as being essential for vision by rearranging the target tissue of the retinal projections in the adult goldfish. In one of his experiments, a rectangular piece of the tectum (the central region receiving direct projections from the retina) was dissected out on the left side, lifted free, and then carefully replaced in the same position. Yoon waited about 6 months and then examined peripherally evoked electrophysiological responses in the reimplanted zone with microelectrode recording techniques. Yoon (1973) was able to demonstrate that the retinal projection of the visual field was "restored to a more-or-less normal topographic pattern [p. 579]," thus confirming an earlier report by Sharma and Gaze (1971). In other words, the regenerating optic nerve fibers in the adult goldfish were attracted to specific positions that appeared to be the same as those found in the intact brain.

If the target tissue (i.e., the tectum) possessed a highly specific chemical marker that attracted regenerating fibers to the appropriate place, a 180° surgical rotation of the tectum should have produced a complete (inversion) of the retinal projection map. When Yoon attempted such rotations, the tectal grafts took less successfully, and only 2 of 41 operated fish proved usable. Despite these problems, when the reimplanted tissue was mapped electrophysiologically in response to visual stimulation, the fish that were usable demonstrated a completely reversed retinotopic ordering of afferent inputs.

Yoon (1973) argues that the specificity of neuromorphological patterning demonstrated by these experiments strongly supports the chemoaffinity hypothesis proposed by Roger Sperry. The tectal tissue does not receive the regenerating fibers passively, but rather there "is an active accomodation which selects appropriate optic fibers to make proper synaptic connections in a consistent topographic order [p. 586]." That is, there is a specific "matching" of inputs with specific target sites, and this is based on some sort of chemical marker that is specific to each element of the system. We should note, at this point, that the specific chemicotrophic markers guiding the growing neurons to their appropriate terminal sites still remain to be identified. Nevertheless, since the fibers do not grow in a haphazard or random fashion, at least not in the mature nervous system, it is difficult to think that such markers are not present.

Quite clearly, the notion of an "alluring" chemical is in itself quite alluring to workers in this field. Yet in spite of evidence like that presented by Yoon and Sperry, Marcus Jacobson (1978) urges caution in considering chemoaffinity as an invariant feature of neural organization.

Jacobson cites an earlier study by Weiss and Taylor (1944), who first cut the sciatic or tibial (both peripheral) nerves of the adult rat and then used a Y-shaped arterial cuff to join the two cut ends. In one stem of the Y they placed the distal nerve stump and in the other they placed a blood clot or tendon. Weiss and Taylor found that abundant regeneration occurred in *both* branches, regardless of whether the neurotrophic substance was present or not.

It should also be remembered that in the Yoon experiment only a few of the many animals used showed successful regenerative outcomes (2 in 41). Jacobson argues that the pathways followed by regenerating fibers can be very tortuous and that many often fail to reach their destinations. Under these circumstances, any correct connections that occur might, in part, be the result of trial and error or chance encounters between regenerating fibers and target neurons. It thus may be that many fibers start out in the early stages of regeneration, but that only those that can eventually make synaptic contacts survive; we then infer order out of randomness and purpose out of chaotic trial-and-error search since we are observing only the outcome rather than the struggle for survival itself.

In adult mammals, there is now considerable evidence which can be taken to suggest that central nervous system regeneration occurs, although the new growth is generally more difficult to detect and less dramatic than in nonmammalian vertebrates. At the present time, it is generally accepted that there can be some regeneration in the transected spinal cords of rats, cats, and dogs after meticulous care, the administration of drugs (e.g., steriods, pyrogens), or ionizing radiation (cf. Clemente, 1964). Under some conditions, the regenerating axons traversing the lesions have even been found to conduct nervous impulses to the other side of the cut (Liu and Scott, 1958; see also Windle, 1955). For instance, Cambell and his colleagues (see Clemente, 1964, pp. 287–288) enclosed the transected spinal stumps in a porous plastic cylinder, which allowed nutrients to pass through it, but which prevented fibroblasts and connective tissue from mechanically interfering with the regenerative process. With the tube oriented longitudinally between the cut ends of the spinal cord, there was some regeneration. This was seen histologically, and electrophysiological analyses showed that the new axons could conduct nervous impulses across the tube. Although the regeneration was much more complete than would be expected if scar tissue and related elements were allowed to form, the rats in this study did not show recovery of posture and locomotion.

Evidence for regeneration in the brain itself is now being reported. In one study, Anne F. Marks (1972), of Johns Hopkins University, lowered a very fine wire loop into the brain of a rat to sever the medial portion of the right medial lemniscus (the pathway that carries somatic information from the spinal cord and lower brain stem to the thalamus). The loop was left in place for 18 days and was removed only after the animal had been killed and perfused. With the use of special stains, Marks was able to observe regenerating axons in the vicinity of the lesion. Some of these fibers penetrated the area between the loop, but the majority avoided the scarred area and traveled parallel to the edges of the injury in the uninterrupted tissue until they could join the medial lemniscus. Overall, the fibers were of uniform diameter and appeared normal in that they showed no variscosities or discontinuities. Marks claims that her work shows that anatomical repair of the mammalian brain may be more common than previously thought, although somewhat difficult to detect. Unfortunately, she did not examine the new synapses nor do any behavioral testing to determine whether deficits followed the lesion and subsided as the regenerating fibers reached their destinations. As she states, ''Unless such synapses and function can be demonstrated . . . the reconstructive regeneration of tracts in the mammalian brain may be a trivial, ultimately useless, phenomenon of great promise [p. 462].''

The development of histofluorescence techniques (Falck, Hillarp, Thieme, and Torp, 1962) represents a great advance in this area since one can now begin to evaluate whether the new synapses are ''functional,'' at least on a physiological level. Histofluorescence allows one to assess the status of neurotransmitters in the newly formed terminals. For example, noradrenaline will fluoresce under certain conditions, and the greater the presence of this transmitter, the more fluorescence there will be. In regeneration studies, heightened green fluorescence would signify that the new fibers are biochemically active. (These techniques can also be used to assess the functional status of axonal ''sprouts'' from intact, uninjured axons, as will be seen in the following chapters.)

Anders Björklund and his colleagues at Lund University in Sweden were among the first to use histofluorescence techniques to examine regenerating axons in the mature mammalian brain. In an early study utilizing these procedures, Katzman, Björklund, Owman, Stenevi, and West (1971) subjected rats to electrolytic lesions in the substantia nigra and the adjacent ventromedial tegmentum and then sacrificed them at varying times after surgery. They found that in rats permitted only a few days for survival there was an intense accumulation of fluorescent catecholamine in the transected axon stumps adjacent to the lesion. Fluorescent swollen cell bodies and coarse, beaded convoluted fibers, characteristic of damaged and dying neurons, were easily identified in the 2–7 day survival groups. In rats killed after the seventh postoperative day, differences in the character of the green catecholamine fluorescence were detected. Here the experimenters observed fine, varicose fibers outlining the electrode track as it entered the area of the lesion, and, within the damaged area, densely woven, fine fibers were observed. These fine fibers were not observed during the short survival period.

Two weeks after damaging the substantia nigra, all of the swollen and distorted neurons had largely disappeared. The damaged neurons were apparently replaced by densely packed, thin fibers growing into the borders of the lesion. There was also an abnormally dense fiber innervation to the blood vessels in the area of the lesion and to areas not usually receiving catecholaminergic fibers. Overall, these findings were interpreted as a clear indication that central catecholaminergic neurons are capable of significant regenerative sprouting.

It is important to ask whether the presence of green fluorescing fibers actually represents the regeneration of central catecholaminergic fibers or whether it could be reflecting offshoots from intact nerve fibers passing near the vacated terminals (i.e., collateral sprouting). The workers at Lund were well aware that both possibilities could be occurring, but concluded that they were observing regeneration, for a number of reasons. First, they point out that the fluorescence seen in the first few days following the damage was confined to the damaged stumps and reflected the damming up of the vesicles carrying the neurotransmitter. Second, they state that the changes in fluorescent activity that occurred with the longer survival times clearly paralleled the "fast outgrowth" of terminals from the severed axons, which permitted the accumulated noradrenaline to migrate to the newly formed endings.

As we stated earlier in this chapter, the question of function, at least with regard to behavior, would appear to be related to whether the reinnervation pattern and its pharmacology match the original properties of the system under study. One way that this can be assessed is by placing different transplants into the area of the transected neurons.

Björklund and Stenevi (1971) transplanted pieces of rat iris (which is partially adrenergically innervated) into the region of the animal's medial forebrain bundle, an area containing both ascending and descending noradrenergic and dopaminergic neurons. The animals with transplants were killed at various stages after surgery, and their brains were examined for evidence of fiber regeneration. At first (3–5 days after transplantation), there was the typical pattern of amine accumulation in the proximal region of the axon stumps. Very delicate "varicose fibers" appeared near the surface of the transplanted iris about a week after the operation, and a week after this, the regenerating fibers entered the iris in specific orientations similar to the normal sympathic innervation seen in the intact eye. With longer survival periods (e.g., 40 days), there were even more dopamine- and noradrenaline-containing fibers present, and these remained in abundance for at least 6 months, strongly suggesting that they were not abortive or feeble attempts at regenerative growth. This is shown in Figure 4.1.

To examine the specificity of the reinnervation further, Björklund and Stenevi (1971) introduced other types of tissue (the mitral valve from the heart, which receives adrenergic input or pieces of diaphragm or uterus, which have little or no adrenergic innervation) into the region of the medial forebrain bundle. The mitral valve transplants showed patterns of innervation that closely resembled those of the normal state. In contrast, regenerating sprouts rarely entered the diaphragm or uterus transplants, but instead grew in a somewhat haphazard manner around the tissue. These findings are illustrated in Figure 4.2 and show that the target tissue may play a role in determining the extent of regenerative growth following injury to the brain and that regenerative connections tend to be affected by chemical properties of the target tissue.

Is the reinnervation of target tissue by the regenerating axonal stumps limited only to adrenergic or dopaminergic fibers? This is an important question because, if true, it would mean that only a relatively limited degree of recovery of function might be expected, if any were to occur at all. If the cholinergic systems of the brain could also be shown to have regenerative capabilities in mature mammalian subjects, a greater degree of functional recovery following central nervous system injury would be expected.

In a recent series of experiments, Svengaardt, Björklund, and Stenevi (1976) once again challenged the widely accepted belief that mammalian central nervous system regeneration is of very limited character. They transplanted cholinergically innervated peripheral tissue into specific brain areas and then determined the rate and extent of reinnervation of axons from the damaged neurons. For this purpose, Svengaardt and his colleagues made autologous transplants (i.e., from the same animal) of iris into either the thalamus and hippocampus or the hippocampal fimbria of adult rats. Visualization of catecholamine and acetylcholinesterase-containing fibers was made under light microscopy with the histofluorescence procedure referred to earlier and with a histochemical stain specific to acetylcholinesterase-containing nerve fibers (Holmstedt, 1957). The iris transplants were made in such a way as to transect the acetylcholinesterase-positive pathways, such as the septo-hippocampal and dorsal-tegmental tracts. As shown in Figure 4.3, the iris was placed in direct contact with transected, presumably acetylcholine-containing fiber stumps.

Within 18–30 days after the operation, Svengaardt and his co-workers (1976) observed that the irises were "richly supplied with new AChE fibers that were *seen to originate primarily from the severed axons* in the septo-hippocampal

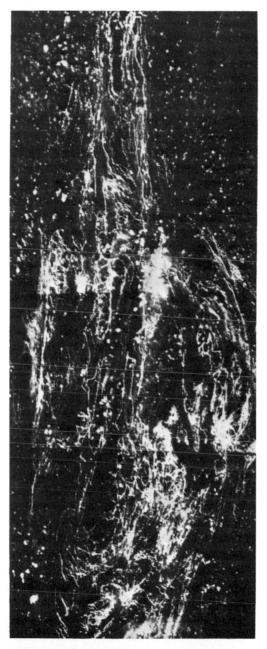

Figure 4.1. *Photomontage of an iris transplant (sagittal section) in the rostral mesencephalon, 6 months after transplantation. The entire transplant is reinnervated by mainly noradrenaline-containing fibers of central origin. (From Björklund and Stenevi, 1971.)*

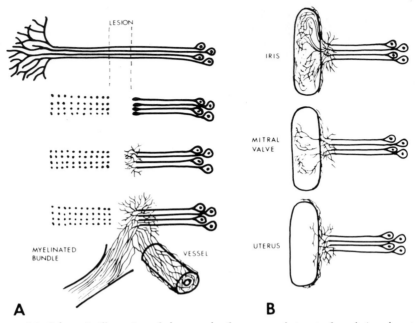

A   **B**

Figure 4.2. *Schematic illustration of the growth of new axonal sprouts from lesioned central adrenergic neurons. (A) After mechanical lesion; (B) After transplantation of peripheral tissue into the site of axonal damage. (From Stenevi et al., 1973.)*

pathways [p. 6]." The pattern of reinnervation in some parts of the iris was strikingly similar to that seen in the normal animal. The authors point out that in the normal iris, adrenergic and cholinergic fibers run together within the same Schwann cell sheaths; and in the iris transplanted to the caudal diencephalon or hippocampus, there is reinnervation by noradrenergic as well as acetylcholinesterase-containing fibers. Svengaardt and his colleagues concluded that regeneration restores the original cholinergic-adrenergic arrangements by following preestablished neural sheaths.

Such observations lend support to the idea that the target tissue (e.g., deafferented area) plays a very important role in guiding and perhaps determining the extent and efficiency of terminal regeneration. If this is the case, then the status and viability of tissue remaining intact after localized injury may be a very important factor in determining whether or not successful regeneration and recovery of function will occur.

Overall, the findings of the workers from the University of Lund seem to provide a strong counterargument to the pessimistic picture drawn by Santiago Ramón y Cajal (1928; Figure 4.4) more than 50 years earlier. Yet, in considering the results just outlined, as well as comparable data on regenerative growth of severed axons in the spinal cord (Björklund, Katzman, Stenevi, and West, 1971),

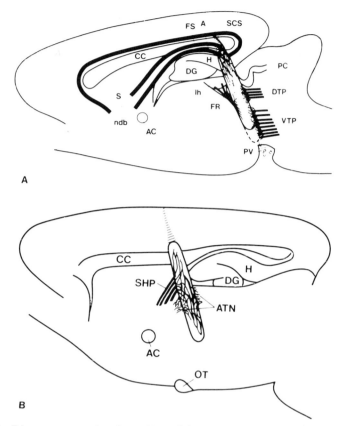

Figure 4.3. *Diagram representing the position of the iris transplanted through the hippocampus into the caudal diencephalon (A) and into the hippocampal fimbria and the anterior thalamus (B). Lesioned AChE-positive pathways are indicated by heavy black lines. Striped area represents the track of the transplantation rod. Abbreviations: A, alveus; AC, anterior commissure; ATN, anterior thalamic nuclei; CC, corpus callosum; DG, dentate gyrus; DTP, dorsal tegmental AChE pathway; FS, fornix superior; FR, fasciculus retroflexus; H, hippocampus; lh, lateral habenular nucleus; ndb, nucleus of the diagonal band; OT, optic tract; PC, posterior commissure; PV, pial vessels; S, septum; SCS, subcallosal stria; SHP, septo-hippocampal AChE pathways; VTP, ventral tegmental AChE pathway. (From Svengaardt* et al., *1976.)*

one must wonder why there are not more reports on functional regeneration in the adult mammalian central nervous system or why there is not a greater degree of functional restitution than is usually observed in clinical settings. The answers to these questions are not clear, although a number of factors must be taken into consideration (for detailed reviews of these problems see Clemente, 1964; Reitan, 1966; Schoenfeld and Hamilton, 1977; Windle, 1955).

In the first place, traumatic damage to the brain rarely, if ever, resembles the neat, clean surgical excision seen in the experimental laboratory. Even under con-

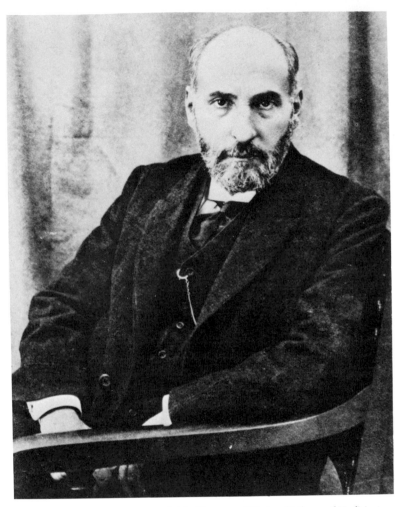

Figure 4.4. *Santiago Ramón y Cajal. (Courtesy of National Library of Medicine)*

trolled conditions, it is difficult to limit the damage to only the desired locus. As a result, haematomas, defective revascularization, and, in the case of accidental injury, infections may all serve to block adequate regrowth from severed stumps. Cerebral damage may also result in mechanical barriers that could limit regenerative growth. In this case, lesions, tumors, penetrating missile wounds, and posttraumatic shrinkage may physically displace and distort the brain so that the regenerating terminals could miss their targets and end in aborted growth. Scar, or necrotic tissue, can also serve to complicate the problem by causing misdirected growth away from the target area; for example, glial inflammatory reactions might inhibit regeneration.

After central nervous system injury, certain nonneural structures may exert strong attractive or trophic influences on regenerating tissues that are not present during normal growth and development. For instance, Anders Björklund and his colleagues (Stenevi, Björklund, and Moore, 1973) mention that many regenerating catecholamine fibers are directed toward blood vessels and away from their "normal" synaptic contacts. Glial cells, such as astrocytes, may also attract growing terminals, which may end by forming neuroastrocytomas rather than reestablishing functional connections. Depending upon the site and the extent of damage, there can also be considerable alterations in the chemical environment of the brain. The growing fibers would almost certainly be affected by these alterations. Thus, if chemotoxins or chemospecificity is changed, the regeneration process could be aborted or completely misdirected (see Cotman and Banker, 1974, for an excellent review of such factors).

Functional regeneration may also be limited to certain neural systems and not to others. This question has not yet received the adequate attention that it deserves, but there is reason to doubt, at least in the adult organism, that all neuronal systems have an equal capacity to regenerate. Svengaardt, Björklund, and Stenevi (1976) suggest that neurons in the central nervous system of mammals can be characterized by one of two responses to axonal damage. One class of neurons seems to show relatively efficient and extensive regeneration, whereas the other class tends to abort the regrowth process. The neurons that show efficient regeneration seem to have long, thin unmyelinated axons. Abortive regeneration, in contrast, seems to be characteristic of long myelinated fiber systems like the retinal projections. Svengaardt et al. (1976) cautiously state that at the present time:

> There are no data, to our knowledge, to exclude that a high capacity for axonal regeneration could be shared by many, or perhaps all, long non-myelinated central systems. From another point of view, however, it is obvious that those central systems, in which a high capacity for axonal regeneration has been demonstrated in the adult mammal (i.e., adrenergic, dopaminergic, serotonergic, and cholinergic systems), can all be regarded as components of the so-called reticular formation, associated primarily with phylogenetically old parts of the brain [p. 20].

In addition, although we have not yet discussed collateral growth (branching of axons in response to injury of other neurons), we can speculate that regenerative growth might be curtailed if axon collaterals from other neurons grow into the area. Suppose that there are intact fibers whose axons pass near to the region into which terminals from the regenerating stumps are heading. If there is collateral sprouting, the collateral projections may reach the target zone before the regenerating fibers, or compete more effectively than they do for vacated receptor sites. As a result, the regenerative growth could be thwarted.

Finally, it should be noted that injury to a particular neuronal group can have more than local consequences. Deafferentation of a given region may, if it is sufficiently extensive, result in transneuronal degeneration (i.e., postsynaptic neural death due to loss of presynaptic inputs) or shrinkage and retraction of the dendritic branches with which postsynaptic contacts are to be established. Under these conditions, if there is any regrowth, it might be abortive since the newly formed terminals would have no target to grow toward.

Neuronal regeneration has a chance element attached to it. Although many terminals start to grow, not all may reach their final destinations, perhaps even too few to mediate behavioral recovery. In this case, the most pessimistic conclusion would be a reaffirmation of Cajal's position that the regenerative process is at best limited, with minimal functional consequences.

When viewed in this context and in the light of the early history of experimentation in this area, it is easy to understand why the behavioral consequences of regeneration have received little attention. At the present time, the rehabilitation therapist would probably be mildly amused to learn that the latest scientific finding is that a part of the eye can be transplanted into the brain. This bleak picture may be subject to sudden change if research continues to show that regeneration is much more pervasive than we currently believe and if the practical significance of enhancing regeneration can be demonstrated.

Efforts to study the behavioral correlates of regenerating neurons would not require tremendous expenditures of time and effort since the paradigms being used by anatomists and biochemists to study regeneration on a neural level are identical to those that would be used to study it on a behavioral level. Here we may begin to ask whether drugs that inhibit scar tissue or promote faster regrowth could aid in the process of recovery from disease of the brain or from traumatic insult. Indeed, until regenerative growth can be related to behavior and understood in terms of the adaptive capacity of the organism, the regeneration now being described will probably continue to be regarded only as an interesting curiosity and an elegant demonstration of the anatomist's technique by those who could best put it to practical advantage.

References

Attardi, P. G., and Sperry, R. W. Preferential selection of central pathways by regenerating optic fibers. *Experimental Neurology*, 1963, 7, 46–64.

Björklund, A., Katzman, R., Stenevi, U., and West, K. Development and growth of axonal sprouts from noradrenaline and 5-hydroxytryptamine neurons in the rat spinal cord. *Brain Research*, 1971, 31, 21–33.

Björklund, A., and Stenevi, U. Growth of central catecholamine neurons into smooth muscle grafts in the rat mesencephalon. *Brain Research*, 1971, 31, 1–20.

Clemente, C. D. Regeneration in the vertebrate central nervous system. *International Review of Neurobiology*, 1964, 6, 257–301.

Cotman, C. W., and Banker, G. A. The making of a synapse. In S. Ehrenpreis and I. J. Koplin (Eds.), *Reviews of Neuroscience* (Vol. 1). New York: Raven Press, 1974, pp. 1–62.

Falck, B., Hillarp, N.-A., Thieme, G., and Torp, A. Fluorescence of catecholamines and related compounds condensed with formaldehyde. *Journal of Histochemistry and Cytochemistry*, 1962, *10*, 348–354.

Guth, L. History of central nervous system regeneration research. *Experimental Neurology*, 1975, *48*, 3–15.

Guth, L., and Windle, W. F. The enigma of central nervous regeneration. *Experimental Neurology*, 1970, Suppl. 5, 1–43.

Holmstedt, B. A modification of the thiocholine method for the determination of cholinesterase. *Acta Physiologica Scandinavica*, 1957, *40*, 331–357.

Jacobson, M. *Developmental neurobiology*. New York: Plenum, 1978.

Katzman, R., Björklund, A., Owman, C., Stenevi, U., and West, K. Evidence for regenerative axon sprouting of central catecholamine neurons in the rat mesencephalon following electrolytic lesions. *Brain Research*, 1971, *25*, 579–596.

Liu, C. N., and Scott, D., Jr. Regeneration in the dorsal spinocerebellar tract of the cat. *Journal of Comparative Neurology*, 1958, *109*, 153–167.

Marks, A. F. Regenerative reconstruction of a tract in a rat's brain. *Experimental Neurology*, 1972, *34*, 455–464.

Meyer, R. L., and Sperry, R. W. Explanatory models for neuroplasticity in retinotectal connections. In D. G. Stein, J. J. Rosen, and N. Butters (Eds.), *Plasticity and recovery of function in the central nervous system*. New York: Academic Press, 1974, Pp. 45–64.

Ramón y Cajal, S. [*Degeneration and regeneration of the nervous system*] (R. M. May, trans.) London: Oxford University Press, 1928.

Reitan, R. Problems and prospects in studying the psychological correlates of brain lesions. *Cortex*, 1966, *2*, 127–154.

Schoenfeld, T. A., and Hamilton, L. W. Secondary brain changes following lesions: A new paradigm for lesion experimentation. *Physiology and Behavior*, 1977, *18*, 951–967.

Sharma, S. C., and Gaze, R. M. The retinotopic organization of visual responses from tectal reimplants in adult goldfish. *Archives Italiennes de Biologie*, 1971, *190*, 357–366.

Sperry, R. W. Effect of 180 degree rotation of the retinal field on visuomotor coordination. *Journal of Experimental Zoology*, 1943, *92*, 263–279.

Sperry, R. W. Optic nerve regeneration with return of vision in anurans. *Journal of Neurophysiology*, 1944, *7*, 57–70.

Sperry, R. W. Restoration of vision after crossing of optic nerves and after contralateral transplantation of eye. *Journal of Neurophysiology*, 1945, *8*, 15–28.

Sperry, R. W. Chemoaffinity in the orderly growth of nerve fiber patterns and connections. *Proceedings of the National Academy of Sciences*, 1963, *50*, 703–719.

Stenevi, U., Björklund, A., and Moore, R. Y. Morphological plasticity of central adrenergic neurons. *Brain, Behavior and Evolution*, 1973, *8*, 110–134.

Svendgaardt, N.-A., Björklund, A., and Stenevi, U. Regeneration of central cholinergic neurones in the adult rat brain. *Brain Research*, 1976, *102*, 1–22.

Weiss, P., and Taylor, A. C. Further experimental evidence against "neurotropism" in nerve regeneration. *Journal of Experimental Zoology*, 1944, *95*, 233–257.

Windle, W. F. (Ed.). *Regeneration in the central nervous system*. Springfield, Ill.: Charles C Thomas, 1955.

Yoon, M. G. Retention of the original topographic polarity by the 180° rotated tectal reimplant in young adult goldfish. *Journal of Physiology*, 1973, *233*, 575–588.

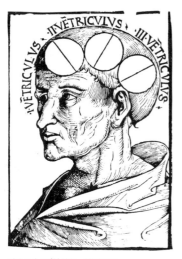

"Anomalous" Growth after Brain Damage Early in Life

It is obviously of great interest to know to what extent the predictable shape and connections of a neuron are determined by its genetic program independent of its physical environment, and then what role the environment plays in molding the neuron's structure and function and by what means it has this effect [Lund, 1978, p. 7].

CHAPTER FIVE

In the previous chapter we examined the case for regeneration in the mammalian central nervous system. However, there are a variety of dynamic events that are known to follow brain damage in addition to regeneration itself. For example, one such change involves the sprouting of new axon terminals from healthy, intact axons. These branches can take over synaptic sites left vacant by degenerating axons that were killed by the injury. As we will see, this is only a small part of the story that is now unfolding. A wealth of new data is now challenging the idea that the mammalian central nervous system is a static entity that is not capable of reorganization or dynamic change after injury.

The belief that there could be more to neuroplasticity than regeneration of damaged axons is not really new, but for all intents and purposes, it has been only during the last 10 years or so that the concept has really caught on. Why are we only now seeing efforts to study "anomalous" and "altered" neuronal projections after brain damage? What can account for the sparcity of research in this field prior to the 1970s and for its great attraction during the last decade? We think that work in this area has been held back for three reasons.

First, until very recently, it was believed that regeneration could not occur in the mammalian central nervous system, at least not in any functional sense. Even now there is very little evidence that regeneration can have major beneficial or adaptive consequences for the organism. This has probably kept many researchers from seriously considering the possibility that there could be other physical alterations of the damaged nervous system capable of mediating or influencing recovery of function.

Second, studying new and anomalous growth in the central nervous system is not an easy task. The job has only recently been made easier as a result of numerous technological advances. In fact, many of the procedures that neuroscientists are already taking for granted represent relatively new achievements. Here we can point to the use of histofluorescence, a type of analysis that we have already looked at in the chapter on regeneration. In addition, there are autoradiographic techniques, which can be used to assess the metabolic activity of specific brain areas in vivo (e.g., 2-deoxyglucose mapping procedures; Sokoloff, 1977), and other techniques (e.g., horseradish peroxidase), which allow us to trace with great precision nerve fibers from the points of termination back to where they originate. Excellent reviews of these methods are available, and many of the procedures can be learned and applied fairly quickly (see for example Jones and Hartmann, 1978).

The third factor that we believe thas retarded development of research in this area is not technological, but philosophical. As mentioned in Chapter 1, scientists have strong predispositions about how the nervous system is organized. One is the belief that the elements comprising the central nervous system are "fixed" and "committed" to specific functions early in life. Another is the assumption that nervous connections are only genetically determined. Both notions have had a tremendous influence on the thinking and research strategies of biologists, predisposing them to search for results that support the paradigms they assume best represent a "truthful" view of nature. Thus, it could be argued that *if* the concept of a "hard-wired" nervous system is reflective of reality, then the only changes that should occur after the period of infancy should be degenerative ones due to diseases or the ravages of time. Obviously, acceptance of such a principle would influence the design of experiments, as well as the selection of relevant data.

This philosophical approach to the mammalian central nervous system should not be viewed as something that arose independently from the histological tools that neuroanatomists have had at their disposal. Until the development of newer techniques, all anatomical examinations of the brain were made in dead tissue, prepared at a single point in time, frozen forever in fixatives, and stained and glued to glass slides for microscopic examination. Geoffrey Raisman (1978), an outstanding British electron microscopist, probably stated it best when he wrote

> It is this very feature of anatomical methodology that has tended to give anatomical observations the appearance of permanence and rigidity. The fact that a synapse exists and can even be photographed in a form in which it appeared at the moment when the animal was killed gives no indication of how long that particular synapse had existed before the moment of death or how long it would have remained had the animal survived [p. 102].

It is now almost certain that anomalous neuronal growth after brain injury occurs in subjects of all ages. Such injury-induced growth can manifest itself in a number of ways. For example, as we have stated, after a part of the brain is damaged, axons passing close to the deafferented zone could respond to the injury by developing and sending "collaterals" to occupy the vacated synaptic sites, while retaining their own synaptic connections. The term most frequently applied to this phenomenon is *axonal sprouting* and the response is thought to be triggered by the absence or removal of the normal afferents to a given area.

We now know that a number of variations on this theme are possible. One that is mentioned by Carl Cotman and his co-workers at the University of California at Irvine is that the terminal endfeet of an intact axon may simply enlarge and establish new synaptic contacts at sites left vacant as a result of damage to another neuron. This phenomenon is usually called *paraterminal sprouting*, and it is distinguished from true collateral sprouting by the location of the branch point—whether it is on the axon itself or in the bouton (terminal) area. It is also possible that

> a reactive fiber which contacts a denervated cell could form new synapses at points of apposition where there were none previously, or the formation of new synapses could follow a shift in position of axon or postsynaptic processes, creating new points of apposition. Axonal growth might not be required. This presently hypothetical possibility has been referred to as contact synaptogenesis [Cotman and Nadler, 1978, p. 241].

Cotman and Nadler (1978) state that it is not easy to distinguish among these possibilities (see Figure 5.1) on the basis of histological examination. They use the general term *reactive synaptogenesis* to refer to all of the different, injury-induced events, a term which seems to have its equivalence in what most investigators simply call *sprouting*.

Does sprouting occur in the intact brain? Probably, but to a more limited extent. Under normal conditions, reactive synaptogenesis may be inhibited by substances released by normal nerve terminals to restrain the growth of adjacent fibers (see Diamond, Cooper, Turner, and Macintyre, 1976). In the presence of

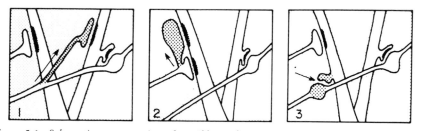

Figure 5.1. *Schematic representation of possible mechanisms in reactive synaptogenesis. Dotted areas (arrows) denote new growth. 1, collateral sprouting; 2, paraterminal sprouting; 3, contact synaptogenesis. (From Cotman, C. W., and Nadler, N. G. Reactive synaptogenesis in the hippocampus. In C. W. Cotman (Ed.),* Neuronal Plasticity, *Copyright © 1978. With permission from Raven Press, New York.)*

injury or early in development, the actions of these growth retardants would be reduced or eliminated, and proliferation from intact neurons would occur, perhaps even aided by growth initiating humoral substances from presynaptic sites (cf. Cotman and Nalder, 1978, pp. 242–246).

Sprouting can occur early in development, while some axons are still in the process of migrating, differentiating, or growing to their target structures. It can also occur later in life when neural projections seem more firmly established and when cell migration and axonal growth toward termination sites are completed.

Trophic activity (i.e., directed growth) during the early stages of development also can take some forms that may distinguish it from plasticity later in life. In particular, as shown in Figure 5.2, if a target structure is severely damaged or totally destroyed in the newborn, axons projecting to the structure may be *rerouted* to new brain areas where they may compete for synaptic space with the terminals of cells that belong there (cf. Lund, 1978). The "rerouting effect" is probably limited to axons that are still in the process of growing, and conceivably the response could also occur with an increase in the number of synapses that these axons would normally show (i.e., reactive synaptogenesis).

While animals and patients are very young, the range and degree of effects observed in response to injury may be greater than it is later in life. If this is the case, one might suppose that the functional consequences of anomalous projections will differ depending on the developmental status of the nervous system at the

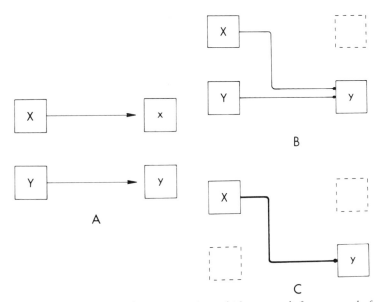

Figure 5.2. *Plan to show abnormal axon connections which may result from removal of a target nucleus, x, with or without simultaneous removal of input, Y. (From Lund, R. Development and Plasticity of the Brain, 1978. With permission from Oxford University Press.)*

time of injury. We will examine some of these effects, first in young organisms and then in mature subjects (Chapter 6), to see if this is so. Let us see whether sprouting and redirected fibers always result in behaviors that help the organism adapt to its environment or whether these phenomena can sometimes be maladaptive and disruptive of normal behaviors.

Some of the most extensive and interesting experiments on the anatomical and behavioral changes that can follow brain lesions early in life have been performed on the golden hamster by Gerald Schneider and his students at the Massachusetts Institue of Technology (Devor and Schneider, 1975; Schneider, 1970, 1973, 1979; Schneider and Jhaveri, 1974; So and Schneider, 1976). The hamster is an ideal subject for research in developmental neuroplasticity because it has a very short gestation period (16 days) and is born with an extremely immature nervous system, which roughly corresponds to that of a 3-month-old human fetus (Schneider and Jhavari, 1974). This similarity to an embryological state means that the hamster's brain can be manipulated postnatally, whereas similar operations would require *in utero* surgery with most other animals. For Schneider's research, the hamster is a good subject because the superior colliculus, which is buried below the cerebral cortex in the adult hamster, has no cortex overlying it in the newborn. This makes it readily accessible to precise ablation. Yet despite the immaturity of the hamster's nervous system at birth, the animal grows rapidly and its brain reaches full size within 3 months. Moreover, because these small animals are usually docile and easy to train, they are also excellent subjects for perceptual, learning, and related behavioral investigations.

In one of Schneider's first experiments, some animals had the visual cortex on both sides of the brain removed shortly after birth, whereas other animals had the same surgery later in life. Both the young and mature subjects showed an almost total atrophy of the dorsal lateral geniculate nuclei, a major receiving area for optic nerve fibers. The neurons in the geniculate died because their projections to the cortex were severed by the surgery. This "dying back" of cells is called *retrograde degeneration,* and it can be used to evaluate the extent of the damage produced by lesions. Schneider also observed that atrophy and neural reorganization in a second area, the superior colliculus, were related to the age at which the hamsters received their surgery. Thus, when lesions are made at 1 day of age, projections from the retina not only go to the most superficial layers of the colliculus, but they also go to the deeper layers that normally would receive corticotectal inputs and project via the lateral posterior nucleus of the thalamus to the cortex. The animals operated on at maturity lacked the anomalous retinal projections to the deeper layers of the superior colliculus and, therefore, a potential alternate route by which visual information could be sent to intact forebrain regions.

But can this anomalous formation of neurons be correlated with performance differences among the groups? Schneider and his students found that the animals operated on at 8 days of age could learn striped pattern discriminations, whereas the hamsters with comparable visual cortex ablations made at maturity failed to learn the task even afer much training. In fact, the animals operated on at maturity performed very badly even though their lesions were smaller than those made in the infants.

In a second set of experiments on other hamsters, lesions were made in midbrain. When the superficial layers of the superior colliculus were damaged at birth, anomalous projections from the retina terminated in the remaining, undamaged lower layers of the superior colliculus—layers that normally receive axons from the superficial layers of this structure. Damage to the colliculus also caused some retinal projections to go directly to the lateral posterior nucleus of the thalamus, where they formed axodendritic synapses, and to the ventral part of the lateral geniculate nucleus, which is also in the thalamus. These two sites also normally receive afferents from the superficial layers of the superior colliculus. This means that after early bilateral removal of the superficial layers of the superior colliculus, the newly formed fibers make contacts further up the track. The retinal fibers are not only rerouted, but they also show greater proliferation of synaptic endfeet, suggestive of axonal sprouting. This is illustrated in Figure 5.3.

This aberrant neural circuitry has also been correlated with behavior. In the first place, Schneider and his colleagues noted that hamsters given lesions as adults, who did not have these anomalous pathways, lose their ability to orient

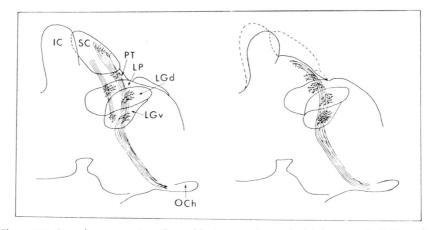

Figure 5.3. *Lateral reconstruction of rostral brain stem of normal adult hamster. (Left) Heavy line depicts schematically the course of a group of optic tract axons and some of their terminations; the tecto-thalamic pathway is shown in similar manner. (Right) Similar view of brain stem of adult hamster that had undergone destruction of the superficial layers of the colliculus in the neonate. Anomalous optic tract connections are depicted by double lines. Abbreviations: IC, inferior colliculus; SC, superior colliculus; PT, pretectal area; LP, lateral posterior nucleus of thalamus; LGd, dorsal part of lateral geniculate body; LGv, ventral part of lateral geniculate body; OCh, optic chiasm. (After Schneider, 1973.)*

(head turning, rearing up, etc.) to the presentation of a highly desirable (for the hamster) sunflower seed. In the second place, the animals given lesions as infants, who *have* these anomalous projections, showed considerable sparing of visually guided behavior, although they were not completely normal in their orientation to visual stimuli in some parts of the visual field (they sometimes overshoot or undershoot the target).

When the tectal damage was bilateral, the behavioral sparing was related to the number of rerouted connections that the hamsters had. If the lesions of the tectum were large enough to prevent fibers from getting to the dorsal midbrain, there was very little sparing of behavioral function; the greater the extent of re-routed projections, the greater the degree of sparing. Schneider and Jhaveri (1974) report that ''the correspondence of the behavioral performance with the retinal projection to the midbrain provides evidence that anomalous axonal connections are responsible for sparing of function [p. 73].''

We think that some of Schneider's most interesting findings emerged when he removed the superficial layers of the superior colliculus on only one side of the hamster's brain. When this was done in newborn hamsters, immature axons coming from the opposite eye not only crossed the midline to terminate in the remaining part of the damaged structure, but they also recrossed the midline in the tectum to end in the ''wrong'' (ipsilateral) superior colliculus. This highly unusual rerouting effect, in which the axons twice cross the midline, seems to be limited to the first 2 weeks of life, but it can be made even more striking if the eye on the same side as the tectal lesion is also removed very early in life (So and Schneider, 1976).

These unilateral tectal preparations (see Figure 5.4) should serve to caution us about jumping to the conclusion that rerouted neural circuitry is always beneficial to the organism. When Schneider took animals with early right side damage and presented them with a sunflower seed in the left visual field, they did not ignore, it, as would be characteristic of adult-operated hamsters, but rather turned away from the food rather than toward it! Thus, the axons that recross to the opposite side of the brain have the capability to mediate some performance, but owing to how the visuomotor system is rewired, the resulting behavior is clearly maladaptive and detrimental to the survival of the animal. Moreover, the hamsters were unable to overcome the deficit by changing their response strategies.

Schneider thinks that his work sheds some light on the possible factors that could govern the growth of axons after lesions. His contention is that basic principles of normal growth and development are involved and that these principles also apply to injury-induced anomalous growth. One principle is that of competition for available synaptic space among growing nerve fibers and a tendency for axons to invade vacated terminal space. Another factor that he mentions is ''a tendency for axons to conserve at least a minimum quantity of terminal arborization [Schneider and Jhaveri, 1974, p. 81].'' The conservation of terminals relates

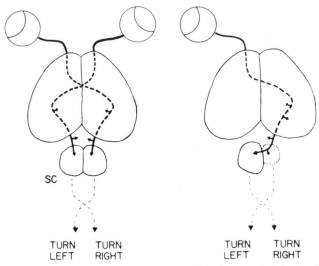

Figure 5.4. *Axonal pathways in the Syrian hamster, critical in the control of visually elicited turning of the head. (Left) Top view of eyes, cerebral hemispheres, and superior colliculi (SC), the latter are displaced caudally for the sake of the diagram. The course and termination of axons of the retinal ganglion cells are indicated by heavy lines and arrows. These axons pass below the forebrain and most cross at the optic chiasm and rise along the surface of the diencephalon (where some axons terminate), finally reaching the SC. Connections in the right SC mediate turning toward the left via descending pathways to the brain stem and spinal cord; similarly, connections in the left colliculus mediate turning toward the right. (Right) Similar view of brain of hamster in which the right eye and the superficial layers of SC were ablated at birth. Axons from the remaining eye not only form anomalous connections in the diencephalon, but also form an abnormal pattern of termination in the midbrain tegmentum, some ending in the area of early surgical damage, others recrossing to the left SC. This leads to the prediction of abnormal turning behavior in response to stimuli in at least part of the left visual field. (From Schneider and Jhavari, 1974.)*

to what Schneider has referred to as a ''pruning'' effect. If some of the branches of an axon are cut, the surviving parts will grow more (hypertrophy) to bring the total volume of arborization back to approximately normal. The other factors mentioned by Schneider are an axon ordering principle, whereby terminals tend to retain their general topographic organization, even if the total synaptic space is reduced, and a mechanical deflection factor, in which fibers can be forced to deviate from their normal course. Schneider contends that the ordering factor should still operate when axons are deflected, but that it might not be able to compensate for too much disarray. Some of these ideas are illustrated in Figures 5.5–5.7.

The visual system is not the only sensory system that can be reorganized when damage is sustained early in life. Marshall Devor (1975, 1976) recently examined the effects of cutting the lateral olfactory tract (LOT) (which contains afferent axons that go to the ventral forebrain, as well as efferents headed back to the olfac-

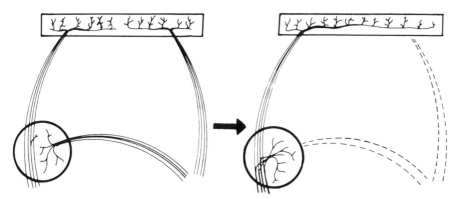

Figure 5.5. *Diagrammatic illustration of the concept of a tendency for axons to invade available or vacated terminal space and compete with other axons for, in some cases, exclusive occupancy. Two hypothetical structures are indicated, each innervated from two sources, but the terminal distribution of one is limited by the presence of the other. This is demonstrated by the consequences of removing one of the sources of input to each structure: the other system then expands its terminal field. (From Schneider and Jhavari, 1974.)*

tory bulb) in newborn and older male hamsters. In the hamster, mating seems to be highly dependent upon olfactory cues. Cutting the LOT effectively eliminates hamster mating if the lesions are made in mature animals and if the transections are complete on both sides of the brain. If the same cuts are made in 3-day-old hamsters, there is considerable sparing of mating behavior later in life. The next step was to determine whether the spared mating was due to anatomical reorganization induced by the injury.

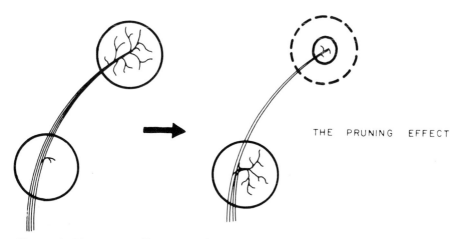

THE   PRUNING   EFFECT

Figure 5.6. *Diagrammatic illustration of the concept of a tendency for growing axons to conserve at least a minimum quantity of terminal arborization. (From Schneider and Jhavari, 1974.)*

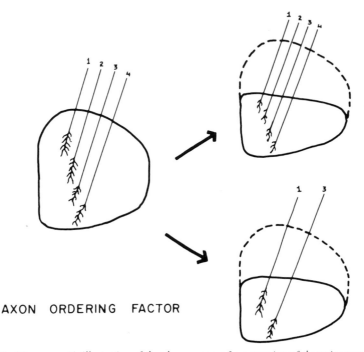

AXON   ORDERING   FACTOR

Figure 5.7. *Diagrammatic illustration of the phenomenon of compression of the retino-tectal map. This could happen if the same groups of axons each terminated in a smaller space (upper), or if distributed axons degenerated in numbers proportional to the reduction in terminal space, leaving the remainder to terminate each with normal-sized end arbors (lower). In either case, the axon groups maintain a normal relationship relative to each other. (From Schneider and Jhavari, 1974.)*

Devor's (1975, 1976) careful analyses showed that when surgery was performed in 7-day-old hamsters, all brain areas distal to the cut that would have received fibers from the lateral olfactory tract were completely denervated. In contrast, if the total transections were made before or at 3 days of age, fibers from the olfactory bulb were able to reinnervate the cortex distal to the cut by sprouting new terminals or by traversing the cut over the cortical surface.

Devor also found extensive neuronal branching when *partial* lesions of the lateral olfactory tract were made in neonatal animals, but in this case the sprouting was more restricted in range, and the most distal (caudal) part of the normal LOT distribution was left barren. Most of the axons did not grow beyond the boundary of the lateral olfactory nucleus to establish connections with remote cortical tissue. The hamsters who received surgery as infants failed to mate under these conditions, despite the fact that the axons in their olfactory systems showed extensive sprouting. Mature hamsters with partial lesions of the lateral olfactory tract retained the ability to mate, presumably because some of their already-established connections with the distal regions were left unaffected by this surgery.

Devor's data on the olfactory system parallel those of Schneider on the visual system in showing a greater capacity for dynamic anatomical reorganization early in life, and in revealing that anomalous projections do have the potential to be beneficial (they can spare both mating and visually guided behaviors). Yet, at the same time, their experiments can also be taken to indicate that sprouting and related kinds of anomalous projections in infancy do not always guarantee a return of normal behaviors. The new projections can mediate maladaptive behaviors like the head turning away from food or nothing resembling the critical behavior at all, as was the case when mating was examined after incomplete lateral olfactory tract lesions in infancy.

It is now clear that aberrant pathways and reactive synaptogenesis in infancy are not limited to the classical sensory systems. A good example of the generality of injury-induced plasticity is provided by Samuel Hicks and Constance D'Amato (1975a, b) of the University of Michigan Medical School. They ablated the motor-sensory cortex unilaterally in very young rats and observed an abnormal, uncrossed corticospinal tract in the medulla and spinal cord that parted from the main tract before it crossed the midline in the pyramids. These newly formed fibers distributed themselves to the reticular formation, trigeminal region, posterior column region, and spinal cord. All of this new growth seemed to occur during the third postnatal week, a period of rapid growth for the fibers in the corticospinal tract. The new pathway could be detected readily in rats given unilateral lesions before the sixth postnatal day, was less prominent when surgery took place on Day 7, and could just barely be detected in 9-day-old rat pups. If the rats were given unilateral lesions in the second week of life, the ipsilateral projections were never observed.

Hicks and D'Amato (1975a) also noted some unusual changes in the sensory-motor cortex itself when the ablations of this region were incomplete:

> One (change) was that what normally would have become the most medial part of the motor-sensory cortex differentiated instead into cingular cortex continuous with the normal cingular cortex. The other (change) was the ingrowth of an extensive number of fibers into layer 1 of this aberrant cortex as well as the normal cingular cortex [p. 22].

Hicks and D'Amato thought that the aberrant developments in the cortex and the formation of a miniature uncrossed pathway that ends in the same nuclei of the medulla and spinal cord that the crossed pathway would have may account for the partial sparing of locomotor abilities that occurs when cortical damage is inflicted in early life. They specifically point to the ability of rats with unilateral lesions to walk and run along narrow elevated pathways and to locomote on a broad track. Age at the time of surgery plays a major role here, with older operated rats often letting their limbs slip and hang over the side of the elevated pathway contralateral to the lesion—deficits much more intense than those seen when animals are operated on in the period immediately following birth (see

Figure 5.8). The latter, for example, would quickly correct slips and would not allow their limbs to dangle over edges for extended periods of time.

Photographic analyses showed that the groups also differed in the character of their stride when running. Normally there is a "foreward thrust of the forefoot, fanning of the digits, and then precise downward placing of the foot, digits first, on the ground [Hicks and D'Amato, 1975b, p. 42]." The animals operated on in infancy continued to show these general characteristics, but those suffering comparable unilateral ablations later in development lost some of the thrust and displayed an abnormally short stride. Hicks and D'Amato (1975b) are aware that although the anatomical and behavioral data are in agreement, they do not necessarily signify causality. Because causality can only be inferred, Hicks and D'Amato conclude on the cautious note that "the uncrossed tract in the animals operated upon as infants, by providing bilateral corticospinal tract representation, might have spared the stride, but this is wholly speculative at present [p. 43]."

The experiments performed on hamsters and rats allow us to make several generalizations about neuroplasticity. First, we now know that damage to the central nervous system in infants and adults does not always result in the same anatomical and behavioral sequelae; in fact, as we have seen, the differences can be rather dramatic. Second, the development of anomalous pathways can coincide, with the emergence of certain behaviors, but unfortunately, anomalous growth may sometimes cause aberrant rather than adaptive behavior. Third, evidence currently available shows that neuroanatomical plasticity is a relatively general phenomenon in the mammalian central nervous system; anomalous growth now has been seen in a number of different areas of the brain.

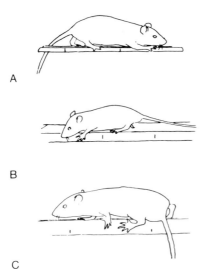

A

B

C

Figure 5.8. *Tracings of rats in movies to represent some of the characteristics of motor-sensory behavioral alterations that resulted from ablating the motorsensory cortex (MSC) or its quadrants. (A) Normal rat, 7-weeks-old, positioning its feet precisely as it traverses a narrow path of two small dowels. (B) A rat, 6-weeks-old, that had its right MSC ablated at birth. The whole left forelimb and left hind toe have slipped off the edge of a broad flat track. (C) A rat, 5-weeks-old, whose postero-lateral quadrant of the right MSC was ablated at birth, applying its left feet in slipshod manner to a narrow path, unable to grasp and hold on well. (After Hicks and D'Amato, 1975b.)*

But how do these findings relate to primates and, in particular, to humans? Patricia Goldman, now at Yale University, has carefully examined this question. Her research with monkeys is based on her conviction that more can be learned about the human condition with these animals than with rats and hamsters. For example, Goldman points out that monkeys, like humans, have an extended period of development, although most of the events concerning neurogenesis and the formation of neuronal connections occur prenatally in both cases.

Goldman has concentrated her efforts on studying the effects of dorsolateral prefrontal cortex lesions. This region was chosen because it has been the subject of intense anatomical and physiological study and because there is very extensive research literature showing that memory and spatial performance are severely disrupted in adult animals with lesions in this area. Furthermore, Goldman views this "nonspecific" association area of the monkey as an excellent model for shedding light on human recovery processes since the best evidence for age-related sparing and recovery of function in humans can be found after damage to association regions where language and cognition can be affected.

In one very unique and technically difficult experiment, Goldman and Galkin (1978) removed fetal rhesus monkeys from the uterus in order to perform surgery on them between Days 102 and 119 of embryonic life. The investigators then carefully ablated dorsolateral prefrontal cortex bilaterally and replaced the fetuses in the womb until they were delivered by Caesarian section at approximately 159 days of gestation.

Most of the monkeys that received this surgery were used for anatomical study, but one, which was operated on embryonic Day 106 (E106), was saved and periodically evaluated on some behavioral tests from the time that it was 1 year of age until it was killed at 2 ½ years of age. The tests used to study this monkey were chosen for their known sensitivity to frontal lobe dysfunction. Goldman and Galkin tested the monkey on (a) a delayed spatial response task; (b) visual pattern discrimination; (c) spatial delayed alternation; and (d) an object discrimination reversal. The behavioral testing of this animal revealed a very dramatic sparing of function. This monkey showed absolutely no behavioral deficits on any of the tasks and may even have performed somewhat better than normal subjects on some of them! This was in marked contrast to the scores obtained on a monkey operated upon on the fiftieth day of postnatal life and, of course, to monkeys that received damage to the frontal cortex as adults.

The anatomical analyses on the animals used in this experiment revealed some very interesting and highly unusual neuronal patterns that were never observed when surgery was performed after the time of birth. One of the most striking and puzzling findings reported by Goldman and Galkin was the unusual (ectopic) growth of new gyri and sulci in the area adjacent to the lesion and also in regions of the cortex far removed from the initial site of injury. For example, Goldman and Galkin noted the appearance of anomalous sulci in parietal, temporal, and occipital areas of monkeys operated on between Days 102 and 106 of embryonic life. The abnormal sulci had cytoarchitectonic and laminar characteristics that were similar to those seen in the normal primate cortex.

When the authors counted neurons to assess retorgrade degeneration in the mediodorsal nucleus of the thalamus, which is the primary projection area to the prefrontal cortex, they obtained more surprising and dramatic anatomical data. The monkey given surgery on embryonic Day 106 had no loss of cells in the parvocellular region of this thalamic nucleus, although its projections were known to have already invaded the frontal region. In contrast, the animal with frontal lesions made on embryonic Day 119 showed some loss of cells, whereas very heavy retrograde degeneration was noted in the subject operated on at 50 days after birth. What might account for the remarkable sparing of neurons in the thalamus? One idea is that the thalamic neurons survive because they are able to send out collateral branches that could establish synaptic contacts elsewhere in the cortex. Another notion suggested is that the neurons in the early stages of development have more collaterals than they really need so that some die off when the appropriate synaptic contacts are made by the bulk of the terminals. When the main axons are cut, the ancillary collaterals survive and grow rather than retract, and this permits the neuron itself to grow and function.

At the present time there is no substantial evidence to show that this ectopic growth and unusual preservation of thalamic neurons resulting from damage to the immature nervous system are responsible for the spared behaviors exhibited by animal E106. The data, summarized in Figures 5.9 and 5.10, are only correlative and circumstantial, but they are the best available at this time. That which is clear is that the Goldman and Galkin findings show a remarkable reorganizational ability in the case of the monkey with early brain damage—an observation that strongly suggests that similar events can be observed in all mammals, that is, that man will not be unique.

We should note that unusual projections can also be observed in the primate brain after *unilateral* lesions even when they are made after embryonic Day 106. In an animal operated upon on embryonic Day 119 for unilateral removal of the dorsolateral prefrontal cortex, for example, there was a cortical projection to a part of the contralateral caudate nucleus that normally has only ipsilateral connections with the frontal areas. The data obtained after unilateral cortical lesions in monkeys seem analogous to those reported by Hicks and D'Amato on rats with unilateral sensorimotor cortex damage.

But what do these anomalous caudate projections represent? Goldman (1978, p. 770) offers three possibilities that reflect how little is known about reactive synaptogenesis and neuroplasticity at the present time:

1. The most obvious possibility is that the anomalous axons belong to . . .neurons that normally issue a minor projection to the contralateral caudate nucleus . . . (that) may expand their terminal fields to occupy vacated synaptic space.

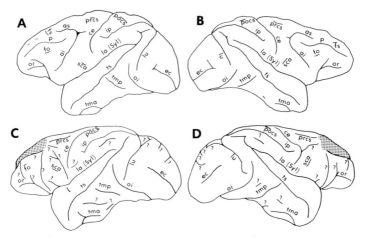

Figure 5.9. *Lateral view reconstructions of left and right hemisphere of a 2½-year-old unoperated monkey (A and B), and left and right hemispheres of the 2½-year-old monkey operated at E106 (C and D). Question marks in C and D are placed adjacent to anomalous sulci. Abbreviations: ai, inferior ramus of arcuate sulcus; as, superior ramus of arcuate sulcus; ce, central sulcus; ec, ectocalcarine sulcus; fo, orbital-frontal sulcus; fs, sulcus frontalis superior; ip, intraparietal sulcus; lu, lunate sulcus; la (Syl), lateral (Sylvian) fissure; oi, inferior occipital sulcus; or, p, parieto-occipital incisure; pocs, superior postcentral sulcus; prcs, superior precentral dimple; sca, anterior subcentral dimple; tma, anterior middle temporal sulcus; tmp, posterior middle temporal sulcus; ts, superior temporal sulcus. (From Goldman and Galkin, 1978.)*

2. The anomalous axons belong to callosal neurons, which, in the absence of homotopic target cells, are attached to and invade the caudate nucleus.
3. Cortico-caudate projections may be bilateral at embryonic stages and . . .many contralateral fibers may fail to contract in the absence of competition from the resected ipsilateral cortico-striatal pathway.

The ways in which an investigator or an investigative team may go about solving problems like this, accepting one theory first and then another theory, can represent a fascinating study in itself. Therefore, before turning to the question of reactive synaptogenesis in more mature organisms, the research and thinking of Raymond Lund and his colleagues should be given special attention.

In 1973, Lund, Cunningham, and Lund examined the distribution and rearrangement of optic nerve terminals in the superior colliculus in groups of white rats that each had one eye removed at different ages from infancy through adulthood. Lund and his colleagues chose the albino rat because the retinas of these animals project very heavily upon the contralateral superior colliculus (as well as upon the dorsal segment of the lateral geniculate body). In this sense, the white rat is like the Siamese cat and other albinos, including man, who typically have almost all of their retinal fibers crossing in the optic chiasma to the opposite side

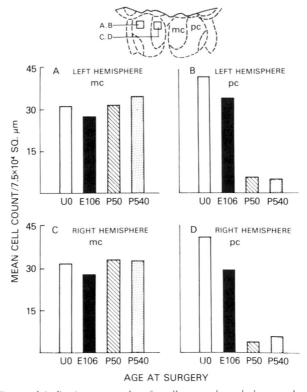

Figure 5.10. *Bar graph indicating mean values for cell counts through the areas denoted by squares on the diagram of the thalamus at the top of the figure. Each mean is based on counts from seven matched sections through the relevant region of the mediodorsal nucleus. Abbreviations: UO, unoperated monkey (2½ years of age); E106, monkey operated at embryonic Day 106 and sacrificed at 2½ years of age; PSO, representative monkey operated at postnatal Day 50 and sacrificed at around 2½ years of age; P540, monkey operated at postnatal Day 540 and sacrificed as an adult. (From Goldman and Galkin, 1978.)*

of the brain, with very few fibers projecting back on the same side as their source of origin (Guillery, 1974; Lund, 1965).

It is well known that, shortly after eye removal, the optic nerve fibers originating from that eye degenerate. If the remaining eye is removed some months later (after the "debris" from the initial degeneration has been cleared) and if the animal is sacrificed very shortly after this, the degenerating retinal pathway from the latter eye can be stained and traced throughout the brain stem to its point of termination.

Lund and his colleagues found that following removal of one eye at birth, the fiber projections from the remaining, intact eye covered the superior colliculus on the same side as the intact eye, as well as on the contralateral side. This is illustrated in Figure 5.11. The size and extent of the ipsilateral projections diminished

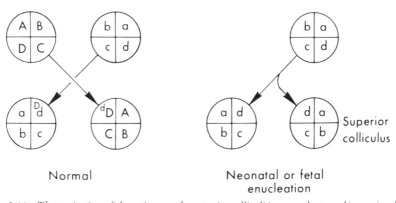

Figure 5.11. *The projection of the retinas on the superior colliculi in normal rats and in rats in which one eye was removed or lesioned early in development. (From Lund, R.* Development and Plasticity of the Brain, *1978. With permission from Oxford University Press.)*

considerably as enucleation was performed later in life up to the tenth postnatal day. After this time, there was no increased coverage of the superior colliculus on the intact side; the animals resembled adult-operated rats in their optic nerve projections to the colliculus. Lund *et al.* (1973) also noted that the uncrossed projections arose from areas of the retina that they thought would normally only project to the opposite side of the brain. What is particularly interesting is that although the projections now covered ipsilateral sites, they managed to distribute themselves as if no error had been made! That is, they formed a topographic retinal map that was a mirror image of the one on the contralateral side.

The phenomenon observed by Lund and his colleagues seemed to be directly related to whether axons were still "en route" to their points of termination at the time of eye removal. That is, the last of the retinal axons normally crosses the optic chiasma no later than the tenth postnatal day. Once the axons crossed the chiasma and established their normal synaptic connections, the neuronal reorganization no longer seemed possible.

The underlying basis of the ipsilateral projection was at first poorly understood. In 1973, Lund, Cunningham, and Lund hypothesized that the abnormal ipsilateral pathway

> may arise as a rerouting of axons which, at the time of the first eye removal had yet to reach the optic chiasm. On reaching the chiasm . . . the normal guidance factors determining that they should cross to the contralateral side are no longer present. Either these axons then distribute some contralaterally and others ipsilaterally or they distribute all to the ipsilateral visual centers [pp. 67–68].

In 1976, using a cobalt tracing method, Cunningham presented data that suggested that the hypothesis mentioned earlier was at best only partially correct. His work indicated that at least a good part of the ipsilateral projection is not due to rerouted axons, but rather to axons *branching* at the optic chiasma while they are still in the process of growth. The ipsilateral innervation, according to Cunningham, could involve not only the branching of neurons that normally would not branch at all, but the formation of more branches from those few neurons that were destined to have bilateral connections. Cunningham points out in this context that the small ipsilateral pathway that is normally seen in rats is in fact formed by collaterals of axons that project to the contralateral side of the brain and is not due to cells that have only ipsilateral projections.

This explanation for the bilateral innervation of the superior colliculus after early eye removal was recently amended by these workers. Land and Lund (1979) took 1-day-old rat pups and injected one of their eyes with horseradish peroxidase, an enzyme that allowed them to "label" the axons of cells situated in that retina. In contrast to adult rats that showed little of the labeled substance in the ipsilateral superior colliculus (where it is confined to the anteromedial region), the 1-day-old rats showed a substantial uncrossed projection across much of this nucleus. This suggested that all areas of the retina are providing an uncrossed projection at birth. Moreover, the pattern resembled that seen after unilateral enucleation in infancy.

Land and Lund report that the uncrossed projection *shrinks* during the first week of life as fibers recede and that by Day 10, the adult pattern is established. They argue that early unilateral eye removal serves to *block the retraction process.* Whether these fibers are branches from axons projecting to the other side of the brain is not clear, but is suggested by the available evidence. Thus, the uncrossed optic projection described by Lund *et al.* (1973) would not appear to be due to rerouted projections, nor to a proliferation of axonal branching at the optic chiasm, but to the prevention of the elimination of uncrossed axon collaterals.

The series of experiments on unilateral eye removal thus reflects how little we still know about the capacity of the brain to adapt to injury, but how far we have come toward a better understanding of this in just a few years. The findings are especially pertinent because they tell us that reactive synaptogenesis, such as that described by Cotman and his colleagues, and rerouted axonal projections, such as the recrossed axons observed by Schneider, may really be only part of the story. The possibility that "plasticity" can also include the preservation of pathways normally destined to die now must also be given serious consideration when examining lesion material. In this context, we can only wonder whether a similar explanation can underlie some of the findings reported by Hicks and D'Amato and those reported by other workers in this field.

Whether the retraction of a pathway is confined to infancy, as was observed in the visual system, or whether it can also take place later in life, is an empirical question that still remains to be answered. We know that the adult mammalian nervous system is itself a dynamic entity that is constantly undergoing change and that here too some events can be exaggerated when significant brain damage occurs. However, as we will see, only collateral sprouting, or more specifically, reactive synaptogenesis has been studied in animals past the period of infancy.

References

Cotman, C. W., and Nadler, J. V. Reactive synaptogenesis in the hippocampus. In C. W. Cotman (Ed.), *Neuronal plasticity*. New York: Raven Press, 1978, Pp. 227–271.

Cunningham, T. J. Early eye removal produces excessive bilateral branching in the rat: Application of cobalt filling method. *Science*, 1976, *194*, 857–859.

Devor, M. Neuroplasticity in the sparing or deterioration of function after early olfactory tract lesions. *Science*, 1975, *190*, 998–1000.

Devor, M. Neuroplasticity in the rearrangement of olfactory tract fibers after neonatal transection in hamster. *Journal of Comparative Neurology*, 1976, *166*, 49–72.

Devor, M., and Schneider, G. E. Neuroanatomical plasticity: The principle of conservation of total axonal arborization. In F. Vital-Durand and M. Jeannerod (Eds.), *Aspects of Neural Plasticity/Plasticite Nerveuse*. INSERM, 1975, *43*, 191–200.

Diamond, J., Cooper, E., Turner, C., and Macintyre, L. Trophic regulation of nerve sprouting. *Science*, 1976, *193*, 371–377.

Goldman, P. S. Neuronal plasticity in the primate telencephalon: Anamalous projections induced by prenatal removal of frontal cortex. *Science*, 1978, *202*, 768–770.

Goldman, P. S., and Galkin, T. W. Prenatal removal of frontal association cortex in the fetal rhesus monkey: Anatomical and functional consequences in postnatal life. *Brain Research*, 1978, *152*, 451–485.

Guillery, R. W. Visual pathways in albinos. *Scientific American*, 1974, *230*, 44–45.

Hicks, S. P., and D'Amato, C. J. Motor-sensory cortex-corticospinal system and developing locomotion and placing in rats. *American Journal of Anatomy*, 1975, *143*, 1–42. (a)

Hicks, S. P., and D'Amato, C. J. Functional adaptation after brain injury and malformation in early life in rats. In N. R. Ellis (Ed.), *Aberrant development in infancy*. Hillsdale, N.J.: Erlbaum, 1975, Pp. 27–47. (b)

Jones, E. G., and Hartman, B. K. Recent advances in neuroanatomical methodology. *Annual Review Neuroscience*, 1978, *1*, 215–296.

Land, P. W., and Lund, R. D. Development of the rat's uncrossed retinotectal pathway and its relation to plasticity studies. *Science*, 1979, *205*, 698–700.

Lund, R. D. Uncrossed visual pathways of hooded and albino rats. *Science*, 1965, *149*, 1506–1507.

Lund, R. D. *Development and plasticity of the brain*. New York: Oxford University Press, 1978.

Lund, R. D., Cunningham, T. J., and Lund, J. S. Modified optic projections after unilateral eye removal in young rats. *Brain, Behavior and Evolution*, 1973, *8*, 51–72.

Raisman, G. What hope for repair of the brain? *Annals of Neurology*, 1978, *3*, 101–106.

Schneider, G. E. Mechanisms of functional recovery following lesions of visual cortex or superior colliculus in neonate and adult hamsters. *Brain, Behavior and Evolution*, 1970, *3*, 295–323.

Schneider, G. E. Early lesions of superior colliculus: Factors affecting the formation of abnormal retinal projections. *Brain, Behavior and Evolution*, 1973, *8*, 73–109.

Schneider, G. E. Is it really better to have your brain lesion early? A revision of the "Kennard Principle." *Neuropsychologia*, 1979, *17*, 557–583.

Schneider, G. E., and Jhavari, S. R. Neuroanatomical correlates of spared or altered function after brain lesions in the newborn hamster. In D. G. Stein, J. J. Rosen, and N. Butters (Eds.), *Plasticity and recovery of function in the central nervous system*. New York: Academic Press, 1974, Pp. 65–110.

So, K. F., and Schneider, G. E. Abnormal recrossing retinotectal projections after early lesions in Syrian hamsters: A critical-age effect. *Anatomical Record*, 1976, *184*, 535–536.

Sokoloff, L., Rievich, M., and Kennedy, C. ^{14}C deoxyglucose method for the measurement of local cerebral glucose utilization. *Journal of Neurochemistry*, 1977, *28*, 897–916.

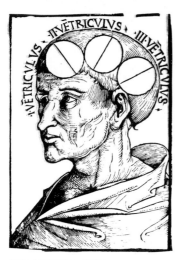

Sprouting and Remodeling in the Mature Brain

Studies on reactive synaptogenesis are not only relevant to an understanding of recovery of function, but probably also reveal important adaptive capacities of normal brain circuitry. . . . It seems likely that in denervation studies we are revealing an extreme expression of the inherent plastic properties of the adult brain [Cotman and Nadler, 1978, p. 264].

CHAPTER SIX

The idea that collateral sprouting may be a fundamental principle of neurobiology and one which is not limited to the period of infancy is not new. In 1885, Exner, on the basis of indirect evidence, postulated anomalous growth following peripheral nerve injury. He thought that if two nerves supplied a muscle and if one of them were injured, the denervated muscle would be resupplied by nerve fibers from the intact spinal nerve (see Figure 6.1). As Mac V. Edds, Jr. (1953) points out in his history of collateral nerve regeneration, "Since intensive study of the motor unit was not to begin for 40 years, it is hardly surprising that this suggestion went unnoticed [p. 260]." Even after Sherrington's formulation of the motor unit concept, it was still widely assumed that "the anatomical relation between a neuron and its associated muscle fibers is constant and unchanging [Edds, 1953, p. 206]."

Exner's "dynamic" position achieved acceptance during the 1940s and 1950s. In this time period, a number of investigators using rats, dogs, and monkeys, produced a remarkably consistent picture supportive of collateral sprouting at the neuromuscular junction.

Exner's concept of collateral sprouting was also supported by early studies on the sensory roots of the spinal cord. Both Nageotte (1906, 1907) and Ramón y Cajal (1928) observed that sensory axons could develop collateral branches even in the absence of trauma:

> It appears to us certain that, by virtue of conditions which as yet are enigmatic, any sensory neurons can temporarily, and in the absence of destructive axonic processes, enter into *neurocladism* (divisory turgescence), emitting appendices that are nervous in character, since they all grow, ramify, and terminate like true axons.

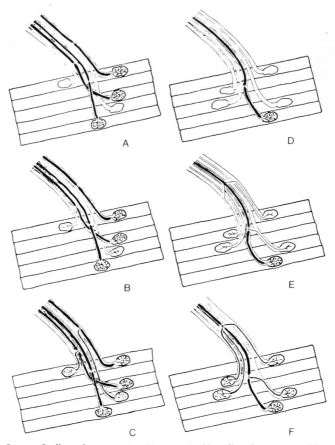

Figure 6.1. *Stages of collateral regeneration. Two terminal bundles of motor nerve fibers undergoing collateral regeneration following partial denervation of their associated muscle fibers. One bundle (A) has lost only two fibers; the other (D) is severely affected, with only one of its five fibers intact. No Schwann cells are shown, but empty neurilemmal tubes mark the original course of degenerated axons. Newly developed collateral branches originate either from old nodes of Ranvier (A and B) or from an internodal region (E). They have penetrated adjacent, empty tubes and reneurotized denervated end plates. In the near-terminal stages (C and F), the branches have matured; eventually, their calibers approach or equal those of parent fibers. Note in (F) that a new node has developed at the level where three branches arise. (From Edds, 1953.)*

Obeying a law that is very evident in the central stump of interrupted nerves, the stimulated cell, as though it foresaw possible injuries and desired better to insure the act of restoration, gives rise to a great number of sprouts. When the stimulus is due to chemical agents incapable of seriously altering the neurone, the resulting neoformation is incongruent and superfluous. . . . When, on the other hand, the neoformation is due to grave pathological causes, such as toxins, traumatic agents, etc., some fortunate sprouts are able to reach the lesion and to repair, more or less imperfectly, the interrupted paths [Ramón y Cajal, 1928, p. 412].

In 1941, Weddell, Guttmann, and Gutman worked on the cutaneous afferent system of the rabbit and demonstrated that the sprouts from intact nerve fibers could invade deafferented regions and account for some recovery of tactile sensations. One important point worth noting is that in the experiments of Weddell and his colleagues, as well as in the other studies mentioned earlier, the subjects receiving peripheral nerve injuries were well past the period of infancy. At least in the peripheral nervous system, researchers have long recognized that collateral sprouting is not confined to the early stages of life. Of course, this does not mean that age-related differences in regeneration phenomena do not exist. In their work on sprouting of the sural nerve of the rabbit, Weddell, Guttmann, and Gutman (1941) stated

> The area of skin supplied by the sural nerve in the rabbit is very small, and, indeed, the process of extension of in-growing fibres from neighboring zones may lead to the almost complete disappearance of the area of sensory loss. . . . In addition, after isolated section of the sural nerve in three very young animals (4 weeks old) it was found that the shrinkage of the area of sensory loss *was more rapid* than in older animals, and the area of analgesia finally disappeared in each case in the absence of regeneration from the proximal stump [pp. 222–223].

During the 1950s, Murray and Thompson (1957) were able to demonstrate collateral sprouting in the superior cervical sympathetic ganglion of the cat and their results were confirmed a bit later by Guth and Bernstein (1961). Nevertheless, Lloyd Guth (1975), in his brief history of research on central nervous system regeneration, reminds us that the phenomenon of collateral sprouting in the peripheral nervous system still seemed to be only remotely related to the problem of regeneration in the central nervous system. But in 1958 things changed. Chan-Nao Liu and W. W. Chambers, of the University of Pennsylvania School of Medicine, published a study which showed that not only could elaborate collateral sprouting be seen in the spinal ganglia itself, but that this phenomenon could also take place directly in the spinal cord of adult cats. This investigation "altered drastically our views of the organization of the central nervous system by revealing for the first time an anatomical plasticity . . . that had heretofore been unsuspected [Guth, 1975, p. 6]."

The Liu and Chambers study actually followed an earlier report by McCouch, Austin, and Liu (1955) in which cats and monkeys with hemisected spinal cords showed presynaptic dorsal root potentials that were suggestive of collateral sprouting. With this to go on, Liu and Chambers took several cats and cut some of the dorsal roots on one side of the spinal cord. Then, after adequate time for removal of the debris (several months), they severed a single intervening or adjacent dorsal root and its matching root on the opposite side of the cord. In other cats, they partially denervated the spinal cord by unilateral section of the corticospinal tract and then after the degenerating axons had been absorbed, they sectioned a pair of dorsal roots. In both experiments the cats were killed 4 days after the second operation, and a silver stain was used to impregnate the degenerating axons resulting from the last surgery.

Liu and Chambers found that the degeneration products were more extensive on the side of the spinal cord that was chronically denervated than on the control side. This indicated to them that in response to the initial partial denervation, the remaining, intact axons (later removed to examine the pattern of degeneration) expanded their coverage, presumably by forming collateral sprouts such as those reported for the peripheral nervous system by Weddell, Guttmann, and Gutman (1941). Liu and Chambers (1958) felt that "the sprouting occurring at the peripheral and intraspinal portions of dorsal root neurons, at terminals of somatic motor neurons, and in preganglionic sympathetic neurons indicates that this is a general phenomenon of all neurons, and therefore collateral sprouting can be anticipated in the axonal processes of purely intracentral neurons [p. 58]."

Despite Liu and Chamber's assertion and some brief statements by Ramón y Cajal (1928), there was still no conclusive proof that collateral sprouting could occur in the brain itself. In 1966, Donald Goodman and James Horel (1966) claimed to show collateral sprouting in the brain. A few years later, in 1969, Geoffrey Raisman's elegant electron microscopic analysis of collateral sprouting following partial denervation of the septal nuclei in adult rats caught the attention of neuroscientists all over the world.

Raisman chose the septal nucleus primarily because it receives afferents from two distinctly different parts of the brain. One set of fibers originates in the hippocampus and travels to the septum via the fimbria. The other fiber system originates in the hypothalamus and travels through the preoptic part of the medial forebrain bundle (MFB). As a first step, Raisman determined the exact pattern of synaptic contacts for each of the two afferent inputs to the septum. His procedure involved making a small lesion in either the fimbria or the MFB and then examining the neurons in the septum a few days later to determine the pattern of degenerative change in the boutons. In this way he was able to show that the axons coming from the hippocampus terminate primarily upon the dendrites of the septal neurons, whereas fibers coming from the hypothalamus are primarily confined to the somata of the same cells.

Once Raisman was able to describe the normal pattern of degeneration, he then created lesions in one or the other of the two pathways. The rats, which were all adults at the time of surgery, were allowed to survive for many months so that any vestiges of axonal debris could be eliminated, and to permit new synapse formation to reach a steady state. At this point Raisman made a second lesion in the remaining pathway to the septum (e.g., if the fimbria were damaged first, the second lesion would damage the medial forebrain bundle), and then sacrificed

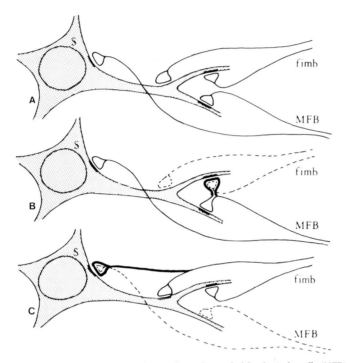

Figure 6.2. *A. In the normal situation, afferents from the medial forebrain bundle (MFB) terminate in synapses on the cell soma (S) and on dendrites. B, Several weeks after a lesion of the fimbria, the MFB axon terminals extend across from their own sites to occupy the vacated sites, thus forming double synapses. (Degenerated connections denoted by discontinuous line; presumed plastic changes denoted by heavy black line.) C, Several weeks after a lesion of the medial forebrain bundle, the fimbrial fibers now give rise to terminals occupying somatic sites, which are presumably those vacated as a result of former lesion. (From Raisman, 1969.)*

the rats 2 days later to study the degeneration pattern of the pathway damaged by the second lesion.[1]

Raisman's results are illustrated in Figure 6.2. He found that after damaging the fimbria in the first operation, fibers from the hypothalamus sprouted new terminals which made contacts on the dendritic sites evacuated by the dying hippocampal projections. Likewise, when the hypothalamic pathways were interrupted first, the fimbrial axons sprouted new terminals, which then came to occupy sites along the cell bodies of the septal neurons. Thus, the initial lesion re-

[1] The short survival period given the rats (2 days) was chosen so that degenerating synaptic terminals could be easily analyzed. Although fibers may remain for many months, degenerating terminals typically are absorbed after just a few days.

sulted in a major reorganization of the synaptic inputs to the septum, with the afferents from the remaining intact system sprouting to occupy sites left vacant by those axons that were severed.

Raisman (1969) suggested that the vacated synaptic sites are simply taken over "by an extension from the nearest axon terminal with a minimum of structural modification required to bring the two surfaces into contiguity [p. 45]." In the case of his own work, the result was "heterotypic" reinnervation; a type of axonal sprouting where the fibers from one system are replaced by the axons of another system—a relatively generalized form of growth (see also Raisman and Field, 1973).

In an attempt to pursue this further, Robert Moore, Anders Björklund, and Ulf Stenevi (1971) replicated and extended Raisman's findings, but used biochemical indices to determine which neurotransmitters were involved in the reorganization process. Moore and his colleagues showed that the hippocampal fibers were cholinergic, whereas those coming from the hypothalamus were noradrenergic. Not only then do the septal neurons receive terminal contacts from different areas of the brain, but they also undergo a change in neurotransmitter stimulation after one of the two incoming systems is injured.

The degree to which heterotypic sprouting can account for recovery of function after brain damage is very poorly understood. As Lloyd Guth and William Windle (1970) expressed it:

> These studies of the ultrastructure of the central nervous system after injury suggest that the presence of denervated tissue constitutes a stimulus for growth, a stimulus so powerful that it induces formation of collaterals from adjacent intact axons that have not only not themselves been cut but that also form synapses at sites they never normally innervate. If, as seems likely, the reinnervation of postsynaptic deafferented sites by collateral sprouts can satisfy this growth stimulus, then in effect the process would deny these sites to the original severed axons. One must, therefore, entertain the possibility that the phenomenon of collateral sprouting can be inimical to complete restitution of the interrupted connections in the central nervous system [p. 9].

There are two important points that need to be considered in the context of these remarks. The first is that sprouting in response to injury does not occur in all loci where it might be expected. This was shown in the Goodman and Horel (1966) experiment cited earlier. They found that the optic tract sprouted into only 2 of 13 potential, deafferented visual system sites after the occipital cortex was damaged on one side of the brain of the rat. Second, most sprouting is probably not heterotypic. For example, Goodman, Bogdasarian, and Horel (1973) found that if they carefully limited the damage to just the optic tract, only axons in the visual system sprouted successfully to fill vacated synaptic sites; anomalous projections from other systems failed to appear. In this case at least, the pattern of axonal sprouting was quite specific, and only those fibers that normally would have innervated the denervated regions showed successful sprouting.

Goodman *et al.* (1973) suggest that priority for "within-systems" sprouting would make the most sense in terms of adaptive behavior and recovery, and that such sprouting "should be most effective in establishing system repair and maintenance or recovery of function when small numbers of neurons of a given system are damaged in the adult brain [p. 41]." Nevertheless, they stress that if within-system sprouting is to occur, the system must only be damaged partially so that remaining, intact neurons could grow into the vacated terminal areas that might otherwise be reinnervated by fibers from a competing neuronal system.

Although the efficacy of within-system sprouting has not been tested directly, the notion fits well with some of the more holistic explanations that have been offered to account for behavioral recovery after brain damage (see Laurence and Stein, 1978; Rosner, 1974, for specific details). When behavioral sparing or gradual recovery follows injury of the central nervous system, some authors have suggested that it is the remaining tissue *within* a given area that mediates the more-or-less efficient pattern of behavior. When the lesions are well circumscribed or partial, the concept of within-systems sprouting as a basis for recovery is very appealing; however, when brain damage is extensive or diffuse, or when a projection is completely or near-totally damaged, limited sprouting of the kind described by Goodman, Bogdasarian, and Horel would probably be insufficient to account for *behavioral* sparing.

Michael Goldberger and Marion Murray of the Medical College of Pennsylvania have also suggested that there may be limits to sprouting following damage to the spinal cord. In their investigations, they cut the lumbar and sacral dorsal roots from the hindlimb of the cat between the ganglion and the spinal cord itself. This operation effectively prevented topographic tactile and cutaneous information from being sent to the brain. With respect to behavior, it meant that any recovery that developed would have to be due to the compensatory use of other neural systems.

Goldberger and Murray first observed the behaviors of their cats and noted that the animals initially showed a complete, flaccid paralysis of the hindlimb on the same side of the body as the transection. This was observed despite the fact that the major pathways to the motor neurons remained intact (i.e., ipsilateral and contralateral descending motor systems, postural reflex systems of the trunk, crossed reflex pathways mediated by contralateral dorsal roots). During the first few days after surgery, the cats dragged their hindlimbs uselessly behind them. Yet, soon after the operation a variety of haphazard and uncontrolled movements began to appear. During this "period of recovery of generalized movements," the cats could not make accurate limb placing responses on even a wide, elevated platform. By the second week after surgery, a number of reflexes mediated exclusively by the ipsilateral descending systems began to emerge but in exaggerated form. They included the scratch reflex, the vestibular placing response, and righting responses when tilted. At about this time, the cats also began to use cues from the trunk (posture, changes in the center of gravity) to guide the hindlimb. Accurate placing of the deafferented limb, presumably based on tactile cues, and the ability to cross a 2-inch-wide runway, soon followed.

After making these behavioral observations, Goldberger and Murray turned their attention to an analysis of the changes in spinal cord anatomy that could account for the recovery seen in the cats. The investigators employed both silver degeneration staining techniques and electron microscopy to evaluate any injury-induced neural reorganization of the spinal cord. It soon became apparent that there was an increase in the density and spread of projections from the descending motor pathways onto the deafferented side of the spinal cord. This sprouting was confined to laminae IV and VIII; the regions of known existing overlap of sensory and motor fibers. Goldberger and Murray (1978) stated that the sprouting "was confined to some but not all of the normal projection fields of the descending systems," and revealed that "the adult sprouting increases an already existing projection rather than creating a new and therefore aberrant projection [p. 78]."

In addition to this increased projection from the descending spinal systems, Goldberger and Murray also found some evidence for sprouting from the dorsal roots of the trunk—fibers seemingly important for the compensatory postural cues that were needed to guide the deafferented limb during locomotion. Together, the sprouting of these two systems may have allowed the animals to overcome their handicaps through the use of a new set of strategies.

One way to test this hypothesis is to damage some of the structures in which the new sprouting is seen. Under these conditions, the recovered behavior should be completely lost. Goldberger and Murray, following this logic, destroyed much of the ipsilateral descending motor system in some of the previously deafferented but "recovered" cats. The second lesion completely abolished the recovered behavior and rendered the limb totally useless for the remainder of the animals' lives. The dorsal roots and descending motor systems contralateral to the damaged side apparently played no role in the recovery of conditioned movement, and the sprouted trunk afferents were incapable of mediating the behavior alone.

The sprouting found by Goldberger and Murray thus was beneficial to the injured cats. Although neuronal reorganization was not accompanied by a perfect return of the original movements, the sprouting did seem to allow existing functions to be strengthened, and permitted some control over limb movements. So, although the "recovered" movements differed in detail from the ones observed prior to surgery, they did allow the animals to achieve some of the same ends, and this in itself must be regarded as a significant accomplishment.

The limited type of sprouting seen by Goodman and his co-workers, and by

Murray and Goldberger, raises a number of important questions about these phenomena and the laws that might govern them. For example, why is sprouting seen in some areas and not in others? Is there a preference for within-systems sprouting? And, are all systems equally capable of sprouting? The answers to some of these questions are coming from a number of different laboratories. With respect to the question of why sprouting is seen in some parts of the brain but not others, Goodman, Bogdasarian, and Horel speculate that tightly coupled systems (systems with strict topographic organization) may not be capable of much sprouting. Attempts to demonstrate sprouting in the cell nest region of nucleus gracilis of the medulla, which is topographically organized, have failed, and sprouting has not been observed in the motor nuclei of the spinal cord. In contrast, adjacent nuclear groups, which are less well organized, seem to be capable of considerable sprouting after injury.

Another observation is that sprouting may be limited to the original projection region in adults. The specificity may be such that sprouts do not grow to adjacent structures, although such anomalous redirection may readily take place in the immature nervous system. Whether the limits to sprouting are determined by proximity or overlap of similar fibers, or whether chemical or morphological preferences limit these outgrowth events is still not known. The "markers" or stimuli that direct axons, as we have pointed out, are still being sought.

Why are some systems more successful in sprouting than others? Goodman, Bogdasarian, and Horel, and Goldberger and Murray, suggest that sprouting may be competitive, and that not all sprouts are equally able to make functional synaptic contacts. Goldberger and Murray (1978) state that:

> When two different but overlapping systems are given access to the same denervated space, one may succeed in forming permanent sprouts at the expense of the other. In fact, one can imagine that in the initial post-lesion period sprouting may be a property of all terminals in the immediate vicinity, but that not all of these sprouts persist. . . . Why one group of sprouts is successful and another is not may have a simple answer. Perhaps persisting sprouts are those which normally occupy sites on the membrane nearest to the denervated spaces, or it may be the post-synaptic receptor which has a mechanism for accepting some sprouting terminals and rejecting others [p. 91].

In addition, the concept of competition among regenerating terminals for vacated synaptic sites raises other possibilities. Goodman and his colleagues (1973) suggest that:

> if one system sprouted first it would occupy some or all available synaptic stations; if axonal sprouts of a later arriving neuronal system were of greater compatability, the higher priority sprouts could fill remaining vacant sites and possibly displace completely or partially the earlier arrivals of low priority [p. 29].

Some of the underlying factors that could be important in determining how and when new synaptic contacts are formed might be mechanical in nature, such as tissue shrinkage and scar formation. These factors could influence and even enhance growth in one direction, and block it in another. The role of glia in the sprouting process could also prove to be significant.

Glial cells are just beginning to receive more attention in terms of the role they may play in providing a milieu favorable to regeneration or anomalous neuronal growth. Prior to the development of synaptic terminals, microglia and reactive astrocytes appear to scavenge and clear the injury-induced neuronal debris so that the newly formed terminals can make their appropriate contacts. It has also been suggested that glia may serve to guide afferents, direct new growth, and stabilize the extracellular environment in preparation for new axonal arborization (Cotman and Lynch, 1976). We will have more to say about the role of glia in recovery from brain damage in Chapter 12.

Many laboratories are now interested in injury-induced sprouting. Nowhere is this more apparent than at the University of California at Irvine where Gary Lynch, Carl Cotman, and their colleagues and students have mounted an elaborate and technically sophisticated program to study the anatomical, biochemical, electrophysiological, and behavioral correlates of sprouting in the hippocampal formation. These workers have found the rat's hippocampus to be particularly well-suited for the study of reactive synaptogenesis because of its unique neuronal organization.

Like the septal region studied by Geoffrey Raisman, the hippocampal formation is often characterized by its two major cell types, the pyramidal cells and the granule cells, each of which has a different distribution within the structure. The pyramidal cells are the major cell population in the hippocampus proper, and the granule cells are the major cell type in the dentate gyrus (see Figure 6.3). The granule cells receive converging inputs from the entorhinal cortex, the septum, and from both contralateral hippocampus (commissural fibers) and ipsilateral hippocampus (associational fibers). Furthermore, the septal and entorhinal afferents are located in different positions on the granule cell dendrites and can also be distinguished from commissural and associational afferents on the basis of their distance from the cell body. Armed with a detailed knowledge of hippocampal anatomy in the normal rat and data showing biochemical differences among some of the inputs, these investigators set out to determine the nature of the changes in neuronal organization that would occur after disruption of the fiber systems projecting to the dentate gyrus.

In one of their first experiments, the Irvine group (Lynch, Matthews, Mosko, Parks, and Cotman, 1972) made unilateral entorhinal cortex lesions in adult rats and then examined the dentate gyrus of the hippocampus for changes in the level of acetylcholinesterase (AChE is the enzyme which is thought to ''neutralize'' the effect of the neurotransmitter acetylcholine). Increased levels of AChE can be

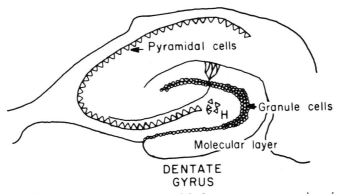

Figure 6.3. *The hippocampal formation consists of the hippocampus proper, where the pyramidal cells are the major cell population, and the dentate gyrus, where the granule cells are the major cell type. Granule cell dendrites ramify in the molecular layer. (From Cotman and Lynch, 1976.)*

taken as evidence of increased acetylcholine activity which would, in turn, reflect the anomalous growth of new fibers into a zone of the dentate, which does not normally receive them. Because the entorhinal projection is primarily ipsilateral, the contralateral side of the brain was able to serve as a control in these preparations.[2]

Lynch and his colleagues thought that the loss of fibers from the entorhinal cortex would trigger the sprouting of nearby AChE-containing fibers, which originate in the septal region of the brain. On the side of the brain opposite to the entorhinal lesion, the outer molecular layer of the dentate gyrus shows only a small AChE response. In contrast, on the same side as the lesion, there is a marked increase in AChE staining, which is apparent within 4 days after the injury. This finding is shown in Figure 6.4, and was taken as evidence that terminals from the normally small septal input to the dentate gyrus had proliferated in response to injury to the entorhinal cortex. A subsequent lesion of the septum caused a sharp loss of the AChE staining in the dentate gyrus, as would be expected if this hypothesis concerning the origin of the new fibers were correct.

What is the nature of the new terminal fields (see Figure 6.5) that develop after entorhinal cortex lesions? New collaterals may form after injury, but it is important to know whether such terminals have morphological characteristics that are similar to those seen in the normal brain. Dee Ann Matthews, Carl Cotman, and Gary Lynch (1976a, b) used electron microscopic techniques to examine lesion-induced synaptogenesis in adult rats that had received unilateral damage to the entorhinal cortex. As shown in Figure 6.6, within 2–4 days following this

---

[2] The advantage of this technique is that the researcher can compare one side of the brain directly to the other. Thus, individual differences can be accounted for and the factors that regulate sprouting can be better understood.

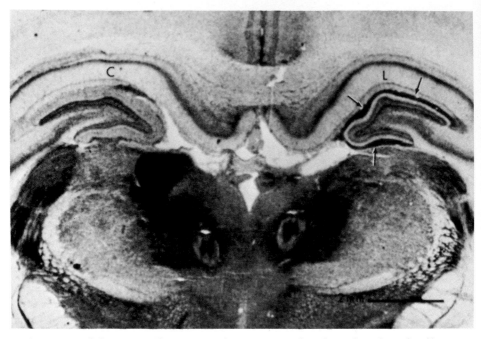

Figure 6.4. *Cholinesterase (ChE) stain in rat hippocampus 40 days after unilateral entorhinal lesion. On the lesioned (L) side, an intense band of ChE is evident in the dentate gyrus (arrows), which is not present on the control side (C). (From Lynch et al., 1972.)*

surgery, the number of intact synapses made by fibers arriving from the entorhinal cortex drops to about 14% of those seen in normal animals, but within 6 months after the surgery, the density of the synapses in the denervated zone is restored to about 80% of the normal complement. This reinnervation process progresses rapidly during the first 30 days after surgery before it slows down. What is important is that the new connections were normal in the sense that they positioned themselves in the same way as the old ones.

Matthews and her colleagues's careful analyses of bouton size revealed that some presynaptic boutons in the reinnervated zone were larger than normal terminals, although they had about the same number of mitochondria seen in normal control tissue. A related difference between normal and reinnervated cases was that the unusually large boutons sometimes made contact with an abnormally large number of different dendritic spines. The functional significance of this finding is not known.

When a granule cell is denervated by a lesion of the entorhinal cortex, is there a dramatic decrease in the number of dendritic sites that have contacts with incoming terminals? What happens to these vacated junctions? Are they reinnervated by new growth or are new synaptic junctions assembled by the hippocampal

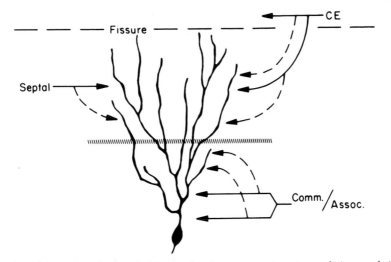

Figure 6.5. *After unilateral removal of the entorhinal cortex, axon sprouting results in a reordering of synaptic inputs on the granule cell dendrites. The commissural (Comm.) and associational (Assoc.) systems appear to expand their terminal fields by about 40 μm into the denervated zone (dashed lines). In the remainder of the denervated zone, septal and residual entorhinal afferents appear to proliferate. (From Cotman and Lynch, 1976.)*

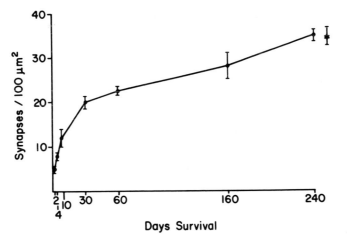

Figure 6.6. *The reappearance of morphologically intact synapses over time in the region of the molecular layer of the dentate gyrus denervated by lesion of the entorhinal cortex. Values are expressed as the mean ± S.E.M. number of synapses per 100 μm^2. The asterisk (versus dots) indicates the density of synapses in control samples. In all those animals that survived 160 and 240 days after the lesion, the lesion completely removed the medial and lateral entorhinal cortex as far ventral as level IX and essentially all of the subiculum, presubiculum, area retrosplenialis and the parasubiculum. (From Matthews, Cotman, and Lynch, 1976.)*

neurons? Matthews and her colleagues (1976b) were able to show that many new postsynaptic sites actually are formed de novo. They state that:

> New assembly as opposed to reoccupation (of previously denervated sites) provides for a greater diversification and formation of functional synaptic contacts with new and possibly different afferents. Newly reassembled sites can be placed in appropriate positions so as to optimize functional capabilities, and a new set of receptors and other molecules related to the postsynaptic response may be created and customized to the new afferents. . . . The production of new synaptic junctions which are typical of the normal molecular layer would indicate that the granule cell retains a capacity, *even into adulthood* to participate in the manufacturing and assembly of these specialized components. In fact, the mature neuron may be constantly establishing new connections at a reduced rate, and *simply accelerate an ongoing process in response to extensive loss* of afferent input created by the lesion [p. 38].

At this point we should mention that even in the hippocampus, sprouting is not seen in all locations, a finding analogous to that reported by Goodman and Horel (1966) and Goldberger and Murray (1978) in other regions of the central nervous system. For example, Lynch and his co-workers (1974) found that, in contrast to the dramatic sprouting from the septum produced by entorhinal cortex lesions, destruction of the hippocampal commissures or dentate gyrus association fibers did not produce any changes in the distribution of septal or entorhinal fibers. This is somewhat surprising because the septal and entorhinal projections make up most of the terminal fields of the inner molecular layer of the dentate gyrus and are immediately adjacent to the deafferented zone. Once again, we have to note that chemical affinities that induce and guide new terminals to their destinations may not necessarily induce new terminal growth in the most appropriate fiber systems. We could speculate that damage to the brain, especially if it is relatively extensive, produces widespread changes in cerebral organization and biochemistry that lead to changes in "functional" hierarchies. Thus if one structure substitutes for another, it may be that structure that is most likely to sprout new terminals, even though it has fewer inputs into the initially intact region, or was spatially further from it.

In any case, although alterations in synaptic morphology and AChE staining in the hippocampus can be taken as evidence for neuronal rearrangement following injury, such data do not speak to the question of whether the newly formed terminals have adaptive significance. To provide such evidence, it would have to be demonstrated that there are both changes in the physiology of the altered system and further, that such changes are accompanied by at least some behavioral recovery of acts that would be impaired after the initial lesions.

As a first step, Gary Lynch, Sam Deadwyler, and Carl Cotman (1973) sought to determine whether the new terminals would show evoked responses to electrical stimulation. In their initial experiments, the investigators removed the en-torhinal cortex in 11-day-old rats. This operation causes the commissural projec-tions to the dentate gyrus to greatly increase and replace the terminal fields that were lost by the initial surgery. In the normal rat, entorhinal projections to the dentate gyrus occupy the outer (molecular) layer while fibers coming from the hippocampal commissures innervate exclusively the inner molecular layer. Lynch *et al.* (1973) point out that there is no overlap between the two fiber systems. After a lesion, the commissural fibers spread into the zone normally occupied by fibers from the entorhinal cortex; but are the new terminals capable of physio-logical excitation?

To answer this question, Lynch *et al.* (1973) examined the animals as adults by slowly lowering a microelectrode through the layers of the dentate gyrus and by recording electrophysiological responses from the granule cells during electrical stimulation of the contralateral hippocampus. The recording electrode was moved in very small steps, up or down, to obtain a response profile that could be compared to that secured from a nonoperated control. The researchers found sub-stantial differences in the electrophysiological patterns between normal and early-operated rats. The short-latency response to commissural stimulation in those rats operated on early in life was observed to spread into the outer molecular layer of the dentate gyrus; a response to stimulation *not* at all seen in adult, unop-erated rats. Lynch *et al.* (1973) take this finding to indicate that the new terminal fields are indeed functional, especially since there were very marked similarities between the wave-forms and latencies of the responses in normal and brain damaged subjects. (We will have more to say on the electrophysiological aspects of functional recovery in Chapter 7.)

The next problem to be resolved is whether or not the new terminals affect be-havioral recovery after injury. In this case, the data are more difficult to interpret because there can be considerable recovery of function in the absence of specific reinnervation (e.g., as in the case where there is complete bilateral removal of structure thought "critical" for mediation of behavioral responses; Chapter 9). Nonetheless, it is important to take a step in trying to resolve the issue by design-ing experiments in which the time parameters of behavioral or physiological recovery coincide with the time it takes for collateral sprouting to be observed.

Jacquelyn Loesche and Oswald Steward (1977) have collected data that they believe reflect on this issue. They compared the rates of recovery on an alternation task between adult rats given unilateral or bilateral lesions of the entorhinal cor-tex, or sham operations. They postulated that if reinnervation of the dentate gyrus following injury has behavioral consequences, then the time course for be-havioral recovery should parallel the time course for postlesion reinnervation. In addition, they suggested that bilateral lesions of the entorhinal cortex would block both the reinnervation and the recovery. Finally, they hypothesized that if such recovery could be found in the unilateral preparations, cutting the fibers from the contralateral entorhinal region would permanently eliminate the ability of the rat to perform this task.

Loesche and Steward first trained their animals to alternate from right to left in a T-maze to obtain food. Once this was learned the animals underwent surgery and were retested after recovery periods ranging from 3 to 40 days. In those rats that had recovered, some were given a second, entorhinal cortex lesion, and others received a transection of the dorsal psalterium, the fiber tract that carries the projections of the contralateral entorhinal area to the dentate gyrus.

As predicted, Loesche and Steward found that the rats with bilateral entorhinal cortex lesions showed a profound deficit that persisted over the entire postoperative testing period. The unilateral animals (after a 3-day recovery period) showed an initial impairment, which began to disappear about 1 ½ weeks after the surgery. Those rats permitted 10 days for recovery showed little if any disruption on the alternation task. When the recovered rats received a second lesion (opposite entorhinal cortex or dorsal psalterium), they developed a severe deficit from which they did not recover during the 1 month period of testing.

Loesche and Steward believe that sprouting from the intact entorhinal cortex provides the best explanation for the recovery they observed. The time course for recovery and sprouting corresponded quite closely in their experiment, and since running speeds and other measures were not impaired, they argue that the effects must reflect more than neural shock.

Because there are so few reports of behavioral recovery that correlate with neuronal sprouting, some of us at Clark University thought that it would be important to replicate the findings of Loesche and Steward to provide more evidence to support the hypothesis that behavioral recovery might have a specific physiological substrate. Thus, in one experiment, Julio Ramirez (1980) used the same anatomical manipulations and behavioral tests employed by Loesche and Steward to examine adult rats given unilateral or bilateral lesions of the entorhinal cortex and then subsequently tested for retention of learned alteration. First of all, Ramirez was able to show that the rats given *bilateral* damage were very impaired on the spatial alternation task compared to those rats given unilateral damage only. In contrast to the report by Loesche and Steward, Ramirez did observe recovery of function when rats with bilateral entorhinal cortex damage were given 30 days of massed-trial postoperative training. Such behavioral recovery is difficult to interpret in the context of a specific, within-system reinnervation hypothesis because all afferents from the entorhinal cortex (EC) are eliminated after bilateral injury.

Ramirez found that the rats with unilateral lesions of the entorhinal cortex performed as well as intact control animals, even with short recovery periods, thus precluding the possibility that sprouting is needed to mediate "spared behavior" in this group of rats. More surprising was the fact that after Ramirez cut the dorsal psalterium in the rats first given unilateral EC lesions, there was still no detectable impairment; once again, the rats were able to perform as well as their intact counterparts on retention testing. Ramirez was forced to conclude that sparing of alternation performance in these animals had little to do with fibers sprouting from the contralateral, intact entorhinal cortex. His data show that the role of sprouting in mediating recovery after lesions in this system is far from resolved.

On the basis of the experiments we have discussed in this chapter, it seems that the synaptic proliferation observed after injury may be an extension of a normal growth process in which neurons are constantly adjusting their terminals to changes in the internal milieu. For example, Goodman, Bogdasarian, and Horel (1973) have discussed the possibility of a continuous remodeling of axonal connections in the normal brain, such that thoughout life there are always some nerve endings that degenerate near adjacent axons, which might have the opportunity to establish new synaptic contacts.

A short time ago, in an investigation that bears directly on this possibility, Descarries, Beaudet, and Watkins (1975) carried out an exhaustive electron microscopic examination of serotonin (5-HT) nerve terminals in adult rat neocortex that had been labeled with ^{3}H/5-HT. They noted that only 5% of the terminals found after extensive sampling had "genuine synaptic relationships." On the basis of this observation, the authors suggested that the morphological characteristics of 5-HT fibers in the cortex are not compatible with a fixed pattern of neuronal circuitry and that there may be a process of continuous translocation and dynamic synaptic reshaping.

Constantino Sotelo and Sanford Palay (1971) also view sprouting after injury as an exaggeration of an everyday phenomenon. They used the electron microscope to show that axons and axon terminals of healthy adult rats undergo degeneration and hypertrophy and are constantly altering their synaptic contacts in the absence of detectable lesions. Sotelo and Palay view the retraction of synapses and the replacement of lost connections as lifelong processes, and not as developmental events or responses that are unique to pathological states. Nevertheless, they raise the interesting point that with the tools currently available to us, it is extremely difficult, if not impossible, to evaluate the functional status of the sprouts that are observed under the microscope. The problems is one of distinguishing "normal" from "degenerative" forms.

Axonal remodeling, which may include sprouts taking over existing synapses, as well as the formation of new synapses (Matthews, Cotman, and Lynch, 1976b) may represent a general state in the nervous system that can be exaggerated under pathological conditions. If this is in fact the case, and if axonal sprouting and new synaptic site formation are the rules rather than the exceptions, attempts to define "fixed" functional circuits by studying small pieces of preserved tissue should be viewed with extreme skepticism. As Raisman (1978) warned, dynamic processes may appear static even though they are not, only because the procedures employed to prepare the material for study merely appear to confer this property upon them.

In closing this chapter, it should be noted that the question of whether collateral sprouting can enhance recovery after brain damage, prevent it, or have no measurable behavioral effects is still not completely resolved. Although the findings of Goldberger and Murray (1978) and Lynch and his colleagues strongly suggest that anomalous growth after injury can have beneficial consequences for the organism, Teuber (1975) points out that sprouting may play a role in the development of spasticity after central nervous system damage (Liu and Chambers, 1958; McCouch, Austin, Liu, and Liu, 1958), as well as in epileptogenesis (Bowen, Demirjian, Karpiak, and Katzman, 1973). Devor and Schneider (1975) hypothesize that adaptive changes could reflect the degree to which collateral sprouts resemble the normal projections to a region, and they stress that these new connections could be maladaptive under some circumstances. One reason for this is that the collateral sprouts may prevent fibers that normally would grow into an area from reestablishing their synaptic contacts. It can also be argued that the new projections could introduce noise into the system. Thus, with regard to the Raisman studies (Raisman, 1969; Raisman and Field, 1973), there is no a priori reason to assume that the medial forebrain bundle inputs to the septum are providing the same information as the hippocampal fibers. If they are not, the result might be the neurobiological equivalent of "jamming," with disruption of the remaining function. Nevertheless, as stressed by most researchers in this area, these ideas are only speculative, and considerably more data will have to be collected before they can be evaluated in a more definitive way.

In the final analysis it seems as if there is considerable neuronal modeling in both intact and brain-damaged organisms, but the last word on the matter is far from in. In adults, Lynch and his associates have demonstrated clearly that such terminal proliferation does exist and have clearly defined some of the morphology related to neuronal plasticity. Whether such proliferation, at least in the adult preparations, can be related to specific functional recovery from injury remains to be determined. The wealth of data and experimentation on neuronal "plasticity" certainly cannot be overlooked, even though we still seem to be some distance from understanding the complex nature of recovery of function in mature organisms. We think that it occurs under some conditions. We can also be certain that proliferative sprouting and neuronal remodeling also occur, but such growth may *not* always be adaptive. The task can be simply stated, but the final goals difficult to achieve: namely to determine in precise fashion, the relation between reactive synaptogenesis and the behavioral sparing or recovery that often follows brain damage.

References

Bowen, F. P., Demirjian, C., Karpiak, S. E., and Katzman, R. Sprouting of noradrenergic nerve terminals subsequent to freeze lesions of rabbit cerebral cortex. *Society for Neuroscience, Third Annual Meeting,* San Diego, California, November 1973, p. 112.

Cotman, C. W., and Lynch, G. S. Reactive synaptogenesis in the adult nervous system. In S. H. Barondes (Ed.), *Neuronal recognition.* New York: Plenum, 1976, Pp. 69–108.

Cotman, C. W., and Nadler, N. G. Reactive synaptogenesis in the hippocampus. In C. W. Cotman (Ed.), *Neuronal Plasticity,* New York: Raven Press, 1978. Pp. 227–271.

Descarries, L., Beaudet, A., and Watkins, K. C. Serotonin nerve terminals in adult rat neocortex. *Brain Research,* 1975, *100,* 563–588.

Devor, M., and Schneider, G. E. Neuroanatomical plasticity: The principle of conservation of total axonal aborization. In F. Vital Durant and J. Jeannerod (Eds.), *Aspects of neural plasticity.* Lyon, France: Colloque INSERM, 1975, *43,* Pp. 191–202.

Edds, M. V., Jr. Collateral nerve regeneration. *Quarterly Review of Biology,* 1953, *28,* 260–276.

Exner, S. Notiz zu der frage von der faservertheilung mehrerer nerven in einem muskel. *Pflüger's Archiv für die gesamte Physiologie,* 1885, *36,* 572–576.

Goldberger, M. E., and Murray, M. Recovery of movement and axonal sprouting may obey some of the same laws. In C. W. Cotman (Ed.), *Neuronal plasticity.* New York: Raven Press, 1978, Pp. 73–96.

Goodman, D. C., Bogdasarian, R. S., and Horel, J. A. Axonal sprouting of ipsilateral optic tract following opposite eye removal. *Brain, Behavior and Evolution,* 1973, *8,* 27–50.

Goodman, D. C., and Horel, J. Sprouting of optic tract projections in the brain stem of the rat. *Journal of Comparative Neurology,* 1966, *127,* 71–88.

Guth, L. History of central nervous system regeneration research. *Experimental Neurology,* 1975, *48,* 3–15.

Guth, L., and Bernstein, J. J. Selectivity in the re-establishment of synapses in the superior cervical sympathetic ganglion of the cat. *Experimental Neurology,* 1961, *4,* 59–69.

Guth, L., and Windle, W. F. The enigma of central nervous regeneration. *Experimental Neurology,* 1970, *5,* 1–43.

Laurence, S., and Stein, D. G. Recovery after brain damage and the concept of localization of function. In S. Finger (Ed.), *Recovery from brain damage: Research and theory.* New York: Plenum, 1978, Pp. 369–407.

Liu, C-N., and Chambers, W. W. Intraspinal sprouting of dorsal root axons. *Archives of Neurology and Psychiatry,* 1958, *79,* 46–61.

Loesche, J., and Steward, O. Behavioral correlates of denervation and reinnervation of the hippocampal formation of the rat: Recovery of alternation performance following unilateral entorhinal cortex lesions. *Brain Research Bulletin,* 1977, *2,* 31–39.

Lynch, G., Deadwyler, S., and Cotman, C. Postlesion axonal growth produces permanent functional connections. *Science,* 1973, *180,* 1364–1366.

Lynch, G., Matthews, D., Mosko, S., Parks, T., and Cotman, C. Induced acetylcholinesterase-rich layer in rat dentate gyrus following entorhinal lesions. *Brain Research,* 1972, *42,* 311–318.

Lynch, G., Stanfield, B., Parks, T., and Cotman, C. W. Evidence for selective post-lesion axonal growth in the dentate gyrus of the rat. *Brain Research,* 1974, *69,* 1–11.

McCouch, G. P., Austin, G. M., Liu, C. N., and Liu, C. Y. Sprouting as a cause of spasticity. *Journal of Neurophysiology,* 1958, *21,* 205–216.

McCouch, G. P., Austin, G. M., and Liu, C. Y. Sprouting of new terminals as a cause of spasticity. *American Journal of Physiology,* 1955, *183,* 642–643.

Matthews, D. A., Cotman, C. W., and Lynch, G. An electron microscopic study of lesion-induced synaptogenesis in the dentate gyrus of the adult rat. I. Magnitude and time course of the degeneration. *Brain Research*, 1976, *115*, 1–21. (a)

Matthews, D. A., Cotman, C., and Lynch, G. An electron microscopic study of lesion-induced synaptogenesis in the dentate gyrus of the adult rat. II. Reappearance of morphologically normal synaptic contacts. *Brain Research*, 1976, *115*, 23–41. (b)

Moore, R. Y., Björklund, A., and Stenevi, U. Plastic changes in the adrenergic innervation of the rat septal area in response to denervation. *Brain Research*, 1971, *33*, 13–35.

Murray, J. G., and Thompson, J. W. The occurrence and function of collateral sprouting in the sympathetic nervous system of the cat. *Journal of Physiology*, 1957, *135*, 133–162.

Nageotte, J. Régénération collatérale de fibres nerveuses terminées par des masseus de croissance, à l'état pathologique et à l'état normal; lésions tabétiques de racines médullaires. *Nouvelle Iconographie de la Salpêtrière*, 1906, *19*, 217–238.

Nageotte, J. Etude sur le greffe des ganglions rachidiens; variations et tropismes du neurone sensitif. *Anatomi scher Anzeiger*, 1907, *31*, 225–245.

Raisman, G. Neuronal plasticity in the septal nuclei of the adult brain. *Brain Research*, 1969, *14*, 25–48.

Raisman, G. What hope for repair of the brain? *Annals of Neurology*, 1978, *3*, 101–106.

Raisman, G., and Field, P. M. A quantitative investigation of the development of collateral reinnervation after partial deafferentation of the septal nuclei. *Brain Research*, 1973, *50*, 241–264.

Ramirez, J. *Behavioral correlates of entorhinal cortex lesions*. Unpublished Master's thesis, Clark University (Worcester, Mass.), 1980.

Ramón y Cajal, S. [*Degeneration and regeneration of the nervous system*] (R. M. May, trans.). New York: Hafner, 1928.

Rosner, B. S. Recovery of function and localization of function in historical perspective. In D. G. Stein, J. J. Rosen, and N. Butters (Eds.), *Plasticity and recovery of function in the central nervous system*. New York: Academic Press, 1974, Pp. 1–30.

Sotelo, C., and Palay, S. L. Altered axons and axon terminals in the lateral vertibular nucleus of the rat. Possible example of neuronal remodeling. *Laboratory Investigation*, 1971, *25*, 633–672.

Teuber, H.-L. Recovery of function after brain injury in man. In *Outcome of severe damage to the central nervous system* (Ciba Foundation Symposium). Amsterdam: Elsevier, 1975, Pp. 159–186.

Weddell, G., Guttmann, L., and Gutman, E. The local extension of nerve fibers into denervated areas of skin. *Journal of Neurology and Psychiatry*, 1941, *4*, 206–225.

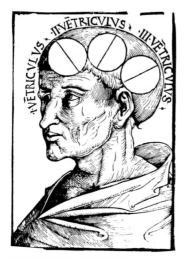

Physiological Plasticity

*Clearly the embryo in differentiating to the speci-
fied adult state has the alternative strategy of either
withering away those branches of axons which fail to
reach the correct target or of physiologically suppressing their postsynaptic effect thereby retaining a
degree of plasticity* [Wall, 1977, p. 371].

CHAPTER SEVEN

In the preceding chapters we described some of the many factors that can
determine the outcome of traumatic injury to the central nervous system. If
nothing else, it should be clear that there is neither a single physiological
mechanism nor a single methodological approach that will lead to a total
understanding of functional recovery from brain damage. Although there are
many changes in cerebral function and anatomy that follow injury, there is no certainty that any of the morphological alterations that do occur are directly related
to functional recovery. When we do try to draw inferences from the experimental
data, it should be remembered that most of the anatomical and structural
evidence for functional "neuroplasticity" rests upon two distinct fields of
endeavor. First, we know from Chapters 5 and 6 that anatomists have
demonstrated the existence of newly formed or deviant pathways as well as increases in terminal proliferation after focal injuries to the brain. Second,
psychobiologists have often been able to show dramatic instances of behavioral
sparing after massive lesions of the central nervous system in developing and adult
organisms. Unfortunately, there is not always an obvious relationship between
the findings provided by the two disciplines. Although some experiments do permit cautious inferences from results obtained in one domain to speculations
about causal relationships in the other, the presence of altered brain circuitry does
not necessarily imply that anomalous growth *causes* functional recovery. More
important, however, is the fact that in adults, there is still relatively little evidence
to indicate that newly formed axons or terminals are physiologically active. It does
not automatically follow that growth induced by injury follows the same laws of

functional organization as neuronal growth during normal development or that such activity, when it is observed, specifically subserves behavioral recovery.

Electrophysiological approaches to assess plasticity are necessary because they provide a direct in vivo measure of injury-induced neuronal growth. Microelectrode techniques can now be used to determine whether individual, newly formed neurons or collateral sprouts are electrophysiologically responsive to stimuli. By making recordings from animals with implanted electrodes, it is also possible to determine if brain damaged animals have a pattern of electrophysiological activity in response to specific stimulation that is systematically different from that of intact control subjects. For example, it might be possible to demonstrate evoked potentials in the visual cortex of intact subjects following retinal stimulation, whereas the same pattern of electrophysiological activity would be induced in more anterior structures in animals with bilateral occipital cortex lesions.

Although such data are not always easy to interpret, they do represent an important link between the domain of static anatomy, which can demonstrate the presence of new pathways in fixed tissue, and behavior.

The first step then, would be to determine the presence of newly sprouted collaterals. The second step requires the demonstration that the new fibers are physiologically active. The third step would be to show that behavioral recovery parallels the development and appearance of physiological activity, and the fourth step would then be to eliminate the new neurons selectively to demonstrate a reappearance of the behavioral deficit. Keeping these four steps in mind, let us now examine some of the research that has attempted to meet these particular goals.

Nakaakira Tsukahara and his colleagues at Osaka University, Japan, have been concerned with the question of synaptic reorganization and functional recovery for quite some time. In one of their earlier studies, these workers traced the main afferent fiber projections to the red nucleus of the brain stem tegmentum. Tsukahara chose this particular region of the brain because the neurons of the red nucleus are large and easily accessible to microelectrode recording and because there is considerable literature on the synaptic organization and electrophysiological properties of these cell membranes (Tsukahara, 1978). The investigators were able to show that there is a very discrete laminar arrangement of the two major synaptic inputs to the red nucleus. In normal adult cats, fiber projections from the sensorimotor cortex terminate on the dendritic portions of the red nucleus neurons, whereas the second major fiber system coming from the deep cerebellar nuclei terminates on or nearer to the cell bodies. If sprouting does occur in the red nucleus when lesions are made in one afferent system or the other, this laminar arrangement would make it easy to detect (see Chapter 6).

Using cats as subjects, Nakamura, Mizuno, Konishi, and Sato (1974) first performed an electron microscopic analysis of the anatomical changes in the red nucleus following damage to its inputs. The anatomists placed unilateral lesions in the interpositus nucleus of the cerebellum and cerebellar peduncle in order to sever all contralateral connections to the red nucleus. About 1 month later, the animals received lesions of the cortex and were then killed after a survival period of several days so that their brains could be prepared for histological analyses. Following the short survival period, Nakamura and his colleagues were able to observe degenerated axon terminals that had numerous contacts with the somata of the red nucleus neurons. Such axosomatic synapses from cortical cells are never seen in cats with intact cerebellorubral afferents. These data were taken to in-dicate that the axons of cells from the cortex that normally ended only on the den-drites of the red nucleus cells sprouted collaterals to make new synaptic contacts on the cell bodies to replace the lost cerebellar projections. What is the evidence that such new terminals are physiologically functional?

If we follow our outline, the next step then would be to examine the "unit ac-tivity" of the newly formed corticorubral synapses that develop after loss of the cerebellorubral pathways. The logic of the experiment is to show that physiologi-cal activity in deafferented subjects occurs in regions of the neuron (or nucleus) that are different from normal animals. However, the properties of the synaptic transmission should be similar to those in normal cats; it would be difficult to conceive of how bizarre postsynaptic potentials would reflect "adaptive" neu-ronal plasticity!

Tsukahara and his colleagues performed an almost exhaustive series of ex-periments in an attempt to determine the specific parameters of elec-trophysiological activity that accompany corticorubral sprouting in adult cats (cf. Tsukahara, 1978). Their technique required several stages of surgery, microelec-trode stimulation, recording, and subsequent histology. First, the interpositus nucleus of the cerebellum was destroyed in one group of adult cats that was al-lowed to survive for varying periods of time. The animals were then prepared for stimulation and recording by exposing their cerebral cortices and implanting in-sulated needles to serve as stimulation electrodes in the corticorubral tract. Glass microelectrodes were then used to record from the soma of the red nucleus neurons. Tsukahara and his associates proposed that if newly sprouted fibers form functional synapses at different sites, the time course of excitatory post-synaptic potentials (EPSPs), recorded at the cell body, would change. (EPSPs are the slow, graded potentials that summate to produce the action potential, or spike, that then travels down the axon in an all-or-none fashion.) Thus, if a ter-minal moves closer to the cell body to replace those that have been lost, the la-tency of the EPSP would be shorter in comparison to that produced by the same cortical stimulation in an animal whose fibers normally terminate on the den-drites.

Figure 7.1 shows some of the changes in rise time of postsynaptic potentials after stimulation in normal cats or after lesions were made in the interpositus

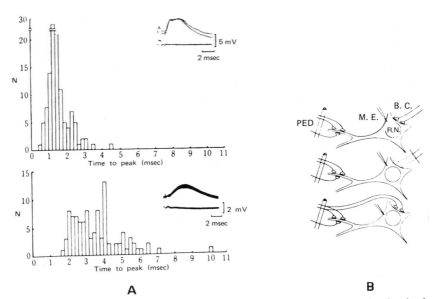

Figure 7.1. *Rise time of the corticorubral EPSPs induced by stimulating the cerebral peduncle after lesion of the interpositus nucleus of the cerebellum. (A) Frequency distribution of the time to peak of the CP-EPSPs in chronic cats (upper histogram) and in normal cats (lower histogram). Specimen records of the intracellular and corresponding extracellular records are shown in the inset of each histogram. (B) Diagram of the experimental arrangement. R. N., red nucleus neurons; B. C., input from IP through brachium conjunctivum; P.E.D., input from cerebrum through cerebral peduncle; M. E., microelectrode. (From Tsukahara, N. Synaptic plasticity in red nucleus. In C. Cotman (Ed.), Neuronal Plasticity. Copyright © 1978. With permission from Raven Press, New York.)*

nucleus. The investigators found that the time-to-peak of the EPSPs induced by stimulation of the motor cortex decreased considerably after a lesion was made in the cerebellum. The decreased latencies of the EPSPs were not seen immediately after surgery, but rather after a 1 or 2 week delay, which would be consistent with the time it usually takes to observe anatomical changes considered to be representative of anomalous growth. Tsukahara takes his data to indicate that new and effective synapses are formed on the somata of the red nucleus neurons in response to interpositus nucleus (IP) lesions.

Although he does indicate that there may be alternative explanations (Tsukahara, 1978), Tsukahara supported his hypothesis by additional physiological studies to determine the functional difference between newly sprouted terminals and "old" ones. Briefly stated, unitary EPSPs in cats with IP lesions can be characterized as two distinct types: (*a*) those with shorter time to peak and larger amplitudes than normal; and (*b*) those EPSPs that were within the normal range. In general, though, the EPSPs of normal cats were smaller in amplitude and had a longer time to peak than the EPSPs of cats with lesions. This would be expected if the newly formed terminals were closer to the soma rather than being located on the dendritic branches. Figure 7.2 demonstrates this phenomenon by showing the differences in amplitude and time to peak of EPSPs in operated (open circles) and normal cats (black circles).

The physiology of postsynaptic potentials has been carefully studied so that the characteristics of the response to repetitive stimulation could serve as an indication of whether the newly formed terminals had response properties similar to normal cells. For example, when a pair of electrically pulsed stimuli are presented in very close order, the EPSP produced by the second of the two stimuli is larger than that produced by the first. This is known as *frequency facilitation*. Murakami, Tsukahara, and Fujito (1977) examined facilitation of EPSPs of red nucleus neurons in cats with and without lesions of the interpositus nucleus. After waiting the appropriate postoperative recovery period and then electrically stimulating the cortex, these investigators showed that the double stimulation

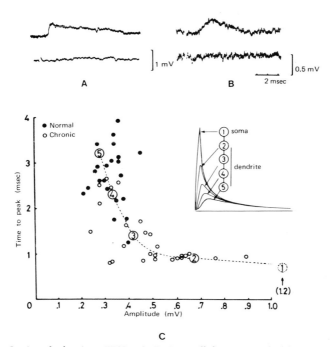

C

Figure 7.2. *Corticorubral unitary EPSPs. A, B: Intracellular EPSP evoked by stimulation of sensorimotor cortex at a rate of 1/sec in a cat with IP lesion 27 days before acute experiment (A), and in a normal cat (B). Upper traces denote intracellular potentials. Lower traces denote extracellular field corresponding to the upper traces. (C) Relation between time to peak and amplitude of the unitary EPSPs. Open circles represent unitary EPSPs of operated cats and filled circles represent those of normal cats. Large open circles represent times to peak and amplitudes of theoretical EPSPs derived by Rall's compartmental model initiated at each compartment of a five-compartment chain. The time course of the theoretical EPSPs generated in these compartments is diagrammatically shown in the inset of the figure. (From Murakami, Tsukahara, and Fujito, 1977.)*

resulted in the same increases in amplitude of the EPSPs in both the normal and brain-damaged cats. The time course of facilitation was also essentially the same for the two groups of animals. Tsukahara's electrophysiological experiments provide strong evidence that reorganization of terminal fields occurs in response to deafferentation in adult cats.

Taken together, these electrophysiological and anatomical experiments show that anomalous growth in the central nervous system of adult animals can be physiologically functional. Still, there is some question as to whether the new growth has *adaptive significance* for the organism. From a behavioral perspective, evidence that animals show behavioral recovery from the lesions of the interpositus nucleus is still lacking.

Tsukahara has reported that preliminary work with innervation of the peripheral nerves after lesions can be taken to indicate that the flexion and extension patterns of forepaw movements resemble, in some respects, those of normal cats. These data suggest that rubrospinal synapses may sprout and be physiologically active, but that behavioral recovery is not complete. The lack of complete recovery should not be surprising since it must be kept in mind that the red nucleus is deprived of its original afferents from the interpositus nucleus. The new terminals arriving from the corticorubral fiber system may be similar to normal end feet, but the "message" they are providing to the red nucleus neurons might be considerably different than that previously received from the cerebellum. Thus, the process of regrowth provides a good example of plasticity in response to injury at the neuroanatomical level, but such "plasticity" could be responsible for maladaptive behavior, a possibility that we raised in the context of other studies on sprouting that were discussed in Chapters 5 and 6.

The functional characteristics of "reactive synaptogenesis" have also been evaluated in a series of carefully designed studies by Gary Lynch, Carl Cotman, and their students at the University of California at Irvine. In Chapter 6, we discussed how the Irvine group demonstrated that neurons in the entorhinal cortex are capable of forming new circuitry in response to brain damage. The next task would then be to determine whether the newly formed terminal fields show any physiological activity characteristic of functional synapses. For the most part, the investigators had an experimental model similar to the one developed by Tsukahara and his colleagues. Like the red nucleus, the dentate gyrus of the hippocampus is a good target structure for the study of neuroplasticity because of its laminar organization and physiological responsivity to electrical stimulation and because the afferents to each layer are reasonably distinct and well known (see Figure 7.3).

In one study, which was briefly mentioned in the last chapter, Oswald Steward, Carl Cotman, and Gary Lynch (1973) made unilateral lesions of the entorhinal cortex in 11-day-old rat pups who were allowed to survive until adulthood. When the rats reached maturity, they received electrical stimulation

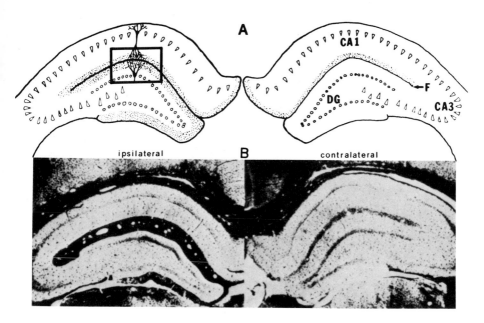

Figure 7.3. *Normal projections of the entorhinal cortex to the hippocampus and dentate gyrus. (A) A schematic representation of the hippocampal formation in coronal section indicates the cellular divisions of the hippocampus (CA1 and CA3) and the dentate gyrus (DG). The orientation of a granule cell of the dorsal leaf, and a pyramidal cell of the CA1 hippocampus is indicated on the left. The terminal field of the normal entorhinal projection is indicated by the dots. (B) The site of termination of entorhinal cortical afferents is indicated by dark staining in a coronal section comparable to that illustrated in A. (From Steward, Cotman, and Lynch, 1973.)*

of the entorhinal cortex contralateral to the early lesion, while extracellular recordings from the dentate gyrus on the damaged side were taken. In the normal rat with no lesion, unilateral stimulation of the entorhinal cortex will cause a strong monosynaptic activation of neurons in the ipsilateral dentate gyrus and a weak response of the pyramidal cells in the hippocampus on both sides of the brain. Short latency responses in the dentate gyrus contralateral to the entorhinal stimulation, which would be indicative of monosynaptic activation, are never seen. These findings are shown in Figures 7.4 and 7.5.

Lynch and his colleagues found that when the entorhinal cortex is damaged very early in life, contralateral entorhinal stimulation produces a short latency response in the dentate gyrus (see Figure 7.6). This response occurs in addition to the normal, long latency discharge and is confined to the granule cell layer. In fact, if the recording electrode is moved even a small distance (50 micra) from the granule cell bodies, the short latency response is lost. In addition, they found that this response could not be evoked by stimulating other parts of the brain and that

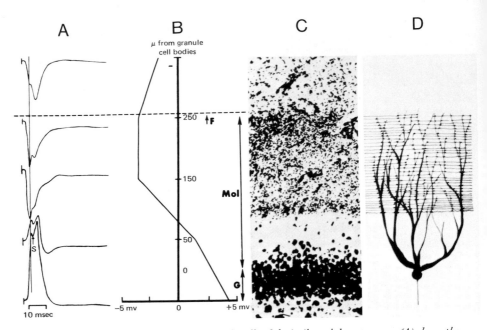

Figure 7.4. *Entorhinal activation of the granule cells of the ipsilateral dentate gyrus. (A) shows the evoked potentials of the dentate gyrus to stimulation of the ipsilateral entorhinal cortex. The evoked potential appears in the dendritic regions of the granule cells (the molecular layer) as a short latency negativity, whereas at the level of the cell bodies, a potential of similar latency, but opposite polarity is recorded. (B) shows a laminar plot of the amplitude of the evoked potential at the latency indicated by the vertical line. Riding on these major potentials is a small spike wave oppositely oriented to the major potential (S). This small spike wave is in many preparations visible only at the level of the cell bodies, as an extracellular negativity. (C) indicates the pattern of termination of entorhinal afferents in the molecular layer of the dentate (Fink-Heimer method). (D) indicates schematically the orientation of an idealized granule cell with respect to the innervating ipsilateral perforant path. (From Steward, Cotman, and Lynch, 1973.)*

even within the intact entorhinal cortex, the locus in which effective stimulation would produce a contralateral response was very limited.

   Steward, Cotman, and Lynch believe that the new potentials were generated from fibers originating in the intact contralateral cortex that now grew over to the opposite side of the brain. By carefully mapping the site of maximal extracellular activity in the portion of the neuropil that receives the reinnervating contralateral sprouts, Steward *et al.* (1973) were able to specify precisely where the new terminal fields made contact with the dendritic branches of the granule cells. As the recording electrode was pushed down through the molecular layer of the dentate gyrus toward the granule cell bodies, a short latency negativity was seen in the outer molecular layer. As the electrode approached the cell bodies, the negativity decreased and then became positive, only to become negative again as the elec-

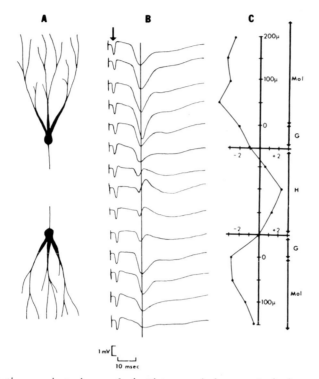

Figure 7.5. *In the normal rat, absence of a short latency evoked response in the dentate gyrus follow-ing stimulation of the contralateral entorhinal cortex. (A) illustrates the orientation of granule cells of the dorsal and ventral leaves of the dentate with respect to a recording electrode advancing through the dentate. (B) illustrates the evoked potentials following stimulation of the contralateral entorhinal cortex. Following the stimulus (arrow), you see no short latency response of the dentate gyrus in-dicative of entorhinal activation regardless of the stimulus intensity employed. The long latency potential shown is evokable only at high stimulus intensities (30–40 V bipolar, 1 msec duration). This long latency potential is recorded as a negativity in the proximal molecular layer (Mol in C) and becomes predominantly a positive potential at the level of the granule cell bodies and hilus; see laminar plot in (C). At the level of the granule cell bodies and hilus, there is in addition a small initial negative deflection in the evoked potential (here at a latency of approximately 11 msec). This negativity is associated with the unitary discharge of cells and is therefore interpreted as a population spike. In (C), the amplitude of the major component of this evoked potential is plotted at the latency indicated by the vertical line. The waveform and location of maximal extracellular negativity of this long latency potential are similar to those of the normal evoked potential to stimulation of the con-tralateral CA3 region, differing only on the basis of latency. Therefore, the long latency potential may be a polysynaptic response in which the final relay is the contralateral CA3 region of the hippocam-pus. (From Steward, Cotman, and Lynch, 1973.)*

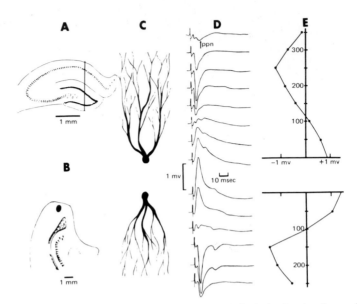

Figure 7.6. *Following lesion, short latency evoked responses in both the dorsal and ventral leaves of the dentate gyrus to contralateral stimulation. Two hundred days after lesion of the ipsilateral entorhinal cortex, the response of the dentate gyrus to stimulation of the remaining contralateral entorhinal area was investigated. (A) illustrates the orientation of the microelectrode penetration with respect to the dentate gyrus. (B) shows a cross-hatched area indicating the site in the entorhinal cortex from which the response shown in (D) was evoked. A small lesioning current was passed through the stimulating electrode at the termination of the experiment. (C) schematically illustrates the orientation of the granule cells of both the dorsal and ventral leaves of the dentate. (D) shows short latency evoked responses following low intensity stimulation of the contralateral entorhinal cortex. The potentials recorded through the hilus are not shown. The amplitude of these potentials is plotted in (E). Note the maximal extracellular negativity in the outer portions of the molecular layer. The uppermost trace of (D) is recorded in the stratum lacunosum-moleculare of the hippocampus, and the longer latency performant path negativity (PPN) is evident at this location. (From Steward, Cotman, and Lynch, 1973.)*

trode entered the ventral molecular layer. ''The negativity in the outer ⅔ of the molecular layer therefore may be used to locate the site of termination of the entorhinal efferents [p. 406].'' The evoked potentials seen in this region correlated perfectly with audioradiographic data suggesting that new collaterals from the intact entorhinal cortex now projected to just this layer of the deafferented dentate gyrus.

The data provided in this sophisticated experiment thus provide physiological evidence for functional sprouting following brain injury. It should be remembered that Steward *et al.* made their lesions in young rats, only 10–11 days old at the time of their first operation. As Land and Lund (1979) have previously indicated, bilateral projections from the contralateral entorhinal cortex may have existed early in life only to shrink back across the midline as the rats approached maturity. The early lesions could have blocked this retraction process. The presence of the "anomalous" terminal fields would then be interpreted as evidence for new growth when in fact, the fibers would have been there all along. This argument is mitigated by the fact that Steward, Cotman, and Lynch (1974) repeated the same basic experiments in adult rats, even including an auto-radiographic, anatomical investigation of the new fiber pathways. Except for slight nuances, Steward *et al.* collected essentially the same data in animals that received unilateral entorhinal cortex lesions as adults. Figure 7.7 shows these results.

The electrophysiological results therefore confirm the anatomical data. Figure 7.8 shows that the reappearance of the evoked potentials to contralateral entorhinal stimulation develop slowly over time and do not reach normal appearance until about 15 days after surgery. According to the investigators, the electrical recordings in all respects appeared to reflect new monosynaptic activation of the dentate granule cells.

Of course, explanations other than sprouting can always be advanced to explain these data, as convincing as they may appear. It may be that the preservation of terminals destined to die is not confined to the period of infancy, but instead can involve different systems and pathways at various times over the course of a lifetime. Goldowitz, White, Steward, Cotman, and Lynch (1975) also showed that there is a very sparse contralateral projection from the entorhinal cortex to the dentate gyrus that is present in normal adult rats. It is therefore possible that following a lesion, the sparse projection is released from suppression and extends to fill the deafferented zone—an important but somewhat less dramatic example of synaptogenesis. Nevertheless, in even their most recent articles (e.g., Steward and Vinsant, 1978), the members of this team reject such notions and argue that the additional connections come from an increased number of neurons that now project contralaterally from the intact entorhinal zone.

If these workers are correct, their findings provide additional evidence that physiologically functional sprouts can emerge in the adult central nervous system, although as we have noted, such sprouting may not necessarily occur in all parts of the brain. Similar attempts to observe crossed-hemispheric sprouting in the visual system once animals reach maturity, for example, have been entirely unsuccessful (Guillery, 1972; Lund and Lund, 1973). But what is particularly interesting about the sprouting seen in the experiments of Steward and his co-workers is that the contralateral entorhinal projections grow as much as 1 mm, and they even cross cellular boundaries (i.e., the hippocampal fissure) to establish synaptic contacts on sites left vacant on the opposite side of the brain. It is as if for some reason the cells closer in proximity to the denervated zones had been inhibited from establishing their own functional sprouts. At present we have no good idea as to why cells in Layer III of the hippocampus do not reinnervate the dentate gyrus,

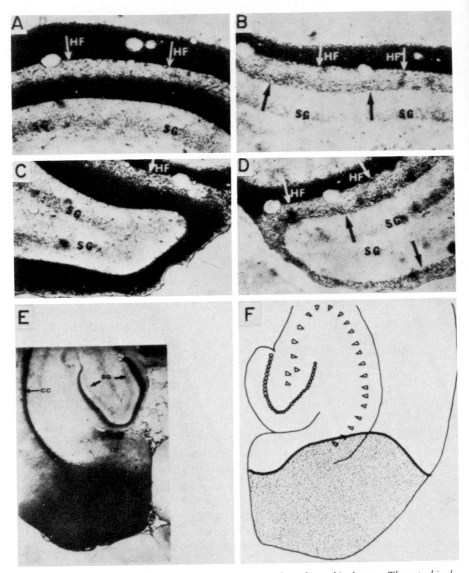

Figure 7.7. *Reinnervation of the dentate gyrus by the contralateral entorhinal cortex. The entorhinal cortex on the right-hand side was ablated, and 60 days later, the projections of the remaining entorhinal cortex were traced autoradiographically. (A) The pattern of entorhinal termination in the ipsilateral hippocampal formation is illustrated. SG indicates the stratum granulare, and HF (see white arrows) shows the hippocampal fissure. (B) The stratum moleculare of the dentate gyrus contralateral to the injection is illustrated. Note the new terminal field of the afferents from the contralateral entorhinal cortex (indicated by the large black arrows). (C) A different portion of the stratum moleculare of the dentate gyrus ipsilateral to the injection is shown. Both dorsal and ventral leaves of the dentate gyrus are visible in this region of the dentate crest (where the dentate gyrus curves around forming the central leaf). (D) A comparable section of the reinnervated contralateral dentate gyrus is*

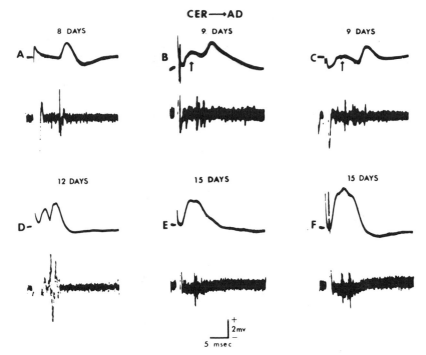

Figure 7.8. *The time course of contralateral entorhinal reinnervation. The recording electrode is situated in the granule cell layer of the dorsal leaf. Evoked potentials and unit discharges are recorded in the denervated area dentata following stimulation of the contralateral entorhinal cortex that remains following ipsilateral entorhinal lesions. (A) 8 days postlesion. This response is comparable to that of the normal dentate to contralateral entorhinal stimulation (cf. Figure 7.6A), and thus there is no evidence of any reinnervation at this time. (B) and (C) 9 days postlesion. Note the hint of a new response in the early portions of the records (see arrows) and note the occasional short latency unit discharge (B). (D) 12 days postlesion. Stimulation here is below threshold for the normal late polysynaptic response. Note the massive new short latency response, which is associated with discharge of the granule cells (indicated by the large population spike). (E) and (F) 15 days postlesion. In (E), stimulation is below threshold for the late polysynaptic response, and the granule cells discharge only once, in association with the new evoked potential, whereas in (F) stimulus intensity is increased above threshold for the normal late polysynaptic response; and under these circumstances, the granule cells discharge twice, once in association with the new short latency response, and once again in association with the normal late polysynaptic response. (From Steward, Cotman, and Lynch, 1974.)*

---

illustrated. Here note that the new terminal field of the contralateral entorhinal afferents is visible in both dorsal and ventral leaves (see large black arrows). (E) The injection site in the entorhinal cortex is evident in horizontal section. In addition, the caudal and ventral hippocampal formation is visible at this level, showing the heavily labeled stratum moleculare of the ipsilateral dentate gyrus. Small arrows, SG, show the layer of dentate granule cells, and cc indicates the heavily labeled lateral margin of the corpus callosum. (F) The extent of the initial lesion is schematically represented in horizontal section. Note that both medial and lateral entorhinal cortices were ablated. (From Steward, Cotman, and Lynch, 1974.)

nor why cells from the nearby presubiculum or parasubiculum do not do so. Instead, fibers coming all the way from the opposite hemisphere establish their contacts here and do so in a highly specific, rather than haphazard manner.

Although the story is still unfolding, the experiments performed by these investigators are providing important clues in the search for the mechanisms that might underlie recovery from brain damage. As noted previously, their findings on the anatomical and physiological plasticity of the hippocampal system have been correlated with a behavioral function, notably alternation performance in a T-maze. Still, a number of questions remain, such as why Ramirez (1980), in a replication of some of these experiments, was able to confirm the apparent sprouting, but unable to correlate it with recovery of function. While the picture of reactive synaptogenesis seems to be one of great precision, we cannot be certain that this is in fact the case. After entorhinal cortex deafferentation, it has been shown that cholinergic afferent fibers arriving from the septum will also proliferate in the deafferented zone. These fibers spread from their normal sites of termination on the proximal dendrites out into more distal regions of the granule cells (see Cotman, Matthews, Taylor, and Lynch, 1973). If it can be assumed that these synaptic contacts are also physiologically functional, then the pattern of postsynaptic activity generated by the new inputs from the septum, coupled with their displacement into different regions of the dendritic branch, would also have to be considered as these data are put into perspective. How all of these new connections interact with each other and with remaining normal contacts is still far from clear. Furthermore, it would seem reasonable to question whether there could possibly be no behavioral consequences of these changes, even permitting adequate time for synaptic stabilization.

Some of the most interesting electrophysiological analyses of the events that follow brain damage have been conducted on the visual system. These studies are particularly informative because much is known about the anatomy and physiology of the visual areas and because the effects of lesions on discriminative behaviors have also been well documented. For example, in most adult mammals, lesions of the visual cortex or upper brain stem often cause severe impairments in visual placing (a suspended animal is gradually moved toward the edge of a table and reaches for it prior to making tactile contact), flicker fusion, movement detection, and brightness discrimination. Yet, very often there is considerable recovery and remastery of the task. In some instances, this recovery appears to be based on the use of cues that differ from those used prior to damage (e.g., luminous flux versus pattern cues on some discrimination), but this is not always the case. What electrophysiological phenomena might parallel behavioral events like these?

Peter Spear, who is now at the University of Wisconsin, and his students and colleagues have been working on this question for a number of years. Spear's group first demonstrated that cats lacking any visual cortex are very impaired in learning a visual task. But despite this handicap, as shown in Figure 7.9, the cats

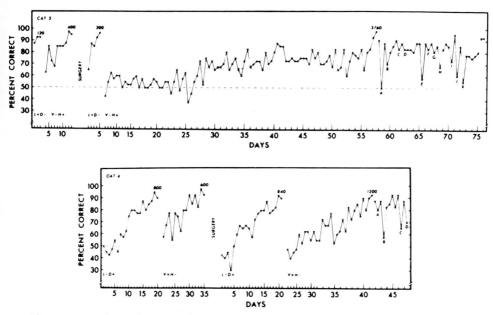

Figure 7.9. *Performance on two-choice brightness (light-dark) and pattern (horizontal-vertical stripes) discriminations by two different cats, before and after visual cortex damage. The cats received 40 training trials per day on each task until they reached a criterion of 90% correct on two successive days. Each point on the curves represents 40 trials. The number above the last point on each curve indicates trials to criterion. The dashed line at 50% correct indicates chance performance for a 40-trial block of testing. The dotted lines at 66% correct and 34% correct indicate the upper and lower limits of th 95% confidence interval for a 40-trial block. Letters below each curve indicate the discrimination task: L, light panel; D, dark panel; V, vertical stripes; H, horizontal stripes. (+) and (−) indicate which stimulus was correct and incorrect in each pair. The cats received damage to areas 17, 18, and 19 at the time indicated by* surgery.

Brightness discrimination: *Cat 3 had initially high performance and cat 4 had initially low performance on this task (LD) preoperatively due to an initial preference for the light stimulus. Nevertheless, the visual cortex damage produced a postoperative loss for both cats. In addition, both cats relearned the discrimination at about the same rate as original learning.*

Pattern discrimination: *The visual cortex damage also produced a loss of the horizontal-vertical stripes discrimination (VH). Nevertheless, both cats showed eventual recovery. However, retraining to criterion required from two to nearly ten times the number of trials required for original learning. When criterion was attained postoperatively, a series of tests was conducted to verify that performance was visually guided and to determine some of the cues utilized. For cat 3, the letter below each point (right end) refers to the following tests: A, bottom halves of both stimulus panels covered; B, top halves covered; C, lateral halves covered; D, medial halves covered; E, bottom halves covered again. Thus, the animal attended to the bottom halves of the stimulus panels, which were near the dishes into which liquid reward was delivered. For letters F–K, light transmission to the stimuli was successively reduced in $\log_2$ steps, thereby decreasing stimulus illumination and contrast. This produced progressive deterioration of performance. Performance returned to criterion when the stimuli were returned to their original contrast and intensity. For cat 4, the following tests were conducted: A, lateral halves of stimulus panels covered; B, bottom halves covered; C, medial halves covered; D, top halves covered. (From Spear and Braun, 1969.)*

can eventually learn to make form and pattern discriminations when brightness differences and subtle changes in the flickering of the stimuli (sometimes used as alternate, but less effective cues) are experimentally controlled (e.g., Spear and Braun, 1969; see also Spear, 1979).

One possible explanation for this behavioral recovery of function is that other brain regions related to the classical visual cortical zones (areas 17, 18, 19) become involved in mediating form discrimination. Of the various structures thought to be important, the suprasylvian gyrus is considered by some to be particularly critical because it is adjacent to the visual cortex in the cat and because it also receives visual inputs and responds with evoked potentials to retinal stimulation, even when areas 17, 18, and 19 are removed. Given these facts, Spear thought that the suprasylvian gyrus would be the most logical substrate for guiding restitution of performance in his cats.

In an initial investigation of this possibility, Wood, Spear, and Braun (1974) ablated the suprasylvian gyrus in adult cats that were trained to discriminate between vertical or horizontal stripes. It was quickly noted that this surgery had virtually no effect on performance of the task. When the same operation was made on cats that had recovered the ability to make visual discriminations following visual cortex lesions, their performance dropped to chance and remained poor throughout testing. This finding was taken by Spear to indicate that the suprasylvian gyrus did, in fact, play a role in mediating performance *after* visual cortex lesions, but not when the visual cortex was intact.

Further analyses, based on anatomical and electrophysiological data, suggested that behavioral compensation may be dependent upon only one part of the suprasylvian gyrus—the lateral region. Baumann and Spear (1977) tested this hypothesis by limiting the damage to just the lateral suprasylvian area in some cats and to other parts of the suprasylvian gyrus in other animals. All of the cats had sustained visual cortex lesions as well. In general, the combined *lateral* suprasylvian gyrus and visual cortex lesions left the cats very impaired on the discrimination, whereas the other lesion combinations did not. This seemed to indicate a very precise localization of the structure mediating restoration of visual function.

Given these findings, it became possible to proceed with the next phase of the experiments, which called for examination of the functional activity of single neurons in the lateral suprasylvian region before and after visual cortex damage. In normal cats, Spear and Baumann (1975) found that approximately 80% of the lateral suprasylvian neurons were sensitive to the *direction* of a moving stimulus and did not respond to stationary stimuli. A much smaller proportion of cells (8%) were movement sensitive, and even fewer responded to lights flashing on and off. The remaining neurons (about 6.5%) seemed to respond to diffuse light or gave indefinite responses to changes in levels of illumination. This can be seen in Figure 7.10.

Figure 7.10. *Summary of response pro-*
perties of lateral suprasylvian visual area
cells in 24 normal cats. (A) Percentage of
cells (N = total number of cells in sam-
ple) in each of the four receptive field
classes described in the text: I, indefinite;
S, stationary; M, movement sensitive; D,
direction selective. (B) Percentage of cells
in each of seven ocular dominance
groups: 1, driven exclusively by the con-
tralateral eye; 2, marked dominance by
the contralateral eye; 3, slight con-
tralateral dominance; 4, driven equally
by both eyes; 5, slight dominance by the
ipsilateral eye; 6, marked dominance by
the ipsilateral eye; 7, driven exclusively
by the ipsilateral eye. In the ocular
dominance analysis, only those cells that
had their entire receptive field within the
approximate binocular overlap field are
considered. (From Spear, 1979.)

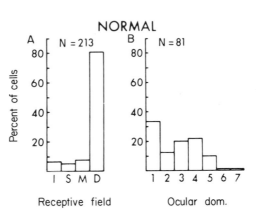

In cats with acute lesions of the visual cortex (areas 17, 18, 19), the neurons in the lateral suprasylvian area were still light sensitive and showed little change in receptive field sizes. Their actual receptive field properties were quite another matter. In the first place, the percentage of directionally sensitive neurons was dramatically reduced (from 80% to 7.5%), whereas the percentage of cells that responded to stationary flashing stimuli increased. In the second place, about 86% of the neurons could now be driven by the contralateral eye, in comparison with only 33% in cats with the visual cortex left intact. These changes were observed from a few hours after surgery to as long as 5 weeks after removal of the visual cortex. These dramatic shifts in activity thus probably represented "the direct effects of removing the visual cortex inputs to the lateral suprasylvian cortex, rather than any secondary effects due to retrograde degeneration in the thalamus or in the lateral suprasylvian cortex itself [Spear, 1979, p. 70]."

When the adult cats were examined 3–7 months later, no additional changes were found in the unit properties of the neurons (Figure 7.11). That is, there was no return to the normal condition, which paralleled the behavioral recovery that was observed in the cats with visual cortical lesions who were allowed to survive for varying periods of time. Since pattern discrimination performance is poor if the suprasylvian area is removed together with, or after, visual cortex ablations, the conclusion drawn from this finding is that the cats had learned to rely on these different lateral suprasylvian unit properties to obtain the needed visual information. Pattern discrimination was possible despite the fact that these cells, with their altered properties, were imperfect substitutes for those normally en-

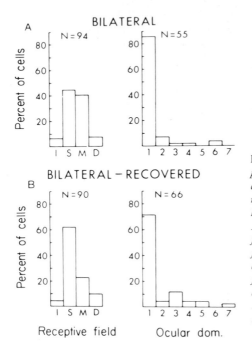

Figure 7.11. *(A) Summary of the response properties of lateral suprasylvian visual area cells in seven cats with short-term bilateral removal of visual cortex areas, 17, 18, and 19. Recording was conducted from a few hours to 5 weeks after the lesion. Compare with data from normal cats in Figure 7.10. (B) Results from five cats with long-term bilateral visual cortex damage. Recording was conducted from 3 to 7 months after the lesion, and all cats learned form and pattern discriminations prior to recording. All conventions are in the legend for Figure 7.10. (From Spear, 1979.)*

countered in intact animals. That is, although the neurons underwent an immediate change in receptive field activity as a result of losing visual cortex inputs, there did not seem to be any signs of further reorganization that could account for the eventual mastery of the pattern discrimination.

A somewhat different picture emerged when cats given visual cortex lesions as neonates were examined as adults. When they were tested they displayed no deficits at all on the pattern problems. Also, unlike adult animals who showed complete retrograde degeneration of the dorsal lateral geniculate nucleus of the thalamus after visual cortex lesions, these cats (operated upon as infants) had many large, healthy neurons scattered through otherwise degenerated portions of this nucleus. These surviving neurons appeared to be physiologically active.

Spear (1979) further noted (Figure 7.12) that neurons in cats with the neonatal lesions showed response properties in the lateral suprasylvian area of the cortex that were essentially *like those of unoperated cats*, even though they lacked visual cortices:

For example, the range of directions of stimulus movement to which they respond (directional tuning) is normal, as is the presence of spatial summation within the receptive field and the incidence of surround inhibition. Very few cells respond as well or better to stationary flashing stimuli as to movement, just as in normal cats. There was no suggestion that the cells became orientation selective or take on any of

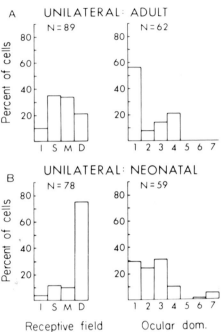

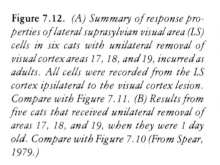

Figure 7.12. *(A) Summary of response properties of lateral suprasylvian visual area (LS) cells in six cats with unilateral removal of visual cortex areas 17, 18, and 19, incurred as adults. All cells were recorded from the LS cortex ipsilateral to the visual cortex lesion. Compare with Figure 7.11. (B) Results from five cats that received unilateral removal of areas 17, 18, and 19, when they were 1 day old. Compare with Figure 7.10 (From Spear, 1979.)*

the properties of the damaged visual cortex. All of the properties are the same as those of the lateral suprasylvian cortex in normal adult cats and are in marked contrast to the damages which occur following visual cortex damage in adults [p. 76].

Putting these findings together, Spear (1979) suggests that removal of the visual cortex in the neonate permitted the development of new, aberrant projections from the dorsal lateral geniculate body to the lateral suprasylvian cortex. Furthermore, these projections allowed the suprasylvian cortical cells to receive information that would normally be transferred to them from the visual cortex. That these ''new'' projections are crucial is seen by the fact that performance drops to chance level if lesions are made in the lateral suprasylvian area that cause the scattered large cells in the dorsal lateral geniculate body to degenerate. Since these projections are not found in adult-operated cats with the visual cortex removed, Spear thought that the increased anatomical projection from the thalamus to the lateral suprasylvian area could only develop during an early ''critical period.''

Of course, we now know that an alternate interpretation of these findings is that the ''new'' projections to the lateral suprasylvian cortex may have been present when the lesions were made in the neonates, but that they failed to retract after visual cortex surgery (Land and Lund, 1979). In either case, however, these experiments show that behavioral recovery on a discriminative task can involve anatomical and physiological events that might not even have been thought possible less than a generation ago. These experiments are significant because they serve as a reminder to us about how little we still know about the response properties of cells after brain damage and how speculative inferences about physiology and function can be when based strictly on anatomical data.

At this point, we should emphasize that not all investigators employing lesion and electrophysiological techniques have found changes as dramatic as those reported in the experiments we have reviewed. In some studies, behavioral recovery has been found to correlate with the presence of electrophysiological activity that does not appear to be any different from that seen prior to insult.

A good example of this can be found in an investigation conducted by Robert Glassman (1971) on adult cats. Glassman evaluated evoked potentials in the sigmoid gyrus of the cortex in response to peripheral electrical stimulation, taught his cats to reach into a narrow tube to obtain food reward, and then created a series of small, punctate lesions in this cortical gyrus. First, he noted a severe but transient impairment in reaching for food after the lesions. Evoked potentials, recorded the same day in sensorimotor cortex surrounding the damaged areas, were eliminated or greatly depressed. Normal electrical activity gradually reappeared in the critical areas surrounding the lesions, and these events were correlated with the ability of the cats to reach into the tube and again obtain pieces of food. Complete recovery of the reaching response was achieved in a few weeks, this being the time that the gross evoked potentials in the undamaged tissue surrounding the lesion returned to "normal." This is shown in Figure 7.13.

We should also mention a recent experiment from one of our own laboratories in the context of behavioral recovery and normal electrophysiological activity. Finger, Simons, and Posner (1978) made bilateral ablations of the sensorimotor cortex of newborn rats and tested the animals in a series of tactile discriminations following a long postoperative recovery period. Although some of the animals operated on in infancy were unable to learn even the simplest of five tactile discrimination problems, most of the rats eventually completed the test battery, and some even performed within the control group range.

In an attempt to account for this variability in behavior, we recorded from single neurons in the vicinity of the lesions. We found that behavioral performance was correlated with the ability to drive individual cortical neurons with electrical and natural stimulation of the body surface (light touch, tapping, brushing the skin). It was not possible to isolate reactive neurons in rats that did not learn any of the discriminations. By comparison, many responsive neurons were readily found in the best tactile learners and most of these cells had receptive fields in the forepaw and mouth regions.

An analysis of firing properties of the neurons in rats given surgery as infants showed that all neurons still had small receptive fields, short latencies, topographical organization, and contralateral innervation. In brief, the neurons

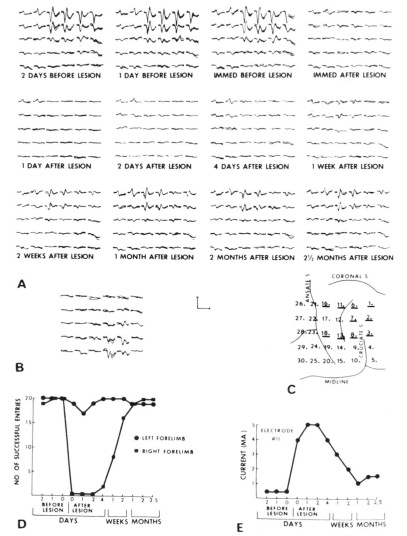

Figure 7.13. *Three measures of deficiency and recovery. (A) Maps of potentials evoked by forelimb stimulation recorded on successive test sessions before and after the lesion was made (positive, upward). Calibrations: 25 msec; 1 mV. (B) Sample map of potentials evoked by hindlimb stimulation before the lesion was made, showing different distribution of responses than that evoked by forelimb stimulation. (C) Exact position of electrodes indicated on tracing of a photograph of the brain, with the points of lesion indicated by underlying. (D) Performance in the food retrieval situation. Left forelimb (●); right forelimb (■). (E) Current required at electrode number 11 to elicit movement. (From Glassman, 1971.)*

did not appear to have any characteristics that distinguished them from the single cells isolated in animals that were given sham operations (skull opening, but no lesions) 1–3 days after birth.

On the basis of these data, it was concluded that tactile learning in the animals with early somatosensory cortical lesions was mediated by spared fragments of a damaged system, rather than by new or unusual connections at the cortical level such as those described by Spear (1979). This contention received additional support when anatomical studies were made of the cortices and thalami of these animals.

Demonstrations of changes in neuronal activity after brain lesions seem especially difficult to understand in the absence of corresponding anatomical data. For example, in one interesting experiment, Stephen Scheff and Dennis Wright (1977) first trained adult male albino rats to make a black versus white visual discrimination for food reward in a T-maze. After doing this, they removed the posterior neocortex from some of the animals in one or two stages (separated by 9 days). About half of the two-stage animals received "retraining" between their operations; the others were left in the home cage.

Scheff and Wright observed that the differently treated groups of rats were all able to relearn the discrimination task, but that only the two-stage group with interoperative training showed a positive saving score on retesting (that is, they took fewer trials to relearn the task than they had taken to learn it in the first place). After all behavioral testing was completed, the experimenters took some animals from each experimental group and after anesthetizing them, mapped cortical evoked potentials to peripheral, visual stimulation in the remaining, intact cortex.

In the serial group that received interoperative retraining, Scheff and Wright found that 70% of the points mapped in cortex contiguous to the area of the lesion (but well outside the visual areas) showed evoked responses. In the animals with single-stage lesions and in the two-stage group that did not receive extra training, evoked responses could only be obtained in 24–39% of the points studied. These authors also noted that the peak-to-peak amplitudes of the gross evoked potentials were significantly greater in the two-stage group given additional training than in the other groups with lesions.

What these evoked potentials may signify remains uncertain, especially since they were so affected by training between the two lesions. Although sprouting might be one explanation for these findings, anatomical confirmation of synaptogenesis was not attempted. Moreover, the events may not have had a time course that would have been suggestive of sprouting, although this is difficult to evaluate because the evoked potentials were only recorded at one point in time— when all behavioral testing had been completed. One possibility that must be entertained, however, is that the evoked potentials in nonvisual areas of the brain represent only a release from inhibition (from the visual cortex), which is in some way catalyzed or affected by visual stimulation or the additional handling that would have taken place during interoperative training.

With regard to the notion of release from inhibition, there is now a considerable body of experimental evidence which seems to show that "latent" synapses do in fact exist in healthy adult animals and that they can become physiologically effective immediately after damage or suppression of other inputs. The switching from one set of inputs to another has been most intensively studied by Patrick Wall and his colleagues at the University College of London (cf. Merrill and Wall, 1978).

In one of his first experiments, he and David Egger (1971) damaged the nucleus gracilis in the medulla of adult rats in order to eliminate the major projection from the hindlimb to the primary somatosensory area of the thalamus (i.e., nucleus ventralis posterolateralis). Following the lesions, Wall and Egger studied the receptive fields of individual neurons in the thalamic area deprived of these projections and compared the receptive field characteristics to those of normal rats. In the normal animals, they found that afferent fibers from the arm are represented in the medial two-thirds of nucleus ventralis posterolateralis (VPL) while the leg occupies the lateral third (Figure 7.14). This fact is demonstrated by gently stimulating these areas of the body and recording the evoked potentials throughout this thalamic nucleus. After lesions of nucleus gracilis, however, forelimb responses were obtained from the hindlimb area (Figure 7.15). That is, following damage to the medullary hindlimb projection, individual neurons in VPL stop responding to stimulation of the hindlimb and instead begin responding only to stimulation of the forelimb!

At first, Wall and Egger thought that the most likely explanation for the orderly expansion of forelimb receptive fields into the hindlimb area was that collateral sprouts had grown from intact projections originating in nucleus cuneatus (the medullary nucleus involved with somatosensory information from the upper part of the body, excluding the face) and had reinnervated the sites left vacant by the damaged axons that had originated from the cells in nucleus gracilis. They based their conclusion upon the fact that the expansion of the receptive fields did not become apparent until a few days had passed after the lesions were made. Wall and Egger also noted that even massive electrical stimulation of the forepaws of intact animals failed to excite the thalamic cells with discrete receptive fields made up of inputs coming from the hindlegs.

A follow-up experiment suggested that sprouting was probably not the underlying mechanism at all. Jonathan Dostrovsky, Julian Millar, and Patrick Wall (1976) first mapped the receptive fields of cells projecting from the body surface to the medulla (gracile and cuneate nuclei) and then carefully identified the (thalamic) locus of the neurons that responded to gentle tactile stimulation of the foot. Neuronal activity from the foot to nucleus gracilis was then blocked for a short period of time by cooling the spinal cord at the lumbar level (L–4). The cool-

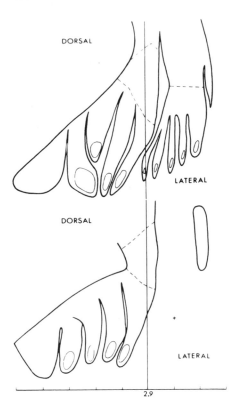

DORSAL

LATERAL

DORSAL

LATERAL

2.9

Figure 7.14. *Transverse map of distribution of receptive fields in the ventral posterior lateral (VPL) nucleus of the thalamus in the rat, 1 day after destruction of nucleus gracilis on one side. The map (above) shows the distribution in the thalamus supplied by the intact dorsal column nuclei with the forelimb representation medial, leg lateral, and body dorsolateral. The* dotted lines *mark the elbow and wrist on arm, and the ankle on leg. The face area is not mapped. The map (below) shows the result of continuing the transverse search plane directly across the midline to the opposite thalamus that is not receiving an input from nucleus gracilis. The arm-hand-finger is similar in both maps. The leg area contained no responding cells in this plane with one exception marked by a* cross. The *horizontal axis marks 200-μm intervals in the mediolateral direction. The* vertical line *marks electrode tracks 2.9 mm from the midline penetrating both left and right thalamic maps. These tracks passed through the lateral arm region in each thalamus and show how similar the two arm regions are. (From* Wall and Egger, 1971. *Reprinted by permission from* Nature, 235, *542–545. Copyright © 1971, Macmillan Journals Limited.)*

ing technique was not only reversible, but it did not have any of the extensive tissue trauma and neural shock associated with it that might be associated with maceration of the roots with a forceps (the technique used by Wall and Egger in their initial study). Under these conditions, the investigators found that most of the cells in the dorsal column nuclei that responded to stimulation of the hind-paw were still capable of ongoing electrical activity, but that hindlimb stimulation was no longer an effective stimulus. As shown in Figure 7.16, when the researchers stimulated other parts of the body in the animals with the cold block, they noticed that some of the cells had acquired new receptive fields (e.g., on the abdomen). Upon removing the cold block, the receptive fields quickly reverted back to the hindlimb, and even intense stimulation of these other body parts was no longer effective.

Because of the rapidity of these changes (a few minutes!), Wall (1977) proposed that there must be "silent synapses" that can carry information from other parts of the body to the medullary hindpaw area. These silent pathways are masked in the normal state by the dominant hindpaw projections. The relatively ineffective synapses are only able to show themselves when the primary connec-

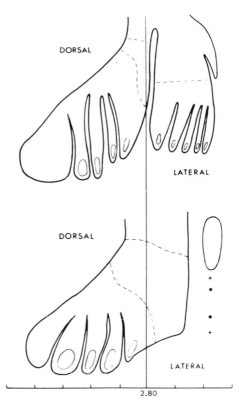

Figure 7.15. *Transverse map of distribution of receptive fields in intact VPL (above) and the map produced by continuing the mapping place across the midline into the opposite VPL studied 7 weeks after destruction of the nucleus gracilis, which projected to this nucleus (below). The* vertical line *marks an electrode track 2.8 mm from the midline, which samples a similar region of the thalamus on the intact side to the vertical line shown in Figure 7.3. The thalamus on the medial side of the line contains a similar map on both the intact and deafferented side. But the region representing the arm, especially the lower arm, has expanded on the operated side to invade a region that responds to leg on the intact side. At the lateral edge of the nucleus, four cells were encountered that responded to body or leg stimulation, but most cells in this region failed to respond to any peripheral stimuli. (From Wall and Egger, 1971. Reprinted by permission from* Nature, *235, 542–545. Copyright © 1971, Macmillan Journals Limited.)*

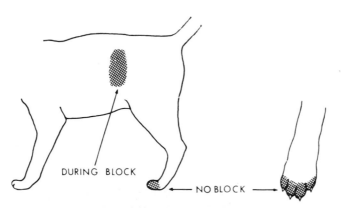

Figure 7.16. *An example of the receptive field of a unit with and without cold block of the cord at L4. During the block the receptive field on the toes was lost and a receptive field on the lateral abdomen appeared. (From Dostrovsky, Millar, and Wall, 1976.)*

tions to the region under study are at least temporarily rendered nonfunctional by blocking the main afferent inputs. Wall believes that this was happening not only in his study with Dostrovsky and Millar with medullary recordings and spinal blockage, but also in the Wall and Egger (1971) investigation in which thalamic recordings were made after the gracile nucleus was damaged.

What are some of the physiological changes that are seen when adult animals are allowed to survive for long periods of time after the dorsal roots are cut to eliminate the hindlimb projection to the central nervous system? Julian Millar, Alan Basbaum, and Patrick Wall (1976) explored this question by first mapping the hindlimb areas of the gracile nucleus of the medulla of the cat. Here the experiments were similar in nature to the work that was just described. Once the somatic map was obtained, the dorsal roots from the hindlimbs were cut. After an 8-month survival period, the cats were reanesthetized and the dorsal column nuclei were again examined electrophysiologically.

In this experiment the most dramatic changes in the receptive field characteristics were the very large expansion of areas subserving the trunk regions, and the accompanying decrease in the somatic representation of the hindlimb. In other words, although neurons in one part of nucleus gracilis only responded to stimulation of the limb and not the trunk in normal cats, the complete reverse proved to be true for cats whose dorsal roots had been cut; that is, these animals had neural units that would only respond to tactile stimulation of the trunk. In addition to this restructuring of the somatic map in response to nerve injury, the investigators observed that a number of the neurons developed double receptive fields that were spatially separated from each other on the animal's body. This was *never* seen in recordings taken from intact cats.

To be sure that the changes seen in the chronic preparations were comparable to those found immediately after surgery, Millar and his co-investigators examined nucleus gracilis 1–12 hours after dorsal root section in another group of cats. For the most part, the changes in the neural response patterns of the cats that had been allowed to survive for long periods of time matched those seen in the same-day preparations. For example, they again found a disappearance of the response to stimulation of the hindleg, and an immediate spread of the trunk area.

Based on these findings, Wall and his associates suggest that anomalous growth, sprouting, shrinkage of neuronal fields, and denervation supersensitivity cannot account for the immediate changes in neural response patterns after the kinds of lesions that they have created. Instead, Wall suggests that when afferents are blocked or damaged, there can be an immediate release of already-present, but latent connections. Nevertheless, as time passes, the altered responses could conceivably become even more efficient as deafferented postsynaptic membranes become supersensitive, or because existing, intact synapses sprout and proliferate over denervated neuronal surfaces.

Insofar as behavior is concerned, one problem that emerges from Wall's work on "latent connections" is that relatively "unmatched" responses seem to be replacing those that were lost. In other words, when neural responses to peripheral stimulation of the foot or toes are replaced by those from the abdomen and when the sensory receptive field of the hindlimb expands after forelimb afferents are lost or blocked, one would be hardpressed to argue for the adaptive significance of stomach replacing leg, or information from the forelimb being replaced by diffuse reactions from a hindlimb. Still, the model of relatively ineffective or latent pathways being unmasked by injury poses interesting and important possibilities for understanding behavior after brain damage and for developing training techniques or physiological manipulations that might "unmask" those silent pathways that could be important in rehabilitation therapy.

To be sure, the spinal cord and the somatosensory pathways provide an excellent model for studying latent synapses, but are there data to indicate that Wall's observations can generalize to other systems? Recent research on kittens that have been raised under monocular deprivation conditions suggests that silent synapses are not confined to the somatosensory system. Here, some experimenters have observed that the cortical receptive fields of an eye deprived of visual stimulation can be dominated by the "good" eye, with no sign of input from the deprived eye until the good eye is removed. In addition, monocular deprivation has been combined with lesions of the central nervous system to unmask these alternative inputs, which are silent under normal conditions.

Looking first at the latter experimental approach, Nancy Berman and Peter Sterling (1976) first deprived cats of visual stimulation in one eye by suturing one eyelid shut when the animals were just 5 days of age (Figure 7.17). After 6–12 months of monocular deprivation, recordings of the responses of individual neurons in the superior colliculus were taken. The deprived eye was opened for these recordings and under these conditions, Berman and Sterling found that most of the units that they encountered in the contralateral superior colliculus were unresponsive to visual stimulation of the deprived eye. Berman and Sterling then made a lesion in the visual cortex, and within an hour, reexamined the same superior colliculus. Now, as can be seen in Figure 7.18, the units responded vigorously to stimulation of the deprived eye and were unresponsive to stimulation from the good eye. As stated by the experimenters:

> The dramatic recovery of the deprived eye following cortical removal cannot result from a sprouting of retinal terminals or some similarly slow process since recovery is essentially complete within 15 minutes. Most probably the recovery depends upon the removal of a cortical inhibitory control over the retinal input [pp. 268–269].

As we pointed out, evidence concerning the presence of latent synapses can also be seen in experiments combining visual deprivation with peripheral lesions. Kratz, Spear, and Smith (1976) sutured one eye of kittens shut until they were at

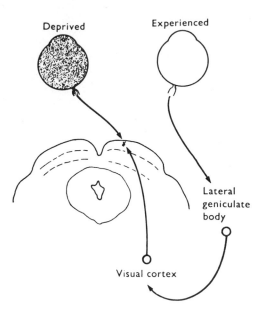

Deprived   Experienced

Lateral
geniculate
body

Visual cortex

Figure 7.17. *Diagram of experimental situation. Left eye, deprived from birth by lid suture, provides direct retinal input to right superior colliculus. Right eye (experienced) provides ipsilateral input to colliculus via geniculo-cortical pathway. In the intact animal most neurones in both colliculus and cortex are activated almost exclusively from the experienced eye. (From Berman and Sterling, 1976.)*

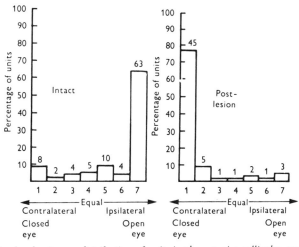

Figure 7.18. *Ocular dominance distribution of units in the superior colliculus contralateral to the deprived eye in five animals before and immediately following removal of visual cortex. Groups 1–7 on the abscissa represent a contralateral to ipsilateral trend in ocular dominance with units in group 1 driven only by the contralateral eye, units in group 4 driven equally by either eye, and units in group 7 driven only by the ipsilateral eye. The numbers above each bar represent the number of units in that group. (From Berman and Sterling, 1976.)*

least 4 months old. Among these animals, they found that only a very small percentage (about 10%) of striate cortex neurons could be driven by stimulation of the deprived eye when it was later opened (in normal cats, about 80% of the cortical cells are binocularly driven). In one group of cats, the experimenters removed the good eye and then recorded immediately from the cortical neurons. In these cats, 29–39% of the cells encountered became immediately responsive to stimulation of the deprived eye. This percentage was comparable to that seen in cats that were examined months after the good eye was eliminated, whereas the deprived eye remained closed. Although the cells driven by the previously deprived eye did have some abnormal characteristics, the data of Kratz and his co-workers show that functional connections remained from the deprived eye to the cortex after selective rearing (monocular deprivation), although these connections could not be seen under normal conditions.

We should also mention some studies that have tried to unmask these silent synapses by pharmacological manipulations. Frank Duffy and his co-workers at the Harvard Medical School (Duffy, Burchfiel, and Snodgrass, 1976; Duffy, Snodgrass, Burchfiel, and Conway, 1976) gave intravenous injections of bicuculline or ammonium acetate to cats that had been monocularly deprived as kittens. Bicuculline is a GABA-receptor blocker, whereas ammonium acetate is an antagonist of synaptic inhibition. Both of these substances produced a sharp but temporary increase in the proportion of neurons that could be activated through stimulation of the previously deprived eye. Furthermore, the previously silent synapses appeared to have more normal properties after drug administration than after removal of the "good" eye.

These data on young cats seem to fit well with Wall's concept of silent synapses. In fact, Merrill and Wall (1978) speculate that silent synapses represent "ghosts of the cell's childhood"; that is, that such connections could be active during very early developmental stages, only to become inhibited or suppressed later on. The visual deprivation experiments strongly suggest that environmental factors can play an important role in determining which connections will become dominant, perhaps as a function of use and disuse. Although the silent connections seem capable of remaining dormant throughout life, the drug and lesion manipulations in the experiments on vision just cited show that under some conditions these connections can be unmasked. We feel that future experiments directed at modifying the functional balance between dominant and suppressed connections may show that certain neuronal systems are even more "plastic" than currently believed—a possibility that should be considered in the light of the fact that the work of Wall and his colleagues was concerned not with neonates, but with sexually mature rats and cats.

The research on latent pathways is really quite new, and there are both practical and theoretical problems that remain to be resolved. Yet, despite some of the limitations that we have discussed, we feel that this area of inquiry represents an important step in trying to develop an understanding of the capacity of the brain to respond to trauma, and how such responses may relate to functional recovery. In the clinic, as we will see later, there is considerable documentation of slow (and sometimes incomplete) recovery from traumatic injury; there is also evidence of relatively rapid recovery (for example, after missile wounds of the head) that would be hard to explain in terms of anomalous growth of new pathways. We can speculate that some recovery of function could well be due to the gradually developing use of already present, but relatively ineffective, pathways and synapses. Indeed, such latent systems may serve the organism by allowing it to develop new tricks or strategies that permit goal attainment. Although morphological changes may be a sufficient condition for functional recovery to occur, it is becoming increasingly clear that it may not be a prerequisite condition. The speed by which some recovery of function occurs (see Chapters 8–10) and the immediate reversibility of impaired neuronal function (Berman and Sterling, 1976; Kratz, Spear, and Smith, 1976) lead us to suspect that alternate neuronal systems may play a very important role.

For practical purposes, the concept of latent synapses deserves more attention since rehabilitation therapy could be directed toward "exposing" and, more effectively, using these previously suppressed pathways. Training, in combination with appropriate pharmacological manipulations (Duffy, Burchfiel, and Snodgrass, 1976), may be one step that can be taken to improve the patient's condition as soon as possible after injury. Such pathways may require immediate activation, lest collateral sprouts suppress them once again. Admittedly, this notion is highly speculative, and much animal research should be attempted before application to the human condition is attempted. Even so, we think that the concept of *latent synapses* should be explored more fully in the context of functional recovery.

In closing this chapter, we want to emphasize again that the electrophysiological changes that follow brain damage are only beginning to be understood. Furthermore, since the *silent synapse* concept appears viable and sprouting does not appear to be limited to neonates, it should only be a matter of time before a wealth of new observations reflecting these events and even more subtle changes are reported with our increasingly sophisticated recording techniques.

References

Baumann, T. P., and Spear, P. D. Role of the lateral suprasylvian visual area in behavioral recovery from effects of visual cortex damage in cats. *Brain Research*, 1977, *138*, 445–468.

Berman, N., and Sterling, P. Cortical suppression of the retino-collicular pathway in the monocularly deprived cat. *Journal of Physiology*, 1976, *255*, 263–273.

Cotman, C. W., Matthews, D. A., Taylor, D., and Lynch, G. S. Synaptic rearrangement in the dentate gyrus: Histochemical evidence of adjustments after lesions in immature and adult rats. *Proceedings of the National Academy of Sciences*, 1973, *70*, 3473–3477.

Dostrovsky, J. O., Millar, J., and Wall, P. D. The immediate shift of afferent drive of dorsal column nucleus cells following deafferentation: A comparison of acute and chronic deafferentation in gracile nucleus and spinal cord. *Experimental Neurology*, 1976, *52*, 480–495.

Duffy, F. H., Burchfiel, J. L., and Snodgrass, S. R. Ammonium acetate reversal of experimental ambylopia. *Paper presented at the Sixth Annual Society for Neuroscience Meetings*, Toronto, Canada, 1976.

Duffy, F. H., Snodgrass, S. R., Burchfiel, J. L., and Conway, J. L. Bicuculline reversal of deprivation ambylopia. *Nature*, 1976, *260*, 256–257.

Finger, S., Simons, D., and Posner, R. Anatomical, physiological and behavioral effects of neonatal sensorimotor cortex ablation in the rat. *Experimental Neurology*, 1978, *60*, 347–373.

Glassman, R. B. Recovery following sensorimotor cortical damage: Evoked potentials, brain stimulation and motor control. *Experimental Neurology*, 1971, *33*, 16–29.

Goldowitz, D., White, W. R., Steward, O., Cotman, C., and Lynch, G. S. Anatomical evidence for a projection from the entorhinal cortex to the contralateral dentate gyrus of the rat. *Experimental Neurology*, 1975, *47*, 433–441.

Guillery, R. W. Experiments to determine whether retinogeniculate axons can form translaminar collateral sprouts in the dorsal lateral geniculate nucleus of the cat. *Journal of Comparative Neurology*, 1972, *144*, 117–130.

Kratz, K. E., Spear, P. D., and Smith, D. C. Postcritical period reversal of effects of monocular deprivation on striate cortex cells in the cat. *Journal of Neurophysiology*, 1976, *39*, 501–511.

Land, P. W., and Lund, R. D. Development of the rat's uncrossed retinotectal pathway and its relation to plasticity studies. *Science*, 1979, *205*, 698–700.

Lund, R. D., and Lund, J. S. Reorganization of the retinotectal pathway in rats after neonatal retinal lesions. *Experimental Neurology*, 1973, *40*, 377–390.

Merrill, E. G., and Wall, P. D. Plasticity of connection in the adult nervous system. In C. W. Cotman (Ed.), *Neuronal plasticity*. New York: Raven Press, 1978, Pp. 97–111.

Millar, J., Basbaum, A. I., and Wall, P. D. Restructuring of the somatotopic map and appearance of abnormal neuronal activity in the gracile nucleus after partial deafferentation. *Experimental Neurology*, 1976, *50*, 658–672.

Murakami, F., Tsukahara, N., and Fujito, Y. Properties of the synaptic transmission of the newly formed corticorubral synapses after lesion of the nucleus interpositus of the cerebellum. *Experimental Brain Research*, 1977, *30*, 245–258.

Nakamura, Y., Mizuno, N., Konishi, A., and Sato, M. Synaptic reorganization of the red nucleus after chronic deafferentation from cerebellorubral fibers: An electron microscope study in the cat. *Brain Research*, 1974, *82*, 298–301.

Ramirez, J. *Behavioral correlates of entorhinal cortex lesions*. Unpublished Master's thesis, Clark University (Worcester, Mass.), 1980.

Scheff, S. W., and Wright, D. C. Behavioral and electrophysiological evidence for cortical reorganization of function with serial lesions of the visual cortex. *Physiological Psychology*, 1977, *5*, 103–107.

Spear, P. D. Behavioral and neurophysiological consequences of visual cortex damage: Mechanisms of recovery. In J. M. Sprague and A. N. Epstein (Eds.), *Progress in psychobiology and physiological psychology (Vol. 8)*. New York: Academic Press, 1979, Pp, 45–83.

Spear, P. D., and Baumann, T. P. Receptive field characteristics of single neurons in lateral suprasylvian visual area of the cat. *Journal of Neurophysiology*, 1975, *38*, 1403–1420.

Spear, P. D., and Braun, J. J. Pattern discrimination following removal of visual neocortex in the cat. *Experimental Neurology*, 1969, *25*, 331–348.

Steward, O., Cotman, C. W., and Lynch, G. S. Re-establishment of electrophysiologically functional entorhinal cortical input to the dentate gyrus deafferented by ipsilateral entorhinal lesions: Innervation by the contralateral entorhinal cortex. *Experimental Brain Research*, 1973, *18*, 396–414.

Steward, O., Cotman, C. W., and Lynch, G. S. Growth of a new fiber projection in the brain of adult rats: Re-innervation of the dentate gyrus by the contralateral entorhinal cortex following ipsilateral entorhinal lesions. *Experimental Brain Research*, 1974, *20*, 45–66.

Steward, O., and Vinsant, S. Identification of the cells of origin of a central pathway which sprouts following lesions in mature rats. *Brain Research*, 1978, *147*, 223–243.

Tsukahara, N. Synaptic plasticity in red nucleus. In C. Cotman (Ed.), *Neuronal plasticity*, New York: Raven Press, 1978, Pp. 113–130.

Wall, P. D. The presence of ineffective synapses and the circumstances which unmask them. *Philosophical Transactions of the Royal Society of London (Series B)*, 1977, *278*, 361–372.

Wall, P. D., and Egger, M. D. Formation of new connections in adult rat brains after partial deafferentation. *Nature*, 1971, *232*, 542–545.

Wood, C. C., Spear, P. D., and Braun, J. J. Effects of sequential lesions of suprasylvian gyri and visual cortex on pattern discrimination in the cat. *Brain Research*, 1974, *66*, 443–466.

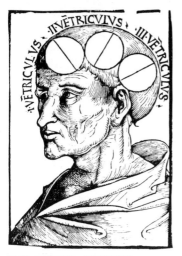

Behavioral Recovery and Development

Unilateral cerebral lesions incurred before age two do not implicate subsequent language development. After age three left hemisphere lesions in the fronto-parietal area cause the patient to lose language temporarily, but soon it is fully reinstated. This impunity last until approximately age 10 to 14 years. At this time and thereafter aphasic symptoms rapidly become more frequent and in about 30% of all cases are irreversible [Lenneberg, 1968, p. 166].

CHAPTER EIGHT

Hans-Lukas Teuber, a well-known neuropsychologist, once stated, "If I'm going to have brain damage, I'd best have it early rather than late in life." This somewhat glib remark reflects the general notion that there is more adaptability to serious head injury in the developing nervous system than there is at maturity.

In the preceding chapters, we noted that anomalous neuronal growth after injury to the central nervous system is more likely to occur in very young subjects. Similarly, some physiological changes that are seen in response to lesions or restricting the sensory environment ("environmental surgery") are more likely to appear when these manipulations take place early in life. On the basis of what we know about "plasticity" from anatomical and physiological studies, we might suppose that the extent of behavioral recovery after central nervous system injury would also depend upon the age of the subject at the time of trauma. Indeed, well before reactive synaptogenesis and silent synapses were even considered, there were data to suggest that early lesions of the brain had less severe effects than comparable lesions made later in life.

Why should localized injury to the brain have different consequences for young, mature, or aged subjects? This is an important question because studying the problem might reveal principles of neuronal and functional organization that could eventually be manipulated to *facilitate* recovery in brain-damaged patients.

Although we have already seen how some factors *intrinsic* to the nervous system (e.g., sprouting, rerouting of fibers) can be important for recovery, we must also consider how experience and training affect the organism's response to early brain injury. In this chapter we will emphasize the *biobehavioral* consequences of early brain damage and describe some of the variables that have been shown to influence behavior following early central nervous system lesions.

Some of the most influential investigations of recovery of function in young animals were performed by Margaret Kennard (1936, 1938, 1940, 1942) who worked at the Yale University School of Medicine. As shown in Figures 8.1 and 8.2, she removed the motor cortex (Brodmann areas 4 and 6) in monkeys and apes of various ages, tested the animals throughout their development, and found that the monkey's ability to use the limbs contralateral to the lesion was related to a number of factors, one of which was age at the time of the operation. She noted that the earlier the lesion, the greater the behavioral sparing. Although there was considerable recovery, Kennard observed that the monkeys with early lesions could still be differentiated from unoperated, age-matched subjects. According to Kennard, the brain-damaged subjects developed some spasticity as they grew older, and they retained mild deficits in purposeful activities such as walking and grasping objects.

Despite these handicaps the animals with early lesions were much less impaired than monkeys given lesions after the first few months of life. The animals with early lesions could walk, climb, feed themselves and perform movements of prehension; behaviors that were *not* seen in monkeys given lesions at an older age. This finding was attributed to a greater capacity for "reorganization" in the developing nervous system. After further research, Kennard concluded that the parietal lobe and the frontal association cortex may be taking over lost motor cortex functions (see Chapter 15, on "vicariation"). However this idea may be viewed today, Kennard's work is extremely important because she focused attention on the fact that the effects of trauma may not be the same for young and mature organisms. To some this implied that brain function must be considered from a developmental perspective in which different stages of organization must *interact* with environmental influences (sensory restriction, trauma, nutritional

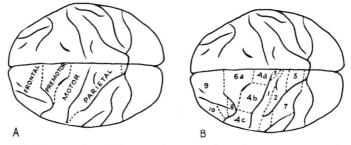

Figure 8.1. *(A) Diagram of cerebral cortex of Macaca mulatta showing approximate boundaries of the areas extirpated: the "motor" regions, that is, motor and premotor areas; and the regions not primarily concerned with motor function, that is, the frontal and parietal areas. (B) Map of the cerebral cortex of Macaca mulatta. (Modification of Brodmann's numerical classification.) (From Kennard, 1938.)*

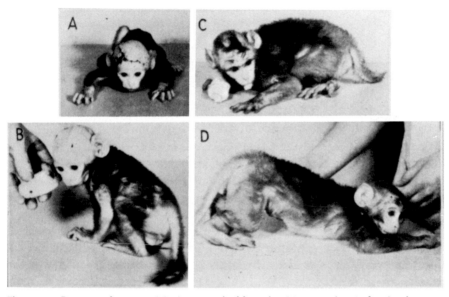

Figure 8.2. *Recovery of motor activity in a 3-week-old monkey* (Macaca mulatta) *after simultaneous bilateral ablation of area 4 and 6. (A) and (B), third postoperative day; (C) and (D), 11 months later. (From Kennard, M. A. Cortical reorganization of motor function: Studies on a series of monkeys of various ages from infancy to maturity.* Archives of Neurology and Psychiatry *1942, 137, 429–430. Copyright 1942, American Medical Association.)*

status, to name a few) to determine the functions of an area; a view, we might add, which is once again becoming acceptable.

Although she had considerable impact on the field of developmental neuropsychology, Kennard's reports were not the first in which someone noted that early lesions can be less deleterious than those occurring later in life. Kennard (1938) herself stated that:

> It has long been recognized that cortical lesions made on young animals have less effect on behavior than have similar lesions in adults of the same species. In 1866, Vulpian, discussing hemidecortication, advised the use of young animals since "they stand the procedure better . . . than do adult animals [p. 677]." In 1875 Soltmann found that puppies deprived of one hemisphere develop a highly coordinated motor performance with little difference between movements of the two sides. And in man it has been consistently observed following birth injuries, or other congenital deficiency of brain tissue, that the degree of motor paresis is often small when compared with the effects of a similar lesion in adults [pp. 490–491].

Kennard's studies, however, stimulated many new attempts to find age-related recovery effects with other lesions and behavioral tasks. For example, Tsang (1937), one of Karl Lashley's students, found that rats that were hemidecorticated at 22 days of age could solve complex mazes faster than adults given the same extent of damage. In fact, Tsang noted that rats operated on in infancy require removal of 50% of the cortex to produce the same extent of impairment seen in brain-damaged adults after only 7.4% of their cortex is ablated. Thirty years later, Tucker and Kling (1967) reported that bilateral lesions of the dorsolateral frontal granular cortex did not severely impair delayed response performance in monkeys operated on in infancy, although the same lesions were severely debilitating to adult animals. Their delayed response task, which has been extensively used to assess the integrity of the frontal lobes in primates, involves putting food in one of two containers while the animal watches, then lowering an opaque screen between the animal and the cups, and, after 4–40 seconds, lifting the screen and allowing the animal to choose between the cups for a food reward. Normal monkeys can remember where the food was last placed, whereas those with frontal cortex lesions usually have great difficulty, except when damage occurs very early in life (see also Kling and Tucker, 1968).

In a related experiment, Bryan Kolb and Arthur Nonneman (1978) have provided data showing that when adult rats are given bilateral lesions of the medial frontal cortex, they cannot easily learn delayed response, spatial reversal, or active avoidance tasks. When the same lesions are created in rats that are only 2, 5, or 9 days of age, they can perform as well on these problems as unoperated control animals. With lesions made at 35–40 days of age, the capacity for behavioral sparing without special training or handling is lost.

Kolb and Nonneman observed that the lesions made in neonatal subjects were much larger than those made in juveniles or adults. Yet, histological analyses of the brains revealed no evidence of retrograde degeneration in the dorsomedial thalamic nucleus of rats operated on in infancy, as long as their lesions did not damage the caudate-putamen complex. Kolb and Nonneman speculated that the dramatic sparing of function following early, but not later, lesions could somehow result from the growth of "sustaining collateral" fibers from the thalamus to intact cortical or caudate areas, a hypothesis similar to that of Patricia Goldman, which we discussed in Chapter 4.

In addition to research on motor and association areas, sparing effects have also been found on relatively simple sensory discrimination tasks. In one case, Benjamin and Thompson (1959) ablated the somatosensory cortex bilaterally in a single operation in kittens and in adult cats. The kittens given surgery on postnatal Day 6 performed very well on a series of rough–smooth discriminations, whereas mature cats given the same lesions failed to master even the easiest problems in the series. But, when required to distinguish between two surfaces differing in degree of roughness, the kittens were as severely impaired as the cats operated on at maturity.

With respect to performance of a task depending upon auditory cues, cats can learn a tonal duration discrimination more rapidly when auditory cortex lesions are made early in life than at maturity (Sharlock, Tucker, and Strominger, 1963). This is shown in Table 8.1 and Figure 8.3.

TABLE 8.1

Trials to Criterion for Cats Learning a Duration Discrimination[a]

Infant-operated		Controls		Adult-operated		Controls	
Cat	Trials	Cat	Trials	Cat	Trials	Cat	Trials
3A[b]	175	3B	120	2A[c]	140	2B	195
11A	125	11B	95	4[c]	160	7	275
12A	160	12B	150	6[c]	170	16	230
35A[b]	140	35B	115	54A[d]	>500	38	150
37A[b]	90	37B	120	57[d]	>500	54B	185
47A	130	47B	110	59[d]	>500		
48A	145	48B	120	60[d]	>500		
49A[b]	220	49B	—[e]				
72A	100	72B	175				
Median	140		120				195

[a] From Sharlock, Tucker, and Strominger, 1963 (*Copyright 1963 by the American Association for the Advancement of Science*).
[b] Lesion large, but not reaching rhinal fissure.
[c] Small lesion confined essentially to AI, AII, and Ep.
[d] Animal failed to reach criterion in over 500 trials.
[e] Died.

Other examples of exceptionally good performance from animals operated on in infancy can be seen in simple sensory discriminations and on higher order perceptual learning tasks. Some of the data can be found in the reports of Akert, Orth, Harlow, and Schiltz (1960); Harlow, Blumquist, Thompson, Schiltz, and Harlow, (1968); Kling (1962, 1965); and Wetzel, Thompson, Horel, and Meyer (1965). Frank Beach (1938), among others, has also shown comparable effects on largely unlearned tasks, such as nest building by pregnant female rats.

We should emphasize that the "Kennard principle" is not restricted to laboratory animals. It can also be seen in humans, especially with respect to the preservation of verbal abilities after damage to the left, or "dominant," cerebral hemisphere. For the most part, adults with left hemisphere injuries develop aphasias of varying severity, according to the extent and locus of the damage. In only a small percentage of the adult population is speech represented on the right

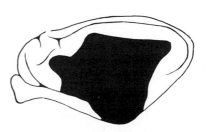

Figure 8.3. *Schematic representation of the lateral cortical surface of the cat brain showing the intended size and location of the lesion. (From Sharlock, Tucker, and Strominger, 1963. Copyright 1963 by the American Association for the Advancement of Science.)*

side, or equally on both sides of the brain (Milner, Branch, and Rasmussen, 1966). In contrast to the language disorders typically displayed by adults with left hemisphere lesions, children with early lesions of the same areas usually develop relatively normal speech and the ability to understand spoken language. This sparing of function is maximal when a child is less than 2 years of age at the time of insult; the capacity for recovery is diminished if injury occurs when a child is older. By the early teens, the adult pattern of language disorders is usually seen, although some symptoms may be less severe.

To account for the difference in linguistic capabilities between patients with early and later injuries of the brain, Brenda Milner (1974), of the Montreal Neurological Institute, has suggested that both hemispheres can mediate language early in life, although probably not to the same extent. As development progresses, the left hemisphere would normally come to inhibit the language mechanisms of the right hemisphere. Hypothetically, this pattern of events is altered when lesions are sustained on the left side of the brain early in life, and the result is that the "disinhibited" right hemisphere takes charge of mediating language functions.

Some studies in which the right hemisphere is rendered nonfunctional by drugs (i.e., sodium amytal injected into the right carotid artery) are supportive of the idea that the right hemisphere mediates language functions when the left hemisphere is damaged in children. There are also data that show that damage to the right side of the brain may have a greater chance of causing *temporary* aphasia in children than in older people (see Hécaen and Albert, 1978, p. 82). Nevertheless, there does seem to be a price extracted for the restitution that children display after left hemispheric lesions. Milner has noted that cognitive functions of both the left and the right hemisphere are generally depressed in these patients (see also Penfield and Roberts, 1959). Milner (1974) postulates that the blunting of verbal and nonverbal IQ scores is due to the "crowding" of too many functions into the intact side of the brain.

One criticism that could be raised concerning the studies showing differences in recovery from left hemispheric damage in children and adults is that the lesions in the two cases are often not very comparable. That is, the children studied in many of these studies have diffuse pathology, seizure activity, or traumatic damage to the brain as a result of falls and related accidents. In contrast, many of the adult patients are stroke victims with relatively focal damage. Still, the fact is that even after complete left hemispherectomy in early life, the capacity for normal language may remain intact. As an example, let us consider a particularly striking case, which was reported by Aaron Smith (1977) of the University of Michigan:

> While preparing this report, I received a call on January 10. The caller was a 29-year-old man who had a *left hemispherectomy* in 1953 at the age of 5 ½ years. Since the Smith and Sugar (1975) report of 15 and 21 year follow-up studies of this patient, he

had been continuing successfully as a full-time industrial executive while completing studies for a college degree, which he expects this June. He said that because of his good grades, he had been invited to continue graduate studies in sociology with a promise of an assistantship appointment. However, he had selected another area and asked if I would be willing to write a recommendation for his graduate training in the new area. "What is the new area?" I inquired. "Library science" [p. 4].

Although it is difficult to argue a point convincingly on the basis of an individual case, other features of this patient's profile should be noted in terms of the degree of recovery achieved. Specifically, although his left hemisphere was ablated, this young man exhibited a WAIS verbal IQ score of 126 and an above-average WAIS performance IQ score 21 years after his operation. On other tests of left and right hemispheric integrity, such as the Raven Coloured Matrices and the Peabody Picture Vocabulary Test, the patient attained scores that were well in excess of the mean found among populations of individuals with both hemispheres intact.

Smith (1976, 1977) stresses that this case, while unusual in terms of the extent of the recovery displayed, is illustrative of how the effects of hemispherectomy differ in children and adults. Adults with left or right hemispherectomies show marked discrepancies between language (left hemisphere) and visuospatial (right hemisphere) skills, whereas in his 16 cases of right hemispherectomy and 24 cases of left hemispherectomy, no glaring, systematic differences or imbalances in language and other cognitive or spatial abilities occurred when surgery was performed early in life.

Findings such as these have led some scientists to conclude that the brain is more "equipotential" early in development than it is at maturity. If its functions are not yet focally localized, neuronal redundancy might be the rule rather than the exception—at least early in life. Remember our earlier discussion of Land and Lund's (1979) finding that early lesions in the visual system *prevent* the "shrinking back" of excess dendritic spines and terminals (Chapter 5). In the neonate, then, the same topographic extent of a lesion may destroy *less* functional neural tissue than the same damage in an adult, and this might account for at least some behavioral sparing.

We can also speculate that very early lesions might permit afferents deprived of their normal target zones to be redirected into areas functionally or anatomically related to the damaged zone (no one really understands what directs differentiating neurons to their appropriate destinations in any case). If the anomalous growth competes successfully for synaptic space, the organism might be able to perform passably, albeit with less efficiency. Moreover, new tricks or new strategies may be developed using alternative pathways and cerebral areas. Even though the new response patterns may not be perfect, they could permit the brain-damaged subject to achieve at least some degree of adaptation to the environment.

Although physiologically based theories are interesting and seem to be receiving more and more adherents, explanations like those based on changes in strategies for approaching a problem should not be overlooked when attempting to account for sparing after early brain damage. At the purely phenomenological level of analysis, it may be that the organism with brain damage early in life simply has more time to learn new habits to cope with its injury and at the same time is less impaired because it does not have to ''unlearn'' strategies of behavior that are no longer adaptive or useful (Finger, Simons, and Posner, 1978). As investigators develop more sophisticated methodologies for examining the effects of brain lesions, it should be possible to distinguish among the various possible explanations for early sparing and recovery, at least in some selected cases.

It is interesting to note that the highly enthusiastic statements that were made during the 1940s and 1950s about the generality of infant recovery effects rarely appear today in unqualified form. One reason for the change in attitude is that over the last few years, some investigators (see Johnson and Almli, 1978) have been unable to find sparing as dramatic as that described by Kennard (1936, 1938, 1940, 1942), Benjamin and Thompson (1959), or Tucker and Kling (1967). Moreover, some early experiments have been criticized for not having two needed control groups—one being animals given lesions as adults and a subsequent recovery period equal to that of the subjects given lesions as neonates. The other important control is to have older animals with brain damage that are tested at the same age as those given the neonatal lesions (see Finger, Simons, and Posner, 1978). More often than not, the recovery periods given to the two brain-damaged groups are not equal.

Histological verification of the early lesions has also been a subject of criticism. Lesion size and configuration of the brain can be markedly distorted after cortical lesions in very young animals (Finger, Simons, and Posner, 1978; Hicks and D'Amato, 1970; Isaacson and Nonneman, 1972; Isaacson, Nonneman, and Schmaltz, 1968; Nonneman, 1970), making subsequent lesion assessment difficult (see Figure 8.4). For example, lesions of the somatosensory cortex and hippocampus ''fill in'' when they are made in infancy, as the brain grows and expands, whereas such ablations in adults typically retain the same configurations months or years after the onset of damage (Isaacson, Nonneman, and Schmaltz, 1968). It is possible that satisfactory performance by animals with early lesions relative to animals operated on in adulthood could also be due to unintentionally spared fragments of target tissue in the younger group that may escape detection with limited or imprecise histological analyses (Doty, 1961, 1971; Finger, Simons, and Posner, 1978; Frommer, 1978).

There is also the possibility that the data from some of the earlier studies on recovery from early lesions were interpreted a bit too optimistically because behavioral testing for deficits was too crude or limited in scope. In fact, *any* research on recovery can be attacked on the grounds that the tests used are not sensitive enough to find deficits. We will address this possibility in a later chapter because

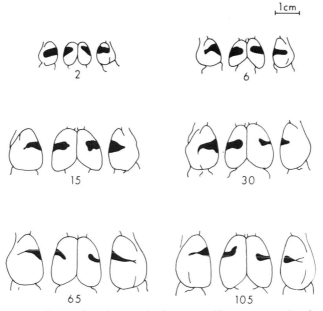

Figure 8.4. *Drawings showing how the superficial neocortical lesions appeared to change as a function of age at the time of sacrifice. These drawings were based on a sample of animals from the population that later was tested on the tactile battery. (From Finger, Simons, and Posner, 1978.)*

the issue does have a certain merit, although such critics sometimes ignore what the tests *do* show. Here, let us just say that some investigators have felt strongly about the problem and have developed their research and theories to come to grips with it by assessing behavior after brain injury for long periods of time and on a variety of different tests.

Robert Isaacson and his students have been particularly critical of the "Kennard principle" because they feel that animals given early lesions and tested in later life are indeed different than "normal" cage-mates, even though they may show some similarities of behavior at first glance. For example, in one series of experiments, Isaacson, Nonneman, and Schmaltz damaged the hippocampi in cats at the time of birth or at later periods of life (6 weeks of age to adulthood) and began behavioral testing on a number of learning tasks when the animals with neonatal lesions were about 1 year of age. For some problems, destruction of the hippocampus in the neonate resulted in less debilitation than when damage was inflicted later in life. This was true on an operant conditioning task in which the cats had to wait for up to 20 seconds between bar presses in order to get rewarded with food. It also was true for a discrimination-reversal task, in which the animals had to give up a previously rewarded response to a stimulus in order to attend to the unrewarded one. In contrast, regardless of when the lesions were done, the brain-damaged cats were very much impaired on passive avoidance (withholding a response) with electrical shock as a punishment for responding. Most importantly, the cats with early lesions developed different patterns of behavior in problem solving than did cats with lesions inflicted later on. In the authors' terms, some tasks were "compensable" after early brain damage and some were not, but the neuronal substrates for these differences are not yet known.

Other researchers have also described recent experiments in which residual deficits following early brain damage were noted (see Johnson and Almli, 1978). Patricia Goldman and Enger Rosvold (1972) studied the effects of large caudate nucleus lesions on delayed alternation performance in monkeys and found no sparing of function after the early lesions. The research of David Johnson (1972) on avoidance responding and social behavior after neonatal lesions of the septum in rats and the experiments of Almli and Golden (1976) on eating and drinking behaviors after early lateral hypothalamic damage in rats also demonstrate a degree of restitution that was far less than expected, with young and old operated animals responding in essentially the same way on most measures.

The seemingly contradictory data characterizing the work on early versus later brain lesions is indicative of the complexity of the perinatal lesion effects. Quite clearly, the consequences of any nervous system injury will result from the interaction of anatomical, environmental, organismic, and task-demand variables. As a result of this complex interplay of many factors, recovery might only be seen under one set of conditions and not another. It might be pointed out that behavioral recovery has been demonstrated more convincingly after cortical rather than subcortical lesions. Other variables that are now receiving attention from researchers interested in early versus later lesions are the characteristics of the task used for behavioral evaluation (Nonneman and Isaacson, 1973), the degree of maturation of the target region and functionally related areas at the time of surgery (Goldman, 1974), the length of the postoperative recovery period (Brunner and Altman, 1974), and the locus and extent of target tissue spared by the lesions (Finger, Simons, and Posner, 1978; Frommer, 1978).

Recently some researchers have claimed that some of the more dramatic instances of sparing after early lesions may diminish partially or completely with long postoperative recovery periods (e.g., Almli, Golden, and McMullan, 1976; Goldman, 1974; Hicks and D'Amato, 1970, 1975). One explanation for the observation that brain-damaged subjects seem to "grow into" deficits as they mature is that the behavioral deficits may appear only at the time when a damaged region would normally begin to mediate the function under study; sometimes months or years after birth. Nevertheless, there are also data showing the opposite; some deficits seen immediately after brain damage recede as the subjects grow older.

Both of these time-dependent changes can be seen in the experiments of Patricia Goldman and her co-workers (cf. Goldman, 1974). They found that ablation of the dorsolateral frontal cortex in neonatal monkeys did not affect performance on a delayed response task when the animals were tested as juveniles (1 year of age). As the monkeys grew older they were retested on the same tasks and severe deficits emerged by the time the monkeys were 2 years of age. By comparison, removal of the orbital prefrontal region in baby monkeys caused severe impairments on a delayed alternation task when the animals were tested at about 1 year of age. By the time the animals were 2 years old, however, this deficit had disappeared. The monkeys then "grow into" or "grow out of" their impairments, depending upon the locus of damage and the time of testing.

Similar phenomena also have been observed in studies with brain damaged children (Teuber and Rudel, 1962), as can be seen in Figure 8.5. The ability to signify (without visual or auditory cues) when a tilted chair is in an upright position may be severely impaired before, but not after, age 11, whereas the capacity to localize the source of a sound under conditions of body tilt may deteriorate at roughly the same age. These effects have been interpreted in terms of structures becoming "committed" to functions as they mature (for example, the dorsolateral frontal cortex may not reach maturity until 2 years after birth in monkeys) and the capacity of other (phylogenetically lower) centers to mediate these functions prior to the time that the damaged structure is "ready" to assume its functions.

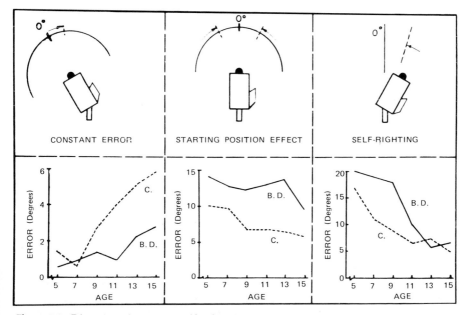

Figure 8.5. *Diagrammatic summary of localization experiments in normal subjects (C) and brain-damaged subjects (B.D.). (From Teuber and Rudel, 1962.)*

Eric Lenneberg (1968) provides an interesting and rather dramatic example of this concept in describing the motor disturbances that occur after cortical lesions in human infants. These lesions (especially those of the parietal lobes) retard the growth of the long bones of the contralateral limbs. What is particularly noteworthy is that damage to the parietal area causes hemiplegia in adults, but when the lesion occurs in infancy there "is no measurable effect whatsoever for at least the first three months—*often much longer.* All four extremities move well and symmetrically at first, and growth is as yet entirely unaffected [pp. 162–163]." Up until about 3 months of age, motor control and growth of the musculature is apparently under the control of brain-stem and thalamic structures. Only when cortical centers begin to exert an influence on behavior of the normal infant do the abnormal signs in the brain-damaged patient begin to emerge, and they are not due to disuse.

At first, the clinical signs are barely noticeable but they grow worse and worse as the child begins to walk. Not only is there stunted bone growth on the opposite side of the body, but signs of spasticity and abnormal reflexes also emerge. As stated by Lenneberg (1968), "One may say that the child with a perinatal cerebral injury only gradually 'grows into his symptoms', and that both lesions and symptoms have their own ramified consequences, often affecting distant structures years after the primary injury [p. 165]."

At this point we might do well to emphasize that living organisms are always in a state of change. Whereas this may be most obvious during early development, even after maturity nothing is really stable. Later in life the changes may be slower and some may tend more toward dissolution rather than elaboration and new growth. Yet, under the appropriate conditions, we can observe anomalous, but nonetheless dynamic, growth in mature and even aged subjects (Buell and Coleman, 1979). Indeed, there is now some evidence that can be taken to indicate that neurogenesis can continue to occur throughout adulthood in rats. Specifically, Michael Kaplan and James Hinds (1977) injected sexually mature (90-day-old) rats with radioactive thymidine because this substance is incorporated into DNA only during cell division and formation. Thirty days later, the animals were killed and their brains examined by electron and light microscopes for uptake of the labeled thymidine into neurons and glia. The analysis showed that there was heavy labeling of neurons in the hippocampus, indicative of cell division and new growth. As stated by these authors, "These results indicate that the old concept that the adult mammalian brain is largely static is no longer tenable [p. 1094]."

Even though neurogenesis in adult humans has not yet been proven, we cannot overlook the fact that dynamic changes in brain-behavior relationships occur throughout the life span and that plasticity, for better or worse, can be manifested long after infancy is over. One indication of this comes from data that show that age-lesion interaction effects can in fact be found with different groups of human subjects that experience brain damage as young adults. Teuber (1975), in his long-term follow-up of Korean War soldiers, observed this on tests of speech, motor functioning, visual field integrity, and somesthesis. In his cases, the greatest percentage of soldiers showing improvement were in the 17–20-year-old range when injured, and the smallest percentage of improved cases belonged to those soldiers who were 26 years of age or older when hit. Soldiers aged 21–25 at the time of trauma constituted an intermediate position. Teuber's observations, presented diagramatically in Figures 8.6 and 8.7, show that the age variable does not become an insignificant factor after the first few years of life.

Another intriguing finding demonstrating the need for a life-span developmental approach to the study of brain function comes from an experiment conducted by one of the present authors a few years ago (Stein and Firl, 1976). In this study very old rats (almost 2 years of age) received bilateral lesions of the frontal cortex. The animals were then tested on a delayed spatial alternation task (go left, go right, go left, etc.) and an active avoidance task. Their scores were compared to rats without ablations and to young, but sexually mature animals with comparable lesions or sham operations.

The surprising finding among the animals with one-stage bilateral lesions was that the aged rats with brain damage learned the spatial alternation task in about the same amount of time that the aged, nonoperated animals needed. Both aged

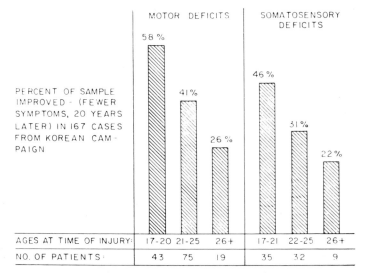

Figure 8.6. *Estimated improvement from initial examination (within days, up to 1 week of injury) and follow-up examination (20 years later) for some body regions (extremities, sides of face) for which symptoms were recorded (reflex changes, paralysis, weakness, motor system); noted sensory losses for somatosensory system. Note advantage of groups with lower age at time of wounding. (From Teuber, 1975.)*

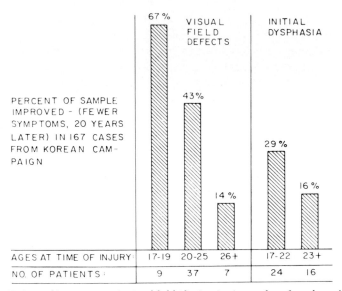

Figure 8.7. *Estimated improvement in visual field (diminution in number of quadrants known to be affected), and in symptoms interpreted as dysphasia, based on comparison of initial reports (up to one week after wounding) and examinations on 20-year follow-up. (From Teuber, 1975.)*

groups were slow in comparison to young normal rats. In contrast, one-stage bilateral removal of the same tissue in the younger group led to severe impairments.

Histological analyses revealed that the frontal cortex lesions sustained by the rats in the different age groups were of comparable size. Stein and Firl then counted the number of intact neurons remaining in the dorsomedial nucleus of the thalamus (whose cells project to the frontal cortex) to determine whether lesions or aging would influence the loss of cells in this region of the brain. As shown in Figure 8.8, they found that the young, unoperated control rats had almost six times the number of intact neurons in the dorsomedial nucleus of the thalamus as did the aged animals; in fact, no differences in the number of neurons were found between old operated and old intact rats. An examination of frontal cortical tissue in the old, unoperated rats also revealed a marked reduction in the number of normal cells.

The behavioral and histological results of this study led Stein and Firl to speculate that the ''functions'' of the frontal cortex may have changed with advancing age and neuronal loss. The reduction of neurons in the thalamus and frontal cortex of nonoperated, aged rats could be an indication that the tissue removed by surgery had been ''functionally dead'' for some time. If this theory is correct, it is hardly surprising that frontal cortex ablation in very old rats appears

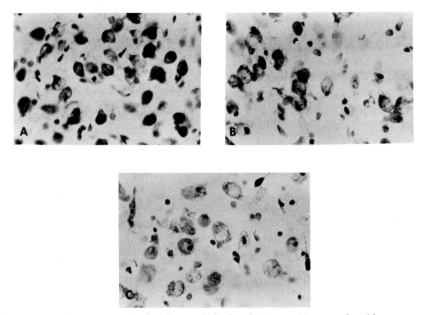

Figure 8.8. *Photomicrographs of nucleus medialis dorsalis (× 175.2) in a 180-day-old nonoperated rat (A), a 575-day-old nonoperated rat (B), and a 620-day-old rat with frontal cortex ablated (C). Note the paucity of Nissl substance, central chromatolysis, poor definitions of limiting membranes, and presence of glial cells in B and C. (From Stein and Firl, 1976.)*

to have different behavioral consequences than identical trauma inflicted earlier in life.

It is interesting to note that Stein and Firl conducted their study without knowing that Richie Russell, a British neurologist, had been thinking along parallel lines when considering certain behavioral differences between children and adults with frontal lobe damage. As pointed out by Teuber and Rudel (1962), Russell (1959) earlier raised the possibility that the frontal lobes may carry on some essential function in children that is no longer critical in adults or that can be mediated by another structure as the developmental process continues. Such an idea leads directly to the hypothesis that under some conditions lesions of the frontal areas may be more deleterious earlier in life than later on. The Stein and Firl experiment, of course, can be viewed as support for this position.

In summary, the fact that some experimenters have demonstrated more complete recovery in young brain-damaged subjects than in subjects with lesions sustained later in life, whereas others present no evidence for better recovery early in life, may be taken to suggest that infant sparing effects cannot be considered either a "myth" (Isaacson, 1975) or a principle. Rather, the truth probably lies somewhere between these two positions. In any case, the important question now becomes: How do we account for the greater recovery or sparing that is often observed in young subjects?

At least two related lines of reasoning may provide an answer to this question. First, the immature brain, being in a state of flux and differentiation, may be less specifically organized and/or more capable of injury-induced growth and reorganization necessary for recovery. If the visual system can be considered as a model, there is good evidence for greater physiological plasticity during certain critical periods of development (e.g., Chow and Stewart, 1972). In Chapter 5 we have seen how events such as anomalous sprouting and failure of axons to retract have been correlated with recovery of function in organisms receiving lesions early in life.

Second, we must consider the possibility that subjects with early brain damage are simply better able to utilize fragments of neural tissue that have been spared by the lesions, or that they have an easier time shifting to new behavioral strategies after their lesions than do organisms that suffer trauma later in life (see Finger, Simons, and Posner, 1978). Even if this should be the case, there remains the critical question as to whether this capacity reflects an age-dependent difference in the anatomical and physiological events that follow brain lesions or whether it represents age-related differences in behavior that might be expected in the absence of brain damage. Could it be, for example, that young organisms are more prone to sample from many different cues in the environment, whether or not they are brain damaged? Do they simply learn to use spared fragments faster than adult animals because they do not have to overcome previous learning sets and well-entrenched habits regarding the way receptors should be utilized?

We will look more carefully at these and related theoretical issues in later chapters. Now it is important to show that striking recovery after brain damage can also be seen in adult organisms.

References

Akert, K., Orth, O. S., Harlow, H. F., and Schiltz, F. Learned behavior of rhesus monkeys following neonatal bilateral prefrontal lobotomy. *Science,* 1960, *132,* 1944–1945.

Almli, C. R., and Golden, G. T. Preweanling rats: Recovery from lateral hypothalamic damage. *Journal of Comparative and Physiological Psychology,* 1976, *90,* 1063–1074.

Almli, C. R., Golden, G. T., and McMullan, N. T. Ontogeny of drinking behavior of preweanling rats with lateral preoptic damage. *Brain Research Bulletin,* 1976, *1,* 437–442.

Beach, F. A. The neural basis of behavior: II. Relative effects of partial decortication in adulthood and infancy upon maternal behavior in the primiparous rat. *Journal of Genetic Psychology,* 1938, *53,* 109–148.

Benjamin, R. M., and Thompson, R. F. Differential effects of cortical lesions in infant and adult cats on roughness discrimination. *Experimental Neurology,* 1959, *1,* 305–321.

Brunner, R. L., and Altman, J. The effects of interference with the maturation of the cerebellum and hippocampus on the development of adult behavior. In D. G. Stein, J. J. Rosen, and N. Butters (Eds.), *Plasticity and recovery of function in the central nervous system*. New York: Academic Press, 1974, Pp. 129–148.

Buell, S. J., and Coleman, P. D. Dendritic growth in aged human brain and failure of growth in senile dementia. *Science*, 1979, *206*, 854–856.

Chow, K. L., and Stewart, D. L. Reversal of structural and functional effects of long-term visual deprivation in cats. *Experimental Neurology*, 1972, *34*, 409–433.

Doty, R. W. Functional significance of the topographical aspects of the retino-cortical projection. In R. Jung and H. Kornhuber (Eds.), *The visual system: Neurophysiology and psychophysics*. Berlin: Springer-Verlag, 1961, Pp. 228–243.

Doty, R. W. Survival of pattern vision after removal of striate cortex in the adult cat. *Journal of Comparative Neurology*, 1971, *143*, 341–369.

Finger, S., Simons, D., and Posner, R. Anatomical, physiological and behavioral effects of neonatal sensorimotor cortex ablation in the rat. *Experimental Neurology*, 1978, *60*, 347–373.

Frommer, G. P. Subtotal lesions: Implications for coding and recovery of function. In S. Finger (Ed.), *Recovery from brain damage: Research and theory*. New York: Plenum, 1978, Pp. 217–280.

Goldman, P. An alternative to developmental plasticity: Heterology of CNS structures in infants and adults. In D. G. Stein, J. J. Rosen, and N. Butters (Eds.), *Plasticity and recovery of function in the central nervous system*. New York: Academic Press, 1974, Pp. 149–174.

Goldman, P. S., and Rosvold, H. E. The effects of selective caudate lesions in infant and juvenile rhesus monkeys. *Brain Research*, 1972, *43*, 53–56.

Harlow, H. F., Blumquist, A. J., Thompson, C. I., Schiltz, K. A., and Harlow, M. K. Effects of induction-age and size of frontal lobe lesions on learning rhesus monkeys. In R. L. Isaacson (Ed.), *The neuropsychology of development*. New York: Wiley, 1968, Pp. 79–120.

Hécaen, H., and Albert, M. L. *Human neuropsychology*. New York: Wiley, 1978.

Hicks, S. P., and D'Amato, C. J. Motor-sensory and visual behavior after hemispherectomy in newborn and mature rats. *Experimental Neurology*, 1970, *29*, 416–438.

Hicks, S. P., and D'Amato, C. J. Motor-sensory cortex-corticospinal system and developing locomotion and placing in rats. *American Journal of Anatomy*, 1975, *143*, 1–42.

Isaacson, R. L. The myth of recovery from early brain damage. In N. R. Ellis (Ed.), *Aberrant development in infancy*. Potomac, M.: Erlbaum, 1975, Pp. 1–25.

Isaacson, R. L., and Nonneman, A. J. Early brain damage and later development. In P. Satz and J. Ross (Eds.), *The disabled learner: Early detection and intervention*. Rotterdam: University of Rotterdam Press, 1972, Pp. 29–44.

Isaacson, R., Nonneman, J., and Schmaltz, L. W. Behavioral and anatomical sequalae of damage to the infant limbic system. In R. L. Isaacson (Ed.), *The neuropsychology of development*. New York: Wiley, 1968, Pp. 41–78.

Johnson, D. A. Developmental aspects of recovery of function following septal lesions in the infant rat. *Journal of Comparative and Physiological Psychology*, 1972, *78*, 331–348.

Johnson, D. A., and Almli, C. R. Age, brain damage, and performance. In S. Finger (Ed.), *Recovery from brain damage: Research and theory*. New York: Plenum, 1978, Pp. 115–134.

Kaplan, M. S., and Hinds, J. W. Neurogenesis in the adult rat: Electron microscope analysis of light radioautographs. *Science*, 1977, *197*, Pp. 1092–1094.

Kennard, M. A. Age and other factors in motor recovery from precentral lesions in monkeys. *American Journal of Physiology*, 1936, *115*, 138–146.

Kennard, M. A. Reorganization of motor function in the cerebral cortex of monkeys deprived of motor and premotor areas in infancy. *Journal of Neurophysiology*, 1938, *1*, 477–497.

Kennard, M. A. Relation of age to motor impairment in man and sub-human primates. *Archives of Neurology and Psychiatry*, 1940, *44*, 377–397.

Kennard, M. A. Cortical reorganization of motor function: Studies on a series of monkeys of various ages from infancy to maturity. *Archives of Neurology and Psychiatry*, 1942, *48*, 227–240.

Kling, A. Amygdalectomy in the kitten. *Science*, 1962, *137*, 429–430.

Kling, A. Behavioral and somatic development following lesions of the amygdala in the cat. *Journal of Psychiatric Research*, 1965, *3*, 263–273.

Kling, A., and Tucker, T. J. Sparing of function following localized brain lesions in neonatal monkeys. In R. L. Isaacson (Ed.), *The neuropsychology of development*. New York: Wiley, 1968, Pp. 121–145.

Kolb, B., and Nonneman, A. J. Sparing of function with early prefrontal cortex lesions. *Brain Research*, 1978, *151*, 135–148.

Land, P. W., and Lund, R. D. Development of the rat's uncrossed retinotectal pathway and its relation to plasticity studies. *Science*, 1979, *205*, 698–700.

Lenneberg, E. H. The effects of age on the outcome of central nervous system disease in children. In Isaacson, R. L. (Ed.), *The neuropsychology of development*. New York: Wiley, 1968, Pp. 147–170.

Milner, B. Sparing of language functions after early unilateral brain damage. In E. Eidelberg and D. G. Stein (Eds.), *Functional recovery after lesions of the nervous system. Neuroscience research program bulletin*, 1974, *12*, 213–216.

Milner, B., Branch, C., and Rasmussen, T. Evidence for bilateral speech representation in some non-right handers. *Transactions of the American Neurological Association*, 1966, *91*, 306–308.

Nonneman, A. J. *Anatomical and behavioral consequences of early brain damage in the rabbit*. Unpublished doctoral dissertation, University of Florida, Gainesville, 1970.

Nonneman, A. J., and Isaacson, R. L. Task dependent recovery after early brain damage. *Behavioral Biology*, 1973, *8*, 143–172.

Penfield, W., and Roberts, L. *Speech and brain mechanisms*. Princeton, N.J.: Princeton University Press, 1959.

Russell, W. R. *Brain, memory and learning: A neurologist's view*. Oxford: Clarendon Press, 1959.

Sharlock, D. P., Tucker, T. J., and Strominger, N. L. Auditory discrimination by the cat after neonatal ablation of the temporal cortex. *Science*, 1963, *141*, 1197–1198.

Smith, A. Differing effects of hemispherectomy in children and adults. *Paper presented at the 84th Annual Meeting of the American Psychological Association*, Washington, D.C., September 1976.

Smith, A. Language and nonlanguage functions after right or left hemispherectomy for cerebral lesions in infancy. *Paper presented at the 5th Annual Meeting of the International Neuropsychological Society*, Santa Fe, New Mexico, February 1977.

Stein, D. G., and Firl, A. Brain damage and reorganization of function in old age. *Experimental Neurology*, 1976, *52*, 157–167.

Teuber, H.-L. Recovery of function after brain injury in man. In *Outcome of severe damage to the central nervous system* (Ciba Foundation Symposium). Amsterdam: Elsevier, 1975, Pp. 159–186.

Teuber, H.-L., and Rudel, R. G. Behaviour after cerebral lesions in children and adults. *Developmental Medicine and Child Neurology*, 1962, *4*, 3–20.

Tsang, Y. C. Maze learning in rats hemidecorticated in infancy. *Journal of Comparative Psychology*, 1937, *24*, 221–254.

Tucker, T. J., and Kling, A. Differential effects of early and late lesions of frontal granular cortex in the monkey. *Brain Research*, 1967, *5*, 377–389.

Wetzel, A. B., Thompson, V. E., Horel, J. A., and Meyer, P. M. Some consequences of perinatal lesions of the visual cortex of the cat. *Psychonomic Science*, 1965, *3*, 381–382.

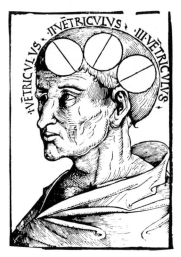

Fast- versus Slow-Growing Lesions and Behavioral Recovery

Before I speak of the several classes of symptoms in cases of intracranial tumours . . . I have to make a statement which may surprise some of you. It is that occasionally there are no symptoms in these cases. And frequently when symptoms are present they are insignificant in comparison with the size of the tumour found post-mortum, or, more correctly speaking, in comparison with what we might theoretically infer from the size of the tumour [John Hughlings Jackson, 1873, p. 139].

CHAPTER NINE

In his book, *The Organism*, Kurt Goldstein (1939), a neurologist with holistic views on brain function, argued that because neuropsychologists are "accustomed to regard symptoms as direct expressions of (brain) damage, they tend to assume that, corresponding to some given damage, definite symptoms must inevitably appear [p. 18]."

In the previous chapter, we have described one condition where brain damage, even when it is quite extensive, does *not* necessarily have lasting behavioral deficits. That is, we noted that there may be a relative lack of symptoms on some tasks when brain injury is suffered early in life. To many investigators, behavioral sparing in brain-damaged young subjects can be traced to the development of new nerve pathways, anomalous growth from existing fibers into deafferented zones, or the rerouting of nerve fibers into other regions following destruction of their primary target areas. Such "dynamic neural reorganization," associated with behavioral recovery, is thought to be possible because the immature brain has not yet become completely differentiated or "committed" to the mediation of specific functions.

The adaptability of the nervous system in neonates may be generally accepted by laymen and experts, but there is more doubt about the capacity of adults to recover from severe brain injury. In fact, it was from the study of adults that lesion-induced symptoms have come to be regarded as the inevitable consequences of brain injury. Over the years, there have been reports documenting the observation that slow-growing lesions (e.g., tumors) cause less impairments and fewer symptoms than damage that occurs more acutely (e.g., gunshot, stroke). For the most part, the cases that violated the principle of "specific lesion-specific symptom'' were dismissed as curious anomalies by scientists and practitioners, rather than being treated as interesting and important phenomena worthy of serious study.

In the laboratory setting, the increasing interest in structural neuroplasticity has encouraged investigators to direct their attention to the question of whether functional recovery after brain injury in adults can be manipulated directly. For example, ''slow growing'' lesions can be created by damaging a part of the brain in an initial operation and then injuring more tissue in subsequent operations, days, weeks, or even years after the first surgery.

In previous review articles, the two of us have described the ''serial lesion effect'' in animals (Finger, 1978; Finger, Walbran, and Stein, 1973; Stein, 1974). This refers to the observation that slow-growing lesions often are not associated with the severe symptomatology seen after of rapid onset. We also pointed out that the effect has been observed not only in experimental preparations (the principal subject of this chapter), but in human patients as well. For example, Walther Riese (1950) opened one of the chapters of his *Principles of Neurology* with a statement that vividly illustrates the fact that the growth rate of brain lesions has been known to be important for symtomatology for at least the last 200 years, although this phenomenon is rarely if ever mentioned in modern textbooks and monographs:

> The time a lesion needs for originating, growing and spreading, is an essential element in cerebral localization. Sudden changes such as traumata, vascular accidents, etc., are most likely to produce symptoms, although sometimes only temporary ones. . . . this chronological factor has not been given the full credit it deserves in our attempts to correlate lesions with symptoms, though as early as 1761 Morgagni mentioned brain lesions of slow onset not associated with paralysis, and though in 1841 Hall made the statement that tumors of the brain ''when developed slowly'' may exist with scarcely any symptom [p. 138].

A related early description of the differences in symptomatology that can emerge with fast- and slow-growing lesions can be found in a report written in 1836 by the French physician, Marc Dax.[1]

The Dax paper has a number of interesting features about it that should not be overlooked by those interested in aphasia or the history of science. In the first place, Dax associated left hemispheric damage with aphasia on the basis of a few

---

[1] This paper, which may contain the first clear statement of the theory of cerebral dominance, was intended for presentation at a regional medical congress at Montpellier, although whether Dax ever presented the report is a matter of controversy (see Joynt and Benton, 1964). The report was brought to the attention of the scientific community after the death of Marc Dax by his son, Gustav Dax, who was also a physician. But by 1865, when the posthumous report appeared, Broca had already presented his findings pertaining to the significance of the left hemisphere for speech functions, and as we know, Broca is usually given full credit for this discovery.

cases involving saber wounds and what appeared to be strokes, but continued to collect material until he could comment on more than 40 cases of aphasia, all of whom had left hemispheric damage. In the second place, Dax emphasized that he had never seen aphasia develop when the right hemisphere alone was damaged and that not all cases of left hemispheric damage resulted in speech disturbances. It was in this context that Dax discussed his observation that lesions that develop slowly are less likely to produce aphasic symptoms. His style of writing about this led us to believe that the differences between fast- and slow-growing lesions were well known in his day and that they represented a widely accepted fact of clinical medicine: "I would not even regard as an exception a disease of the left hemisphere without an alteration of speech, particularly if the disease were slight or if it had developed slowly [p. 852]."

Modern investigators have had little difficulty confirming Dax's contention concerning fast- and slow-growing lesions and aphasia. In reviewing his own case studies on neurological patients with similarly localized lesions differing in speed of development, Walther Riese (1948) himself remarked, "Sudden lesions, i.e., those of greatest momentum, are most likely to produce aphasia, although only transitory in uncomplicated cases. In lesions of slow momentum, speech may be preserved either throughout the whole history, or at least, for a long time [p. 75]."

Any discussion of the importance of the speed of lesion growth would be incomplete if John Hughlings Jackson's name were not mentioned. On the basis of his own clinical observations and the work of others, Jackson (1835–1911; Figure 9.1) never ceased to emphasize that mass × velocity ("mv") must be considered in any attempt to understand brain lesion effects. He noticed that lesions resulting from sudden hemorrhages were much more likely to have striking deficits than those due to "developing softenings" of the brain, and it was Jackon who coined the term *effect of momentum of lesions* to describe these phenomena. Jackson (1879, 1894), however, also commented upon another real difference between lesions of rapid and slow momentum: When symptoms eventually appeared in the slow momentum cases, they generally were more enduring than the symptoms that followed rapidly evolving lesions. One possible explanation for this is that slow growing lesions may have to be much larger and more widespread than those of rapid onset before they cause some of the same symptoms. They may also be associated with less neural "shock."

Other data on adult human patients showing that symptoms are dependent upon the momentum of the lesions as well as on their locus in the brain can be found in the writings of Jackson's contemporaries, especially Constantin von Monakow (1897, 1914), who is best known for his theory of "diaschisis" (Chapter 13), and Henry Head (1926), a founding father of the new structure-oriented neurology.

It is hard to say exactly when findings analogous to these clinical observations

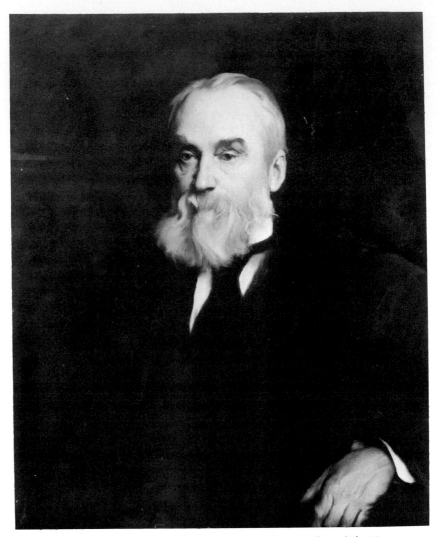

Figure 9.1. *John Hughlings Jackson.* *(Courtesy of Royal College of Physicians)*

were first observed in laboratory animals, but it would be reasonable to guess that serial lesions were initially used because they resulted in lower mortality than would be expected after large, one-stage lesions. For example, in 1824 Flourens wrote that he could keep decorticate birds alive for considerable lengths of time provided that he removed small amounts of tissue in a series of operations, rather than ablating all of the cortex at once. More than 100 years later, Lashley (1929) turned to the same technique when he had to ablate more than 50% of the neocortex of his rats. Lashley performed his smaller ablations in a single operation, and many of his graphs dealing with lesion size and maze performance are seriously confounded in this regard (Finger, Walbran, and Stein, 1973). Kleitman and Camille (1932), who were contemporaries of Lashley and pioneers in the field of sleep research, also relied on serial ablations of the cerebrum because massive one-stage lesions usually killed the dogs that they needed for their experiments.

Perhaps the most striking example of differences in survival rates between animals with fast- and slow-growing lesions is provided in the 1959 report by John Adametz, which we discussed in Chapter 1. As we noted, Adametz gave 80 adult cats large electrolytic lesions of the midbrain reticular formation. When this was done in a single operation, the animals fell into deep coma, and despite intensive efforts to save them, most of the cats died within a few days. When the lesions were spaced 1–2 weeks apart, even though there were up to eight separate surgeries, the animals arose shortly after each operation and were soon able to walk, feed, and groom themselves.

> After the 2nd operation the animals again were able to eat unaided upon the 1st postoperative day, despite the fact that they now had an aggregate of lesions approximating those described above for the 1-stage comatose animals. From that time on their recovery progressed somewhat more slowly, but beyond comparison with the recovery rate of any animal in which bilateral lesions had been made at one sitting. Two months postoperatively several of these animals nearly approached normal except for movements upon horizontal ladders. . . . They pursued mice, could jump a distance of several feet, and groomed themselves regularly. All were alert and constantly interested in their surroundings. At no time after the first few days was a significant disturbance of the normal sleep–waking cycle observed [p. 88–89].

This type of sparing (and even normal learning scores) after extensive reticular formation lesions has now been confirmed in reports from at least two other laboratories (Kesner, Fiedler, and Thomas, 1967; Lourie, Vanasupa, and O'Leary, 1960). The replicability of these "anomalous" findings contrasts sharply with the still prevalent notion that the reticular formation is "necessary and essential" for mediating normal arousal and wakefulness!

At this juncture it should be stated that there are many ways to produce lesions in two or more stages, although two paradigms seem to dominate the serial lesion literature. The most popular method involves making a lesion on one side of the brain, allowing a number of days or weeks to pass, and then producing a matching lesion on the opposite side. The less frequently used alternative to the successive unilateral lesion procedure involves the placement of incomplete lesions on both sides of the brain in the first operation and enlarging the bilateral lesions to full size in a second operation some time later. Both procedures are shown in Figure 9.2. As previously stated, however, two-stage lesions represent only one strategy, and as seen in the work of Adametz (1959), there really is almost no limit

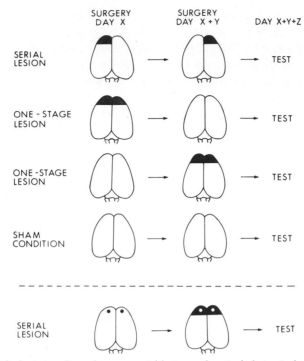

Figure 9.2. *The basic paradigms for many serial-lesion studies. Each design includes a group with sequential unilateral lesions, a group without ablations, and two groups with one-stage bilateral lesions; one matched in time to the first operation sustained by the serial group, and the other matched to that group's second operation. Modifications of this design may include elimination of the latter group (see text), the addition of lesion "control" groups, and preoperative and/or interoperative testing for some or all of the animals in each group. The time period between the lesions is usually referred to as the interlesion interval (ILI). (From Finger, 1978.)*

to the number and configuration of surgeries that can be performed on a single animal.

A good example of a complex multistage procedure can be seen in one of our own reports (Rosen, Stein, and Butters, 1971). Monkeys were given four operations, each spaced 3 weeks apart. Each surgery involved the removal of one bank of one part of the monkey's frontal lobe (sulcus principalis), and on each succeeding operation, the side and the bank were changed. The first operation involved the removal of the lower bank in the left hemisphere. The upper bank of the right hemisphere was ablated in the second operation. After going back to the left hemisphere and then to the right hemisphere, the surgeries were completed. The animals then were compared to monkeys with one-stage lesions of the same region. Rosen *et al.* found that the monkeys sustaining serial lesions made many fewer errors on a battery of spatial discrimination tasks than did the animals with one-stage operations. An added surprise came when the monkeys' brains were examined histologically; the animals with serial lesions had much larger lesions than the one-stage animals who, in fact, were much more impaired behaviorally. The additional damage in the "multistage" group was caused by adhesions and bleeding—complications which resulted from multiple surgical entries in the same wound area.

Some researchers have been critical of reports of serial lesion effects, because they feel that there have been problems in choosing an appropriate "one-stage" lesion group for comparison. One of us (Finger, 1978) previously stated

> Take as representative a study in which the two-stage animals experience successive unilateral lesions spaced 30 days apart, with testing on a discrimination problem starting 20 days after the last surgery. If the one-stage animals also have a 20-day postoperative recovery period, it can be claimed that the serial animals are at a distinct advantage since one side of the brain in that group has 30 additional days for recovery. In contrast, if the one-stage animals are given 50 days for recovery, this being equal to the recovery time from the first lesion of the two-stage animals, the one-stage subjects will have the advantage since the two-stage group will have some target tissue damaged with considerably less time for recovery [p. 139].

One solution to this problem is just to give the one-stage animals the advantage of a recovery period timed from the first surgery of the two-stage animals. If a serial lesion effect *still* emerges, its robustness can be emphasized since the postoperative recovery conditions favored better performance by the one-stage animals. The merits of various serial lesion techniques have been examined by Finger (1978) in review in which he showed that greater sparing of behavior after serial lesions is usually observed even under the comparison condition that favors the opposite result. Cases of one-stage animals performing better than serial animals, if they exist, are rare indeed, although in some studies both one-stage and multistage animals have performed equivalently.

We think that the range and diversity of serial lesion effects show quite clearly that more than just the opportunity to survive surgery is at stake. In short, sparing of function has been found in tests of motor capacity, in simple sensory discriminations, such as light–dark discrimination; in complex learning tasks; in the sphere of homeostasis (eating and drinking); and in a host of motivational and emotional indices. Some examples of the differences between animals with one-stage and multistage lesions are at least as striking as the data collected by Adametz on reticular formation lesions and sleep and wakefulness.

In many cases, textbooks examining the role of the motor cortex in the production of movement and related behaviors typically state the Brodmann areas 4 and 6 are critical for normal movement. Early papers by Karplus and Kreidl (1914) and McKinley and Berkowitz (1933) described the ataxia that follows these lesions, and reports such as theirs typically contain photographs of monkeys with massive bilateral damage centered in the motor cortex lying immobilized on the bottom of their cages. These animals are not able to walk, stand, or even right themselves after simultaneous bilateral lesions of the motor cortex at maturity. In contrast to this picture of severe debilitation, Ann Marie Travis and Clinton Woolsey published an article in 1956 demonstrating good sparing of motor functioning following *total* removal of the motor cortex on both sides of the brain in their monkeys. To accomplish this the researchers had to do a large number of surgeries spaced over a period of many months. When this was done, the monkeys *never* lost the ability to right, feed, or walk, although intensive care had to be provided to them immediately after some of the operations. In two notable cases, Travis and Woolsey slowly extended the lesions to the point where the monkeys were completely decorticated. Even under these conditions, one of the monkeys could still sit up, right itself and walk soon after the last operation, (which was more than 2 years after its first surgery), and its hopping and grasping reflexes remained unimpaired. The other monkey needed more assistance when walking, but still exhibited motor abilities far exceeding those previously reported with one-stage animals sustaining much smaller lesions.

Even performance on a perceptual task can be affected by the manner in which surgery is performed. A perceptual learning study by Harlow Ades (1946) is particularly notable in this regard. Ades planned to make bilateral one-stage ablations of visual areas 18 and 19 in a group of monkeys. With one subject, the surgery had to be terminated after one hemisphere had been damaged. Following a short recovery period, this monkey was retested on a series of visual discrimination tasks. Ades found that the animal's preoperatively acquired size, shape and color discriminations were perfectly retained. Eighteen days after this first operation, Ades then removed the parastriate cortex on the opposite side of the monkey's brain. Unlike the other monkeys that performed poorly after their bilateral extirpations, the animal with serial lesions again showed perfect retention on all of the tasks. Intrigued by this remarkable performance, Ades and Raab (1949) essentially replicated the experiment in another study that required the monkeys to distinguish between an upright and an inverted "F." The "anomalous" performance of the lone monkey was now seen in a whole *group* of animals purposely given serial lesions. The critical features of this experiment are shown in Figures 9.3–9.6.

Since the two-stage animals in Ades's initial studies received more training than the one-stage animals (extra trials were provided during testing in the "interlesion interval"), it still was not possible to say whether the behavioral sparing that he reported was due to serial lesions, to additional training, or to an interaction of these two factors. A third experiment soon was published and provided support for the idea that the spaced operations were mainly responsible for the spared visual behaviors. In this experiment, John Stewart and Harlow Ades (1951) studied the effects of temporal lobe lesions on auditory discrimination in

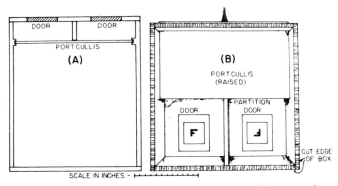

SCALE IN INCHES -

Figure 9.3. *Diagram of test box. (A) Flow plan. (B) Front of inside of box as seen by animal. (From Ades and Raab, 1949.)*

adult monkeys. They varied the length of the interlesion interval and gave only some of the animals interoperative training. Their data showed very clearly that an interval of 7 days between surgeries was all that was required for the serial lesion effect to appear and that interoperative testing did not contribute to the sparing observed in the animals with serial lesions (see Finger, 1978, for a more complete discussion of these experiments).

The range of serial lesion effects is still further illustrated in another study (Stein, Rosen, Graziadei, Mishkin, and Brink, 1969). This experiment involved groups of adult rats with one-stage bilateral or sequential unilateral lesions (25–30 day interlesion interval) of the frontal cortex, hippocampus, or amygdala. The animals were tested on a variety of tasks chosen for their demonstrated sensitivity to the effects of one-stage lesions in these brain areas. In brief, the "one-stage" animals displayed the expected deficits on the learning problems, which included light–dark discrimination and reversal, passive avoidance, and delayed alternation. In contrast, as shown in Table 9.1, the rats with serial lesions performed as well as the control animals on all the measures. Equally dramatic sparing has been reported in other studies assessing behavior after staged limbic system lesions (e.g., McIntyre and Stein, 1973; Patrissi and Stein, 1975; Schulze

Figure 9.4. *Smoothed curve (obtained by rolling averages of 3 days' scores of performance before and after bilateral extirpations of areas 18 and 19. In 30 trials, a score of 23 is 3 standard deviations beyond chance. Note: 1 denotes average of 130 trials in old training box. (From Ades and Raab, 1949.)*

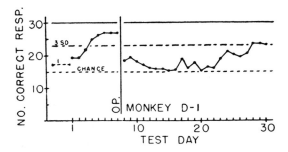

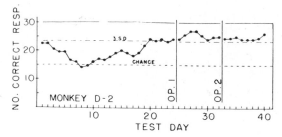

Figure 9.5. *Smoothed curve of performance before, between, and after unilateral extirpations of areas 18 and 19. (From Ades and Raab, 1949.)*

and Stein, 1975), including some experiments on monkeys (e.g., Butters, Butter, Rosen, and Stein, 1973; Rosen, Stein, and Butters, 1971).

   In reviews of the serial lesion literature, the present authors and their co-workers (Finger, 1978; Finger, Walbran, and Stein, 1973) have emphasized that not all results have been as clear as these and that some studies have failed to show differences between ''one-stage'' and ''multistage'' subjects (Dawson, Conrad, and Lynch, 1973; Ettlinger and Kalsbeck, 1962; Hart, 1980; Isaacson and Schmaltz, 1968). This does not mean, however, that serial lesion effects are due to artifact, poor experimental design, or chance. In fact, where replications or additional groups have been used to bolster weak experimental designs, serial lesion effects typically have still appeared. As an example of this from one of our own laboratories, rats with one-stage or two-stage lesions of the somatosensory cortex were tested on a battery of ''rough'' versus smooth discriminations (Finger, Marshak, Cohen, Scheff, Trace, and Neimand, 1971). The rats with one-stage bilateral lesions were barely able to reach criterion on these tests when they were given 35 days for recovery. Animals with sequential unilateral lesions, with a little over a month between surgeries and 35 days to recover from the last operation, scored as well as control animals on the battery. This is shown in Table 9.2. When it was realized that the one-stage animals may have performed worse than the rats with serial lesions because they did not have equivalent recovery times (the serial animals had 35 more days to recover from their first surgery), additional groups of

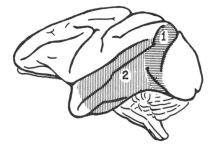

Figure 9.6. *Lateral view of macaque brain showing area of preoccipital cortex removed (area #1). (From Ades and Raab, 1949.)*

Table 9.1

Number of Trials to Criterion in Tasks Performed by Rats with Lesions of the Frontal Cortex[a]

	Delayed spatial alternation (mean)	Light–dark discrimination reversal (mean)	Light–dark discrimination (mean)	Simultaneous discrimination (mean)
Group 1-S	300.0	313	278.5	120.0
Group 2-S	150.0	121	124.0	79.4
Group UC	104.6	132	148.0	73.0

Note. Groups with one-stage lesions are labeled 1-S; groups with two-stage lesions are labeled 2-S; unoperated controls are labeled UC.

[a]After Stein *et al.*, 1969.

one-stage animals were tested (Finger and Reyes, 1975). The new data showed that the deficits displayed by the ''one-stage'' rats were still prominent months and years after surgery, whereas the animals with serial lesions were able to perform reasonably well on the tactile discriminations within a few weeks.

Some attempts are now being made to account for the fact that serial lesions are associated with fewer or milder deficits than ''one-stage'' lesions in some experiments and equivalent deficits in other experiments. These studies are confirming that just producing lesions in stages is no guarantee that serial lesion effects will emerge. That this should be the case should be clear from the Stewart and Ades (1951) experiment that we just discussed. As we pointed out, they found that 7 days between surgeries was necessary to obtain a serial lesion effect (good retention of previously learned discrimination) and that with shorter interlesion intervals, their animals performed as poorly as the one-stage subjects.

Still, as more studies on the subject began to appear, it soon became evident

Table 9.2

Means Number of Days to Criterion for Animals in Four Surgical Groups That Were Tested on Each of Five Tactile Discriminations[a]

Discrimination	Somatosensory cortex: one operation (*n* = 13)	Somatosensory cortex: sequential unilateral operations (*n* = 9)	Control: one operation (*n* = 7)	Control: two operations (*n* = 7)
1	25.38	18.77	14.57	17.14
2	11.38	7.67	6.86	5.71
3	18.00	7.33	4.57	4.29
4	15.69	3.89	3.00	3.57
5	20.62	5.00	10.71	5.29

[a]After Finger *et al.*, 1971.

that the phenomenon of recovery was *not* going to be so easily predicted. This is illustrated by the observation that the effective (7-day) interlesion interval in the Stewart and Ades (1951) experiment proved to be too short in at least two other serial lesion studies. Patrissi and Stein (1975) for example, found that rats with 10 days between successive unilateral lesions of the frontal poles were statistically comparable to one-stage rats on a spatial alternation task (go left, go right, go left, etc.), but that animals with 20 or more days between their lesions performed as well as sham-operated animals (see Figure 9.7). In a related study from a different laboratory, good sparing on a passive avoidance measure was found among mice with 21 days between successive unilateral lesions of the frontal areas, but not in other animals that were permitted only 7 days to recover from the first of their two surgeries (Glick and Zimmerberg, 1972). Although the interlesion interval is certainly an important variable in serial lesion studies, and one which might account for some failures to find serial lesion effects, it is not so easy to generalize results from one study to another. Rather, the time between operations appears to be a factor that is at least partially dependent upon the other variables that are being manipulated, such as the size and placement of each lesion, the training history of the subjects, and age of the animals at the time of surgery.

One pertinent finding in this regard is that a reasonable level of sensory stimulation during the interlesion interval can be important in determining the results of some of these experiments. This was first demonstrated by Donald Meyer, Walter Isaac, and Brendan Maher (1958). They gave rats sequential unilateral lesions of the visual cortex after the animals first learned to avoid shock by running at the onset of a light. Some of the rats spent the 12-day interoperative interval in

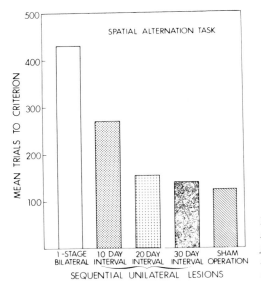

Figure 9.7. *Performance of rats with simultaneous or sequential lesions of the frontal cortex or sham operations on a spatial-alternation problem. (Data of Patrissi and Stein, 1975; from Finger, 1978.)*

their lighted home cages, but others were kept in darkness during a ''recovery'' period. Meyer and his colleagues found that the serial lesion procedure was effective in sparing the learned habit if light were permitted between surgeries. The light-deprived animals with serial lesions performed very poorly in comparison to the group with serial lesions permitted light. This can be seen in Figure 9.8.

Two other factors that must be considered when analyzing serial lesion data are task difficulty and the ordering of the lesions. Although task difficulty has received little in the way of systematic attention from workers in this field, there is little question about the importance of this variable. Two recent studies from one of our laboratories at Washington University bear on this factor. Each assessed the tactile discriminative ability of rats given large lesions of the somatosensory cortex: The age of the animals, the lesions, and the paradigms were the same, but in one case the tactile problem was one which took naive, unoperated rats 40 days to master (Simons, Puretz, and Finger, 1975), whereas in the other, animals without lesions were able to meet the same criterion in 15 days (Finger and Simons, 1976). The serial lesion effect failed to appear on the difficult ridge-smooth discrimination, and all animals with lesions in this experiment performed much more poorly than the control animals. But on the easier discrimination, the rats with serial lesions were comparable to the sham operated rats, whereas only those with one-stage lesions were impaired.

The ordering and configuration of lesions also can play a role in determining symptomatology. In one such case, Isseroff, Leveton, Freeman, Lewis, and Stein (1976) gave rats bilateral hippocampal lesions in stages, with some animals first receiving bilateral, dorsal hippocampi removals, whereas others had the ventral

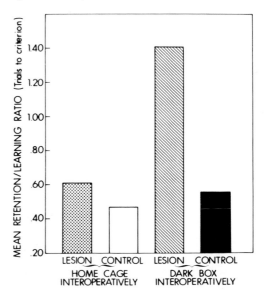

Figure 9.8. *Performance of rats with serial lesions of the visual cortex or sham operations on a brightness-avoidance problem. Some animals were kept in darkness and others were kept in their home cages (light–dark) between surgeries. (Data of Meyer, Isaac, and Maher, 1958; from Finger, 1978.)*

hippocampi damaged first and then the dorsal, and so on. Still other groups had the dorsal and ventral hippocampi operated upon on one side of the brain before both structures were destroyed on the opposite side of the brain. When the rats were tested on a spatial reversal task (after learning to run to one of two positions, the positive and negative sides were switched), these investigators found significant differences depending upon how the serial lesions were made, even though all animals eventually had bilateral lesions of both the dorsal and ventral hippocampi that looked alike.

Some of the other factors that could influence the outcomes of serial lesion studies are the duration of the postoperative recovery period (Reyes, 1977), the type of training during the interlesion interval (Dru, Walker, and Walker, 1975), the administration of drugs between operations (Cole, Sullins, and Isaac, 1967; see Figure 9.9), and the amount of tissue removed in each operation. These variables are discussed in great length in the reviews by Finger, Walbran, and Stein (1973), Stein (1974), and Finger (1978), where it is stressed that the weighting given to each of these factors is in part dependent upon the other conditions in the experiment.

Still, serial lesion effects appear to be rather robust; they have appeared both cortically and subcortically, and in a variety of species including monkeys, cats,

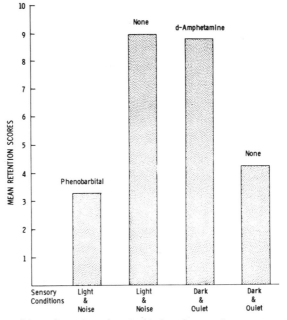

Figure 9.9. *Effects of d-amphetamine, phenobarbital, and sensory input on postoperative retention of a previously learned habit. (From Cole, Sullins, and Isaac, 1967.)*

rats, mice, fish, and birds. Perhaps the most impressive aspect of the sparing and recovery associated with serial surgery is that two-stage or four-stage lesions would hardly be considered examples of "slow-growing damage" by clinical neurologists who describe the growth patterns of tumors and diseases in their papers. At this point in time, the real question is, therefore, not whether lesion momentum effects exist, but *why* they exist.

Just why do serial lesions usually cause less problems for the organism than one-stage damage? An honest answer is that we really do not always know. Although both physiological and behavioral explanations for the serial lesion effect have been advanced, it is not always simple to distinguish among the various possibilities or to determine which events are causal and which are only correlative. With this in mind, let us look at some of the ideas that people in this field are presenting and attempting to evaluate.

In a previous review (Finger, Walbran, and Stein, 1973), we tentatively suggested that axonal sprouting might play a role in the sparing seen with slow-growing lesions. However, it now seems highly unlikely that this can be the whole story since at least in laboratory investigations the lesions wind up being both bilateral and very extensive. This means that homologous, intact neuronal fibers (from the side of the brain that is spared in the first operation) that could conceivably sprout into denervated zones would be lost in subsequent operations. Therefore, any functional sprouting in the adult would have to come from and/or project to nonhomologous zones, there to compete with the normal complement of synaptic terminals—a response that we have repeatedly stressed might not be adaptive. In fact, even if we could conceive of a situation like somatic cortex damage causing spared sensory afferents to project more densely from the thalamus to the so-called "motor" cortex, there would still be the issue of why this should only occur in the serial lesion animals and not in the simultaneous lesion groups. At the present time, the notions of within-systems and alternate-system sprouting, as they relate to serial lesion phenomena, certainly need more attention. These ideas are important because their potential ramifications are enormous; they would bear on concepts of cerebral organization and would also be factors to be considered when developing treatment programs for brain damaged individuals.

A second physiological notion worth considering is that serial lesions could conceivably produce less *transneuronal* degeneration than extensive simultaneous damage. No one knows why degeneration at a distance occurs, but gradual cerebral insult may be an important factor to consider along with the possibilities of reduced vascular inflammation and glial scarring. An initially small region of lesion-induced necrosis may have less deleterious consequences for behavioral sparing than a large zone, characteristic of single-stage, bilateral surgery, simply because the toxic by-products can be phagocitized rapidly and removed more easily.

The momentum of a lesion might also differentially affect the levels of neuro-transmitters in the remaining areas of the brain. For example, John Morrison, Mark Molliver, and Reinhard Grzanna (1979) made small lesions of the frontal cortex in rats and then used immunohistofluorescence techniques to examine the disruption of noradrenergic innervation of the cerebral cortex following the lesions. The authors observed widespread denervation extending over the entire cerebral cortex. These findings were similar to those reported in an earlier article by Pujol, Stein, Blondaux, Pettijean, Froment, and Jouvet (1973), which described how lesions of the raphé nucleus cause alterations in catecholamine synthesis in sites far removed from the site of the damage. If there is an attempt by the organism to reestablish some neurochemical "steady state" after injury, then a series of small injuries could be more conducive to recovery than a massive onslaught (e.g., the feedback mechanisms controlling neurochemical regulation might still partially function). Thus, when the second lesion of a series occurs, the system is already or nearly stabilized. Different systems, depending on the complexity of their interconnections, the types of neurotransmitter involved, the vascularization, and so on, would require more or less time for restabilization. This is why no *one,* specific "critical period" can be defined and why recovery of function following some serial lesions may not be seen until long after *all* surgery is completed (e.g., Isseroff *et al.,* 1976).

There have even been suggestions that the blood supply to an area can account for some serial lesion phenomena. A short time ago, Robert Treichler (1975) of Kent State University repeated the experiments of Rosen, Stein, and Butters (1971) in which adult rhesus monkeys were given one-stage or multistage lesions of the frontal cortex. To reiterate, in the earlier study, the animals with serial lesions were much less impaired on a battery of learning tasks than those with one-stage lesions. Treichler confirmed this general finding, but noted that the ordering of his lesions greatly affected his results. Two-stage lesions with the first ablation performed above sulcus principalis resulted in greater sparing than staged lesions with the lower bank of this sulcus removed first.

One explanation that was proposed for this unexpected ordering effect was that the upper bank lesions had little effect on the blood vessels in the sulcus, whereas lower bank lesions resulted in much greater vascular involvement. This involvement could well have affected the blood supply to the upper bank. When upper bank lesions are performed before lower bank lesions, the consequences of the two surgeries are indeed staggered, whereas when lower bank lesions occur first, the upper bank is also functionally affected—the result not being terribly different from one-stage ablations of both banks.

In addition to speculations like these on the physiological "bases" for recovery, some authors proposed more phenomenological explanations for momentum-of-lesion effects. Given the fact that so little is known about how recovery of function occurs, there is no reason to reject such concepts offhandedly since they could provide experimental models for further research.

Quite some time ago, Clifford Morgan (1951) suggested that brain damage inflicted early in life gives the organism more time to develop the appropriate strategies for coping with the new set of demands made upon it. Because its habits are not completely formed, it can adapt more easily to the altered perceptual environment it faces upon emerging from surgery. We think that the same might be true for serial lesions inflicted upon adults. For example, say we create a unilateral or partial lesion of the motor cortex. Most of the system is intact so the "emergence trauma" (Fuller, 1967) should be less severe than if the area were entirely eliminated. During the interoperative interval, the organism could be developing new response strategies, perhaps less efficient, but nonetheless capable of allowing it to attain its goals. This may be one reason why interoperative stimulation or training has beneficial consequences, even though eventually the subject is required to perform after *bilateral* removal of a brain region. Perhaps John Hughlings Jackson (1881) put it best when he made an analogy to governments that are rapidly toppled as opposed to those that are slowly changed.

> Were the highest governing people in this country suddenly destroyed, we should have to lament the loss of their offices. . . . We should also have to lament the now permitted anarchy of the now ungoverned people consequent on that loss. . . . But . . . if, in this country, the highest governing peoples were slowly removed . . . the rest of the country would not be, or would be only slightly anarchial. The lower governing bodies would, being then highest, gradually become efficient substitutes for general purposes [pp. 399–400].

Ideas such as less emergence trauma with serial lesions are indeed intriguing and perhaps even applicable to all learning tasks since performance must inevitably depend not only on sensory input and motor output, but on attention, motivation, and emotion—factors that conceivably could be differentially affected in subjects with serial or one-stage lesions who must face slowly or radically altered worlds after these respective surgeries. Confusion and emotionality could even prevent rats from rapidly switching to remaining alternate visual mechanisms for performing pattern discriminations after damage to primary visual cortical areas (Barbas and Spear, 1976).

Still, cue and strategy selection models and factors such as attention, motivation, and emotionality cannot account for all serial lesion effects. This should be apparent when we think back to Adametz's cats surviving massive reticular formation lesions and showing normal sleep and wakefulness cycles in comparison to comatose animals who suffered one-stage lesions. The limitation of such models can also be seen in other studies that deal more with homeostatic mechanisms than with complex learned behaviors. For example, a few years ago, some of us

(Fass, Jordan, Rubman, Seibel, and Stein, 1975) decided to examine food intake and weight regulation in rats with one- or two-stage lesions of the lateral hypothalamic area (LHA). In general, bilateral LHA lesions produce aphagia and adipsia, and most rats die without intensive postoperative care. We measured body weight regulation and food and water intake after *unilateral* LHA lesions and noticed that our rats showed an initial decline in weight compared to control animals. Within a month, the unilateral LHA rats regained and increased weight to the same extent as normal rats. In contrast, the "one-stage" rats showed the "classic" LHA syndrome. When we created a contralateral LHA lesion in the former group some 30 days later, we expected to see a reappearance of the deficit that perhaps would be more severe since the lesion would now be bilateral. To our surprise, the rats with the serial, bilateral LHA lesions continued to regulate weight and eat normally.

One very speculative way of interpreting data like these is to postulate that during the interoperative interval, the intact contralateral area could have altered its contribution to central nervous system function (as a result of the initial surgery) since damage to it did not provoke any additional symptoms or exacerbate those previously observed. Furthermore, one might be tempted to suggest that other areas could have taken over the "functions" of the damaged area in the reorganizational process (see Chapter 16).

Because we know so little about structure–function relationships in the intact brain, hypotheses like these are exceedingly difficult if even possible to test, a point to which we will return in later chapters of this book. Still, some individuals claim to have found physiological "evidence" of such reorganization within the context of the serial lesion paradigm.

In one such case, Stephen Scheff and Dennis Wright (1976) tested rats for retention of a black–white discrimination after they were given serial or one-stage removals of the visual cortex. They noted that interoperative training was necessary to obtain sparing of function in the animals with serial lesions. Interestingly, Scheff and Wright also found new evoked responses to light in the cortex contiguous to the damaged zone in those rats that showed behavioral recovery. With this to go on, the authors suggested that cortical reorganization follows serial but not one-stage lesions.

It will not be hard for the reader to detect that we really are limited in our ability to provide a monolithic explanation for the serial lesion phenomenon. Obviously, as with any type of brain damage, there will be many factors that can influence behavior after brain injury. We do not know about the specific physiological substrates of recovery because so little research has been directed toward unravelling the solution to the puzzle. However, we now have seen that definite symptoms need not always appear after brain lesions in infants or adults, and this is by no means trivial.

Whatever its basis might be, these studies are telling us that the mammalian central nervous system has a tremendous capacity to adapt to change that does not end with the period of infancy. They are also telling us that traditional means of associating different functions with each and every brain area and subarea in unique and invariable ways may be misleading. The important point is simply that if a structure has some unique well-defined function, it should not matter if the structure is damaged all at once or over a period of weeks—the function should be lost. Since these serial lesion studies have shown us that many of the so-called "critical" functions of particular brain areas are not really critical at all, we are forced to ask whether the findings are anomalous, wrong, or spurious, or whether our theories of brain organization and associated function must be questioned. Could the message be that our logic has not been perfect when it has come to assigning functions to structures and that we still have a long way to go before we understand how the brain works? We will examine this position and all its ramifications in much greater detail in a future chapter. Next, however, we will look at the role of the environment in affecting recovery from one-stage lesions. Here we will see one line of evidence showing that even with massive, acute damage, sexually mature subjects can sometimes still show considerable recovery.

References

Adametz, J. H. Rate of recovery of functioning in cats with rostral reticular lesions. *Journal of Neurosurgery*, 1959, *16*, 85–98.

Ades, H. W. Effects of extirpation of parstriate cortex on learned visual discrimination in monkeys. *Journal of Neuropathology and Experimental Neurology*, 1946, *5*, 60–66.

Ades, H. W., and Raab, D. H. Effects of preoccipital and temporal neodecortication on learned visual discrimination in monkeys. *Journal of Neurophysiology*, 1949, *12*, 101–108.

Barbas, H., and Spear, P. Effects of serial unilateral and serial bilateral visual cortex lesions on brightness discrimination relearning in rats. *Journal of Comparative and Physiological Psychology*, 1976, *90*, 279–292.

Butters, N., Butter, C., Rosen, J., and Stein, D. G. Behavioral effects of sequential and one-stage ablations of orbital prefrontal cortex in the monkey. *Experimental Neurology*, 1973, *39*, 204–214.

Cole, D. D., Sullins, W. R., and Isaac, W. Pharmacological modification of the effects of spaced occipital ablations. *Psychopharmacologia*, 1967, *11*, 311–316.

Dawson, R. G., Conrad, L., and Lynch, G. Single and two-stage hippocampal lesions: A similar syndrome. *Experimental Neurology*, 1973, *40*, 263–277.

Dru, D., Walker, J. P., and Walker, J. B. Self-produced locomotion restores visual capacity after striate lesions. *Science*, 1975, *187*, 265–266.

Ettlinger, G., and Kalsbeck, J. E. Changes in tactile discrimination and in visual reaching after successive and simultaneous bilateral posterior parietal ablations in the monkey. *Journal of Neurology, Neurosurgery and Psychiatry*, 1962, *25*, 256–268.

Fass, B., Jordan, H., Rubman, A., Seibel, S., and Stein, D. G. Recovery of function after serial or one-stage lesions of the lateral hypothalamic area in rats. *Behavioral Biology*, 1975, *14*, 283–294.

Finger, S. Lesion momentum and behavior. In S. Finger (Ed.), *Recovery from brain damage: Research and theory.* New York: Plenum, 1978, Pp. 135–164.

Finger, S., Marshak, R. A., Cohen, M., Scheff, S., Trace, R., and Neimand, D. Effects of successive and simultaneous lesions of somatosensory cortex on tactile discrimination in the rat. *Journal of Comparative and Physiological Psychology*, 1971, 77, 221–227.

Finger, S., and Reyes, R. Long-term deficits after somatosensory cortical lesions in rats. *Physiology and Behavior*, 1975, 15, 289–293.

Finger, S., and Simons, D. Effects of serial lesions of somatosensory cortex and further neodecortication on retention of a rough–smooth discrimination in rats. *Experimental Brain Research*, 1976, 25, 183–197.

Finger, S., Walbran, B., and Stein, D. G. Brain damage and behavioral recovery: Serial lesion phenomena. *Brain Research*, 1973, 63, 1–18.

Flourens, P. *Recherches Expérimentales sur les Propriétés et les Fonctions du Système Nerveux dans les Animaux Vertébrés*. Paris: Crevot, 1824, Pp. 85–122. Translated and reprinted in G. von Bonin, *Some papers on the cerebral cortex*. Springfield, Ill.: Charles C Thomas, 1960, Pp. 3–21.

Fuller, J. L. Experiential deprivation and later behavior. *Science*, 1967, 158, 1645–1652.

Glick, S. D., and Zimmerberg, B. Comparative recovery following simultaneous- and successive-stage frontal brain damage in mice. *Journal of Comparative and Physiological Psychology*, 1972, 79, 481–487.

Goldstein, K. *The organism*. New York: American Book Company, 1939.

Hart, B. L. Sequential medial preoptic-anterior hypothalamic lesions have same effects on copulatory behavior of male cats as simultaneous lesions. *Brain Research*, 1980, 185, 423–428.

Head, H. *Aphasia and kindred disorders of speech*. Cambridge: Cambridge University Press, 1926.

Isaacson, R. L., and Schmaltz, L. Failure to find savings from spaced two-stage destruction of hippocampus. *Communications in Behavioral Biology*, 1968, 1, 353–359.

Isseroff, A., Leveton, L., Freeman, G., Lewis, M. E., and Stein, D. G. Differences in the behavioral effects of single-stage and serial lesions of the hippocampus. *Experimental Neurology*, 1976, 53, 339–354.

Jackson, J. H. Lectures on the diagnosis of tumours of the brain. *Medical Times and Gazette*, 1873, 2, 139ff.

Jackson, J. H. On affection of speech from disease of the brain. *Brain*, 1879, 2, 323–356.

Jackson, J. H. Remarks on the dissolution of the nervous system as exemplified by certain post-epileptic conditions. *Medical Press and Circular*, 1881, 1, 329ff.

Jackson, J. H. The factors of insanities. *Medical Press and Circular*, 1894, 2, 615–619.

Joynt, R. J., and Benton, A. L. The memoir of Marc Dax on aphasia. *Neurology*, 1964, 14, 851–854.

Karplus, J. P., and Kreidl, A. Über total Exstirpationen einer und beider grosshirnhemisphären an affen (*Macacus rhesus*). *Archiv für Physiologie* (Leipzig), 1914, 38, 155–212.

Kesner, R. P., Fiedler, P., and Thomas, G. J. Function of the midbrain reticular formation in regulating level of activity and learning in rats. *Journal of Comparative and Physiological Psychology*, 1967, 63, 452–457.

Kleitman, N., and Camille, N. Studies on the physiology of sleep. VI. The behavior of decorticated dogs. *American Journal of Physiology*, 1932, 100, 474–480.

Lashley, K. S. *Brain mechanisms and intelligence*. Chicago: University of Chicago Press, 1929.

Lourie, H., Vanasupa, P., and O'Leary, J. Experimental observations upon chronic progressive lesions of the brain stem tegmentum and midline thalamus. *Surgical Forum*, 1960, 10, 756–760.

McIntyre, M., and Stein, D. G. Differential effects of one- vs. two-stage amygdaloid lesions on activity, exploratory and avoidance behavior in the albino rat. *Behavioral Biology*, 1973, 9, 454–466.

McKinley, J. C., and Berkowitz, N. J. Ridigity following ablation of the motor cortex in monkeys. *Journal of Nervous and Mental Disease*, 1933, 78, 604–626.

Meyer, D. R., Isaac, W., and Maher, B. The role of stimulation in spontaneous reorganization of visual habits. *Journal of Comparative and Physiological Psychology*, 1958, 51, 546–548.

Morgan, C. T. Some structural factors in perception. In R. R. Blake and G. V. Ramsey (Eds.), *Perception: An approach to personality*. New York: Ronald Press, 1951, Pp. 25–55.

Morrison, J. H., Molliver, M. E., and Grzanna, R. Noradrenergic innervation of cerebral cortex: Widespread effects of local cortical lesions. *Science*, 1979, *205*, 313–316.

Patrissi, G., and Stein, D. G. Temporal factors in recovery of function after brain damage. *Experimental Neurology*, 1975, *47*, 470–480.

Pujol, J. F., Stein, D. G., Blondaux, C., Pettijean, F., Froment, J. L., and Jouvet M. Biochemical evidence for interaction phenomena between noradrenergic and serotonergic systems in the cat brain. *Frontiers in Catecholamine Research*, 1973, *3*, 771–772.

Reyes, R. *Effects of interlesion interval and postoperative recovery period on recovery of function following serial lesions of somatic cortex in rats*. Unpublished doctoral dissertation, Washington University, 1977.

Riese, W. Aphasia in brain tumors. *Confinia Neurologica*, 1948, *9*, 64–79.

Riese, W. Principles of neurology in the light of history and their present use. *Nervous and Mental Disease Monographs*. New York, 1950.

Rosen, J., Stein, D., and Butters, N. Recovery of function after serial ablation of prefrontal cortex in the rhesus monkey. *Science*, 1971, *173*, 353–356.

Scheff, S., and Wright, D. C. Behavioral and electrophysiological evidence for cortical reorganization of function in rats with serial lesions of the visual cortex. *Physiological Psychology*, 1976, *5*, 103–107.

Schultze, M., and Stein, D. G. Recovery of function in the albino rat following either simultaneous or seriatum lesions of the caudate nucleus. *Experimental Neurology*, 1975, *46*, 291–301.

Simons, D., Puretz, J., and Finger, S. Effects of serial lesions of somatosensory cortex and futher neodecortication on tactile retention in rats. *Experimental Brain Research*, 1975, *23*, 353–366.

Stein, D. G. Some variables influencing recovery of function in the rat. In D. G. Stein, J. Rosen, and N. Butters (Eds.), *CNS plasticity: Recovery of function*. New York: Academic Press, 1974, Pp. 373–428.

Stein, D. G., Rosen, J. J., Graziadei, J., Mishkin, D., and Brink, J. Central nervous system: Recovery of function. *Science*, 1969, *166*, 528–530.

Stewart, J. W., and Ades, H. W. The time factor in reintegration of a learned habit after temporal lobe lesions in the monkey (*Macaca mulatta*). *Journal of Comparative and Physiological Psychology*, 1951, *44*, 479–486.

Travis, A. M., and Woolsey, C. N. Motor performance of monkeys after bilateral partial and total cerebral decortications. *American Journal of Physical Medicine*, 1956, *35*, 273–310.

Treichler, R. F. Two-stage frontal lesion influences upon severity of delayed-response deficit. *Behavioral Biology*, 1975, *13*, 35–47.

von Monokow, C. *Gehirnpathologie*. Vienna: Hölder, 1897.

von Monokow, C. *Die lokalisation im grosshirn und der abbau der funktion durch kortikale herde*. Wiesbaden: J. F. Bergmann, 1914. Translated and excerpted by G. Harris in K. H. Pribram (Ed.), *Mood, states and mind*. London: Penguin, 1969, Pp, 27–37.

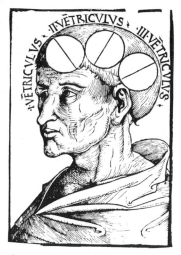

Environmental and Experiential Determinants of Recovery of Function

Education consists of modifications in the central nervous system. For this experience, the cell elements are peculiarly fitted. They are plastic in the sense that their connections are not rigidly fixed, and they remember. . . . By virtue of these powers, the cells can adjust themselves to new surroundings [Donaldson, 1895, p. 336].

CHAPTER TEN

Henry Donaldson, for some years a member of the faculty at Clark University, and later in his career, professor of neurology at the University of Chicago, made the above statement during a time of considerable scientific turmoil, especially when it came to the issue of the relative contributions of heredity and environment in determining behavior. While some individuals stressed the role of lineage in accounting for particular abilities and capacities, others emphasized the importance of experience in guiding the development of a wide range of attributes, and even some of the same traits (e.g., musical abilities, mathematics) that their contemporaries were quick to interpret as due to heredity. Especially in America, where "everyman," in principle, could attain the highest pinnacles of success, there was "a firm belief in the almost limitless efficacy of education [Oppenheim, 1979, p. 533]." The exercise of the "mind" through education and enrichment was likened to the exercise of muscles and glands. If the latter were enlarged by repeated use, could not the brain be expected to respond in similar fashion?

Henry Donaldson was more than a passive observer and commentator when it came to the "nature versus nurture" debate. One of the first attempts to determine whether experience could affect the brain was his case study of Laura Bridgeman (see Oppenheim, 1979). At 2 years of age, she suffered a severe attack of scarlet fever and subsequently lost her ability to see and hear. There were also severe impairments of smell and taste. Despite these terrible handicaps, Miss Bridgeman learned to communicate through sign language, and during her extraordinary lifetime was the author of a journal, three autobiographical sketches, and numerous poems and letters. Upon her death, at 60 years of age, Donaldson undertook the first known systematic attempt to evaluate Laura's brain in order to determine whether the sensory deprivation she suffered could be correlated with anatomical alterations. Donaldson found marked abnormalities in the auditory and visual areas; anomalies that he attributed to years of sensory restriction and disuse (Donaldson, 1891).

The question of the role of the environment in guiding behavior never really lost its emotional charge, especially in the United States with the rise of Behaviorism at about the time of World War I.[1] Nevertheless, more attention was not given to brain changes that might be affected by the nature and degree of the environmental stimulation until 1949 when Donald Hebb, of McGill University, conducted an informal experiment in his own house that pointed to the potential importance of experiential factors in determining "intelligence." In a sense, Hebb looked at the other side of the coin when he asked whether performance could be *improved* by providing laboratory rats with more than a routine existence of semi-isolation in small, barren metal cages.

In his famous monograph, *The Organization of Behavior* (1949), Hebb reviewed and interpreted his maze learning experiment:

> Two litters were taken home to be reared as pets. . . . While this was being done, 25 cage-reared rats from the same colony were tested. When the pet group was tested, all 7 scored in the top third of the total distribution for cage-reared and pets. More important still, the pets improved their relative standing in the last 10 days of testing. . . . one explanation of the better scores of the pets is just that they were tamer, more used to handling, and less disturbed by testing. But if this were so, the longer the cage-reared animals were worked with, the closer they would come to the pet group, as the cage-reared became tamer with prolonged handling. On the contrary, the pets improved more than the cage-reared. This means that *the richer experience of the pet group during development made them better able to profit by new experiences at maturity—one of the characteristics of the "intelligent" human being* [pp. 298–299].

Hebb's rather informal study, and the ideas and conclusions about neural connectivity that he went on to draw from it, clearly challenged the imagination of many scientists and professionals who were quick to agree with him about the potential importance of his findings. But could Hebb's behavioral results be confirmed under more highly controlled testing conditions? And would data from white rats really be applicable to certain human situations, such as the conditions

---

[1] John B. Watson, the founder of *Behaviorism* in 1913, flatly denied the existence of native intelligence, instincts, and "gifts" of nature. He claimed that special talents are strictly the result of environment and training. It is in this context that he came forth with his famous quotation (1925): "Give me a dozen healthy infants, well formed, and my own specified world to bring them up in and I'll guarantee to take any one at random and train him to become any type of specialist I might select—doctor, lawyer, artist, merchant-chief and, yes, even beggar-man and thief, regardless of his talents, penchants, tendencies, abilities, vocations, and race of his ancestors [p. 82]."

under which children were being cared for in foundling homes, orphanages, and hospitals?

To answer questions such as these, a number of systematic experiments were performed. In one study (Forgays and Forgays, 1952) young laboratory rats were assigned to small or large laboratory cages. Some animals were also permitted access to "toys" and objects that could be seen, manipulated, crawled through, and explored. Sixty days later, all of the animals were tested on a series of relatively simple mazes, like those shown in Figure 10.1, to determine whether there would be changes in learning as a function of the different environments. In confirmation of Hebb's results, the rats brought up in the larger cages proved to be better maze learners than those raised under more restricted conditions, and the animals in the large cage group that also had access to the additional toys and objects were the best performers of all.

Although findings such as these are most powerful and replicable when "enrichment" takes place just after weaning, problem-solving performance may also be affected by the level of environmental complexity that is experienced even before the time of weaning (see Denenberg, Woodcock, and Rosenberg, 1968) and sometimes even much later in life. Moreover, findings comparable to those on rats have now been reported with a wide variety of other animals that are commonly used in laboratory investigations. And, as one might predict, household pets, such as cats and dogs, have now repeatedly been found to be superior learners to animals raised in university and medical laboratories under more confined conditions (cf. Beach and Jaynes, 1954; Thompson and Grusec, 1970).

These behavioral observations do have relevance to man. For instance, in 1966, it was reported that children who were given mobiles and brightly colored patterned sheets and bumpers on their cribs and who received increased handling displayed successful visually guided reaching for targets approximately 45 days

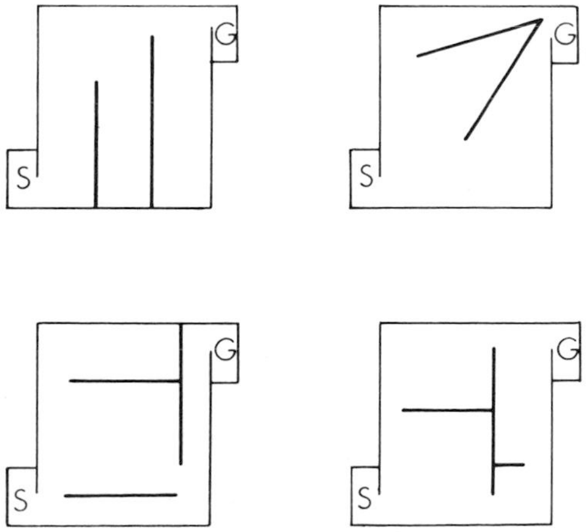

Figure 10.1. *Four mazes from the series described by Hebb and Williams (1946). These mazes have been used to study the effects of environmental complexity on problem-solving abilities. Rabinovich and Rosvold (1951) modified the patterns and standardized the procedures for testing rats in these mazes. (S, start area; G, goal box.) (From Finger, 1978.)*

sooner than children who formed less stimulated control groups (White and Held, 1966). In addition, in one notable study, a small group of children was taken from a rather "sterile" foundling home and placed with mentally retarded girls in a setting where they received physical care, love, attention, and stimulation. At the time the children left the foundling home, where only physical care was really provided, their IQ's were in the 60s. Intelligence test scores rose to relatively normal levels as they matured in the more stimulating environments, and many years later these children were for the most part leading normal, productive lives. By comparison, most of the unfortunate children who did not get to leave the foundling home had to be cared for in institutions of one sort or another as adults (Skeels, 1966).

Research like this, and studies in which institutionalized children are assigned "foster grandparents" (Salz, 1973) have shed some light on a syndrome called *hospitalism,* that is, the failure of babies to thrive in institutions. This syndrome was first attributed to poor nutrition and then to infection, although it now seems to be due primarily to inadequate stimulation, manipulation, and contact; conditions that can be improved by changing the nature and the quality of the environment. In America, as early as 1915, Henry Chapin urged that babies, if at all possible, should be "boarded out" in homes rather than being kept in institutions (see Bakwin, 1949). His idea now seems to have strong empirical support.

The assertion that the nature and level of environmental stimulation can modify the anatomy and physiology of the brain also has received broad, new support. This support has come from experiments in which the effects of rearing and housing under "enriched," as well as restricted, conditions are compared to the consequences of experiencing "standard" laboratory environments.

William Greenough and his students at the University of Illinois have been very active in assessing some of the anatomical correlates of environmental complexity. In a series of relatively recent papers, they reported that rats raised in stimulating environments show increased dendritic branching in selected cortical and subcortical sites relative to animals raised under more typical laboratory conditions (Greenough, 1975). The Illinois group also observed that animals from "enriched" environments have larger synaptic boutons than control animals (West and Greenough, 1972). Earlier studies had shown that significant differences in cortical depth and weight are also usually found between these different environmental groups (e.g., Bennett, Rosenzweig, and Diamond, 1969).

The physiological changes that accompany enrichment have been emphasized by a multidisciplinary group of workers from the University of California at Berkeley, headed at the present time by Mark Rosenzweig. These investigators found differences in RNA–DNA ratios between enriched and more restricted animals, as well as a wide variety of brain emzymatic differences (acetylcholinesterase levels, etc.) that appear to reflect various environmental conditions (Bennett, Diamond, Krech, and Rosenzweig, 1964; Rosenzweig, 1971; Rosenzweig, Bennett, and Diamond, 1972). The Berkeley investigators have always maintained that the brain changes that they are studying are not just due to some artifact, such as the enriched animals having an opportunity for greater activity. Instead, they stress the importance of *active interactions* with the enriched environment itself. These workers also argue that many of the brain changes that accompany enrichment are not confined to cases where stimulation is provided very early in life, although it is possible that *some* of the anatomical changes may be age-dependent (see Greenough, 1975). In the context of their own maze learning studies and all of the other work in this field, the results of these experiments provide strong support for the contention that the central nervous system can be modified by the environment, and for the idea that subjects raised under different conditions differ both behaviorally and biologically.

The fact that environmental complexity can affect anatomy, physiology, and behavior is not just of passing interest to individuals concerned with recovery of function after brain damage. The question that is being raised is whether the environment can also modify certain brain lesion symptoms and syndromes and whether it can enhance or retard the recovery process (see review by Finger, 1978). After all, if it can be accepted that the brains of two individuals differ in terms of such things as the size and number of synapses, why should it be assumed that these two subjects will respond in precisely the same ways to brain damage? But is there good evidence to suggest that environmental complexity can account for some of the "individual differences" that are observed in our clinics and hospitals? And are we at a stage where environmental factors can lead to certain predictions about how particular individuals might be affected by specific brain injuries?

The experimental literature on the interaction between the level of environmental stimulation and the response to brain damage is still very small, but it is suggestive. In short, the environmental variable has been examined at least a few times in each of three different contexts, and the results, although not uniform, show that it clearly can be a significant factor in understanding the diversity of responses to brain damage. The paradigms illustrating this have involved (*a*) environmental enrichment prior to brain damage, a situation in which the "protective" role of the environment is assessed; (*b*) enriching the environment after brain damage to see if it can be a "therapy" for brain dysfunction; and (*c*) providing different environments between successive lesions to see how this might affect the "serial lesion effect," which was examined in the previous chapter. These designs are shown diagramatically in Table 10.1.

The "protective" value of environmental enrichment in cases of brain injury was first studied by Charles Smith (1959). One group of rats was reared in a large arena containing tunnels, barriers, and various objects that they could manipulate and explore. Another was housed individually in small "isolation" cages, typical of most laboratory colonies. After being kept under one or the other condition from 18 to 90 days, some were subjected to lesions of the anterior or posterior cortex. When the previously enriched and restricted groups subse-

Table 10.1
Three Basic Designs for Assessing the Effects of Environmental Variables on Brain-Lesion Syndromes[a]

Prelesion manipulation	Postlesion manipulation	Serial-lesion manipulation
Different environments	Identical environments	Identical environments
↓	↓	↓
Surgery	Surgery	Surgery 1
↓	↓	↓
Testing	Different environments	Different environments
	↓	↓
	Testing	Surgery 2
		↓
		Testing

[a]From Finger, 1978.

quently were tested on a series of mazes (Hebb and Williams, 1946), Smith found that the groups given enrichment made fewer errors on the problems than those who were restricted and that many of the animals with cortical lesions that were permitted enrichment performed *even better than control subjects* without brain damage that were reared in the small, isolated cages. This can be seen in Figure 10.2.

A few years after this report appeared, Kenneth Hughes (1965) showed that the protective potential of enrichment was not restricted to cases of cerebral cortex damage. He performed an experiment roughly comparable to that of Smith, but one in which he limited the stimulating environment to a 27-day period starting immediately after weaning. When Hughes then damaged the dorsal hippocampus, he found the lesion effects to be less severe among the enriched animals. Unlike Smith, his operated animals did not perform in the control group range. In fact, as shown in Figure 10.3, the different environments hardly affected control group performance in this study, but this may have been due to the simplicity of the task for unoperated animals in general.

Other investigators have now shown that the beneficial effects of preoperative enrichment are not just limited to maze learning. This was demonstrated by Peter Donovick and his co-workers (Donovick, Burright, and Swidler, 1973) in an experiment involving rats that sustained lesions of the septal forebrain. These investigators first reared rats from 25 days of age in enriched or isolated environments and then gave some septal lesions. The brain-damaged rats from the unstimulating conditions were found to drink and explore less than those that were housed in the enriched environment. However, on a spatial alternation task,

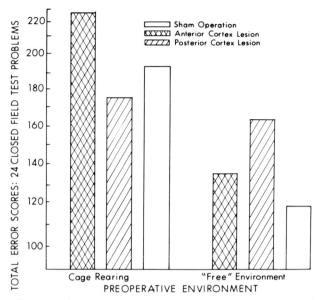

Figure 10.2. *Performance of six groups of rats on the Hebb-Williams test of "animal intelligence." Data taken from Smith (1959). (Although most animals in each group were operated upon on Days 95–100, some had surgery on Days 20–25. Smith pooled this factor when presenting the data shown here since age differences failed to approach statistical significance.) (From Finger, 1978.)*

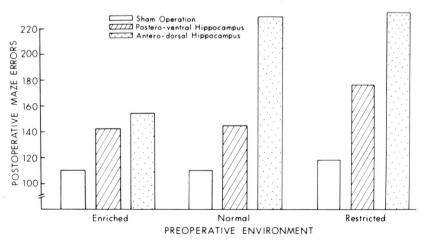

Figure 10.3. *Performance of nine groups of rats on a series of Hebb-Williams mazes. (Data taken from Hughes, 1965; from Finger, 1978.)*

there was no particular benefit to being raised in the enriched condition prior to septal surgery.

More recently, Michael Lewis (1975) noted that manipulation of environmental complexity could produce differences in emotionality (biting, vocalizing, responsiveness to handling, etc.) and weight gain in rats with large, one-stage lesions of the hippocampus. But he, like Donovick and his co-workers, reported little effect of enrichment on a spatial learning task.

In summary, the hypothesis that enrichment prior to brain injury can be "protective" has good support from studies examining maze learning and motivational and emotional factors. The failures to find any effects of complex environments on some learned behaviors (spatial alternation) in brain-damaged animals is noteworthy, but such failures must be considered in the context of additional variables, such as the task and age of the subject, and more importantly, the size and locus of the lesion. Such factors could override any of the beneficial effects of the exposure to complex environments, but as of yet, variables like these have not received much attention as elements in their own right in these experiments.

Enhanced sensory stimulation following brain damage can also be an effective therapy under the right conditions, and possibly because of its potential for clinical treatment, postoperative environmental manipulations have been studied a bit more than preoperative environmental factors.

Because the young brain generally is more responsive to experiential manipulations, Saul Schwartz (1964) created posterior cortical lesions in 1-day-old rats and then placed the animals in complex environments until they reached maturity. The rats were then tested on the Hebb-Williams maze series that others had used in the "protective" paradigm, and performance was compared to littermates reared under more isolated housing conditions. As shown in Figure 10.4, Schwartz found that the brain-damaged rats placed postoperatively in the complex environment were superior in learning to traditionally reared littermates. As had been noted by Smith, using the "protection" paradigm, the rats with lesions that were placed in the complex environment early in life performed even better than *unoperated* rats that were reared under more barren conditions.

Is the same degree of protection afforded to subjects placed in complex environments following brain damage at maturity? This important question was explored by Bruno Will and Mark Rosenzweig in 1976. Rats were given occipital cortex lesions or sham operations when they were 4 months old and then were housed in large group cages with a variety of stimulus objects or in small individual cages that minimized perceptual learning and motor exploration. The rats remained in their complex or isolated environments for 2 months and then were tested on the Hebb-Williams problems. Will and Rosenzweig found that postoperative exposure to the enriched conditions significantly improved the scores of both the brain-damaged and control groups. A short time later, Bruno Will and his colleagues in Strasbourg, France extended this finding to rats operated upon at 30

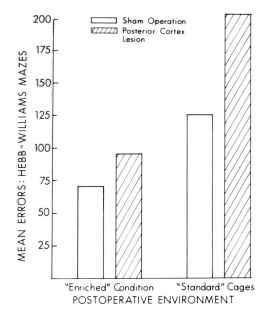

Figure 10.4. *Data collected by Schwartz (1964) on housing rats postoperatively in one of two environments prior to testing them on a series of maze problems. (From Finger, 1978.)*

days of age (Will, Rosenzweig, Bennett, Herbert, and Morimoto, 1977). These workers showed that 2 hours per day of postoperative enrichment is sufficient to produce effects as large as those seen with continuous exposure to complex environments. In the latter study, rats with posterior cortical lesions benefitted more than the sham operated animals from the enrichment experience.

Kelche and Will (1978) have now examined the effects of enrichment on maze learning after hippocampal lesions in adult rats. They damaged the dorsal hippocampi of 120-day-old rats, placed them in enriched or impoverished environments for 60 days, and then tested the animals on twelve Hebb-Williams maze problems. Nonoperated rats learned the tasks faster than those with lesions, but rats exposed to the complex environment following surgery were much better than brain-damaged rats *not* given the "therapy." This is shown in Figure 10.5.

Although these findings support the contention that postoperative enrichment can facilitate recovery from brain damage, there have also been failures to find any beneficial effects of exposure to stimulus complexity among brain-damaged animals. For instance, the performance of adult rats with posterior cortical lesions is not improved when the animals are required to discriminate among different visual patterns (Bland and Cooper, 1969, 1970). In general, it seems that complex environments can best facilitate recovery from brain damage on maze learning tasks where the subject can use multiple cues and strategies to reach a goal. When the task requires a specific sensory modality, such as discriminating between visual patterns, exposure to enriched environments is less successful. One of us recently proposed that "nonspecific environmental enrichment may be

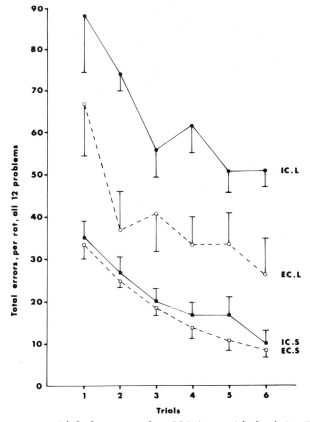

Figure 10.5. *Errors across trials for four groups of rats. IC.L, impoverished × lesion; EC.L, enriched × lesion; IC.S, impoverished × sham operation; EC.S, enriched × sham operation. (Reprinted with permission from Kelche, C. R., and Will, B. E. Effets de l'environnement sur la restauration fonctionnelle après lésions hippocampiques chez des rats adultes.* Physiology and Behavior. *Copyright 1978, Pergamon Press, Ltd.)*

affecting a general factor or a host of specific factors which may relate to the 'general adaptive capacity' of the organism; i.e., its ability to respond appropriately to, and to cope with, a variety of situations and problems of a general nature [Finger, 1978, p. 314]."

Thus, large or complete lesions occurring in specific, sensory areas of the central nervous system would prevent organisms from using the only sensory channel providing information relevant to solving the problem—as could be the case with tactile or pattern discriminations. But in a maze learning situation, animals often use a variety of intra- and extramaze cues (e.g., proprioceptive, vestibular, olfactory, and visual) so that a focal cortical lesion will not completely eliminate the various sensory systems. Under these conditions, the brain-damaged animals that had the enriched experience may be able to switch strategies and sensory cues more readily than would their counterparts raised in isolation who might explore less, and exhibit a greater tendency for perseveration in such a situation.

We must also consider the issue of task difficulty in evaluating the influence of exposure to complex environments, or any other factor for that matter, on recovery from brain injury. For example, in the learning part of the study by Donovick, Burright, and Swidler (1973), the spatial alternation task was so difficult for the rats with septal damage that there was very little above-chance performance among any of the animals with lesions, whereas in the learning part of the study by Lewis (1975) most of the rats with hippocampal lesions were performing as well as the unoperated control animals, regardless of whether they were raised in enriched or deprived environments. These results can be taken to imply that the effects of enrichment are also dependent upon task difficulty (and locus of lesion), with the best chance of a lesion–environment interaction effect occurring when the task is neither too easy nor too difficult for the brain-damaged animals.

As mentioned previously, environments can also differ during the "interlesion interval" of a two-stage operation (see Chapter 9). Stimulation here has also been reported to facilitate recovery from central nervous system injuries, and deprivation between surgeries is now known to impair such recovery. In some cases, differences have been found with no more than simple changes in illumination. Yet even this manipulation seems to have significant consequences. As we have seen, Donald Meyer and his associates (Meyer, Isaac, and Maher, 1958) conditioned rats to jump across a barrier when a light was turned on and found that one-stage, bilateral lesions of the posterior cortex eliminated this behavior. But when the lesions were made in two stages and the animals were kept in a lighted room between the two operations, the habit was not lost even after the second operation. (Rats given two-stage lesions and kept in the dark were as impaired as one-stage operated animals.) Meyer's study clearly shows that serial lesions can facilitate recovery, but only when combined with adequate environmental stimulation, in this case, room illumination.

In a related experiment by Dru, Walker, and Walker (1975), adult, hooded rats were also subjected to two-stage lesions of the visual cortex. One group of animals was permitted 4 hours of unrestrained movements in a patterned visual environment during the interoperative interval of 11 days. A second group of rats received the serial surgery and was kept in the dark; a third was given diffuse light; and a fourth was passively transported through the patterned environment for the 4-hour period. After this experience, all of the animals were trained on a horizontal versus vertical stripe discrimination task. In brief, only the rats that could freely move about the patterned environment showed recovery of visual functions; the animals passively exposed to this environment were just as impaired as rats kept in the dark. Thus, passively experiencing a complex environment may not be sufficient for recovery of function. This, in fact, would be predicted on the basis of the biochemical and anatomical findings obtained by Ferchmin, Bennett, and Rosenzweig (1975). Using "observer" rats, they found that active contact with the enriched environment was necessary for the brain changes associated with enrichment to appear.

We cannot specify the degree to which enrichment effects in laboratory rats have their parallels in the human clinical literature. Harry Harlow (1949), of the University of Wisconsin, once argued that experiential factors could account for individual differences among people with arteriosclerosis, and, citing some data collected in 1935 by Gilbert, he took the position that educated people may show less deterioration with advancing age than uneducated people. However, Sidney Weinstein and Hans-Lukas Teuber (1957) examined Army Intelligence Test scores of soldiers before and after brain damage and were unable to support the hypothesis that the men with the most education would show the smallest declines in intelligence after injury, so the question still remains open.

Until recently, one of the major difficulties in attempting to assess the effects of experience on recovery from brain damage in people seems largely to have been overlooked. Specifically, nonstimulating environments rarely, if ever, exist in isolation from other factors that are also known to affect brain and behavior. For example, one variable that typically interacts with environmental deprivation in people is poor nutrition, and studies that attempt to separate undernutrition and environmental effects are not very common. Such factors, along with increased susceptability to diseases such as gastroenteritis, typically form a "poverty syndrome" that is associated with fewer brain cells, smaller brain size and weight, apathy, and mental deficiency, at least when young children are affected (see Winick, 1976). Some of these effects are shown in Figures 10.6 and 10.7.

The entangling interaction of environmental with nutritional factors can be seen in an investigation by M. B. Stoch and P. M. Smythe (1963) which, unfortunately, is written and frequently cited as if malnutrition were the only determinant of the results. These investigators attempted to compare South African children with a history of malnutrition to those with no such history. Although the investigators were able to match the different nutritional groups in terms of age, race, and sex, the children in the two groups still differed in terms of the level of education of the parents, socioeconomic status of the family, and in that only the better nourished group attended an all-day nursery. Stoch and Smythe observed differences in head circumference (which they associated with brain size), body weight, height, and intelligence test scores and claimed that they were due to nutrition during infancy. But, as we have seen, some of these effects could also be due to obvious differences in the quality and levels of environmental stimulation. It is highly probable that both nutritional and environmental factors combined to produce the severe deficits seen in this study.

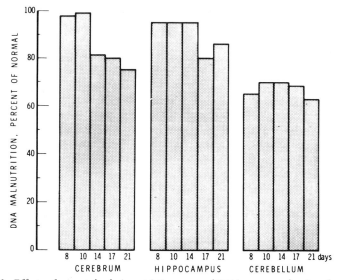

Figure 10.6. *Effects of neonatal caloric restriction on total DNA content of various brain regions. (From Winick, W.* Malnutrition and Brain Development, 1976. *With permission from Oxford University Press. Reprinted from Federation Proc. 29:1510–1515; 1970.)*

Is it really possible to keep nutrition constant while the environment varies, or the environment constant while nutrition varies, in studies of human behavior? Probably not to most people's satisfaction, but one strategy that has been employed in this endeavor involves the testing of two or more children from the

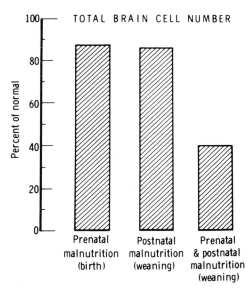

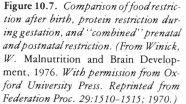

Figure 10.7. *Comparison of food restriction after birth, protein restriction during gestation, and "combined" prenatal and postnatal restriction. (From Winick, W.* Malnutrition and Brain Development, 1976. *With permission from Oxford University Press. Reprinted from Federation Proc. 29:1510–1515; 1970.)*

same family where only one has been affected by undernutrition. This approach can be seen in a number of reports (e.g., Hertzig, Birch, Richardson, and Tizard, 1972; Richardson, Birch, and Hertzig, 1973). One of the findings to come out of these investigations is that even with nutritional "rehabilitation," the behavioral and biological effects *of early malnutrition* may persist for many years and, in some cases, throughout life. Still, there are problems with even this research strategy. In particular, malnourished children may spend a fair amount of time in institutions and be kept from interacting with friends and family, or, if kept at home, they may be so apathetic that they may not be capable of actively interacting with individuals or the potentially stimulating environment. Even with siblings as matched controls, environmental differences could still be contributing to the results of these studies in a significant way.

Research on undernourished families, where both nutritional and environmental stimulation are inadequate, has to be of great interest to all of us because of the wide extent of the problem, the suffering involved, and the tremendous burden that society must absorb in terms of welfare, institutionalization, special schooling, and an ultimately diminished labor force. For these reasons in particular, various therapeutic interventions have been attempted to enhance recovery in these unfortunate cases. We now know, for instance, that the severity of the behavioral and biological effects of starvation can be lessened if adequate nutrition is resumed while the brain is still rapidly growing, that is, during a critical period early in life.

With these children, adequate nutrition, as a therapy, may be only one component of an effective treatment program. Observations of undernourished children are now showing that recovery can be greater when adequate nutrition is combined with a stimulating environment and that some behavioral effects previously attributed to malnutrition alone can be at least partially offset by rich environmental stimulation at the time of, or soon after, the period of undernutrition.

In one study, the effects of the early malnutrition complex were almost completely overcome when Korean infants were adopted into high socioeconomic families in the United States (Winick, Meyer, and Harris, 1975). Moreover, during the Dutch famine of 1944–1945, diets were restricted to as little as 25% of the normal number of calories, but children born during the famine were found to have normal intelligence test scores when they were screened for the Army 19 years later (Stein, Susser, Saenger, and Marolla, 1972). Presumably, the stimulation that these children received helped them to compensate for their nutritional deficiencies.

In the laboratory, where nutritional and environmental factors can be better controlled, Gilfred Tanabe (1972), of the University of Hawaii, restricted the diets of female rats by 50% throughout the prenatal and nursing periods. (This amount of undernutrition can markedly affect the brains of the pups.) He then put half of the undernourished young animals in enriched group cages for about 1 month, after which all animals were placed in individual holding cages. At 100 days of age, the rats were tested on the Hebb-Williams series of mazes. It was found that the malnourished animals that were exposed to the enriched environments outperformed their matched counterparts. As stated by Tanabe, "These results clearly indicate that offspring maze deficiencies due to prenatal and postnatal maternal food restriction can be remedied in an enriched environment [p. 224]." Tanabe's general findings have also been seen in experiments from other laboratories, including some in which enrichment was given at the same time as the postnatal undernutrition (Levitsky and Barnes, 1972; Wells, Geist, and Zimmerman, 1972). Together, these investigations suggest that good nutrition and stimulating environments combine to produce the healthiest organisms and that the effects of malnutrition can at least in part be overcome with *environmental* "therapy" that begins relatively early in life.

It now seems clear that the environment is an important factor that can affect the results of brain lesion studies, whether the lesions are acute, as those made when ablating parts of the cortex in laboratory animals, or more naturally occurring events, such as those that are associated with early malnutrition. Nevertheless, why nonspecific environmental stimulation should be both protective and therapeutic is an unresolved issue. As noted earlier, some researchers working with laboratory animals seem to believe that the structural and biochemical changes that follow enrichment play a role. The opinion shared by many of these investigators is that the enriched subjects have developed functional neural circuitry that the restricted subjects do not have and that this enables them to outperform their counterparts on a variety of problems. The additional circuitry may provide them with a greater capacity for reorganization after brain lesions, or, as most people now believe, it may allow these subjects to utilize existing connections, established independently of the injury, to perform better on certain kinds of tasks.[2] Whatever explanations might be given for the results in these ex-

---

[2] Although anatomical and biochemical changes have been associated with enrichment, other explanations must also be considered when attempting to account for the findings with brain-damaged subjects. It is possible to argue that the only reason that these subjects do better is because they have richer learning histories, which include "elements" that can transfer directly to the testing situations. In the animal field, for example, a simple maze might seem more familiar to a rat raised in an enriched environment containing walls, barriers, and tunnels that can be explored, than it would to a rat raised in a barren cage whose past history might not include any objects to manipulate and examine. This being the case, the enriched animal would be able to draw upon its learning history to master the problem rapidly whereas no such advantage would be conferred upon the restricted animal (see Finger, 1978). In addition, differences in emotionality have been noted between enriched and restricted subjects of many species, including man, and these factors could play a role in how a subject performs in learning and novel situations. In this context, notions such as Fuller's (1967) *emergence as stress* concept may shed some light on the behavioral data without reference to anatomical and physiological differences that may, in fact, exist among the groups.

periments, it is clear that nonspecific environmental enrichment can, under certain conditions, aid in the recovery process, or, if one wishes to take the opposite view, that barren, unstimulating conditions can limit the recovery potential of the organism.

In the larger scheme of things, enriched environments and nutritional histories represent only two kinds of experimental factors that can account for differences in performances after brain damage. Although our purpose is not to review every experiential variable that has the potential to affect brain damage and recovery, mention should be made of at least a few of the other factors that have been studied.

The degree to which material is learned prior to brain damage represents one such factor, and in one aspect of this literature, the key words, which appear to be used interchangeably, are *overlearning* and *overtraining*. The use of either of these words means that after a reasonable criterion for mastery of a task has been achieved, additional trials are required of the subject. For example, learning may be defined as being able to recite a poem two times in a row without a single error. Overtraining in such a situation may involve the addition of 20 or 50 or 100 more recitations of the poem after the criterion has been attained. Actually, overtraining can be defined in two different ways, and giving a constant number of postcriterion trials represents just one of the procedures that can be used. The other is to give an additional percentage of trials after criterion is met, so that slow learners may have more actual trials during the overtraining period than fast learners. Thus, if one subject takes 25 trials to learn and another takes 30, 100% overtraining would involve giving the first subject an additional 25 trials and the second subject an additional 30 trials. Two hundred percent overtraining would mean that 50 and 60 trials are given, respectively.

Investigators interested in learning phenomena have repeatedly shown that overtraining often leads to better retention than just training to a criterion of mastery, and with animals, it also seems to permit more rapid habit reversals than training to criterion (cf. Mackintosh, 1974; Paul, 1965; Sperling, 1965). But how might this affect the performance of brain damaged subjects? Could overtraining be doing something like permitting greater and more widespread duplication of the memory so that the probability would be greatly reduced that memory would be affected by a limited, focal lesion? Or could it in some unknown way be permitting easier access to the same memory stores that nonovertrained subjects might have?

As it presently stands, we do not know the answers to these questions, although, in at least a few cases, brain lesion effects have been circumvented or lessened as a result of preoperative overtraining. Kao Liang Chow and James Survis (1958) and J. L. Orbach and R. L. Fantz (1958) reported that overtraining strongly aids visual retention following temporal neocortical ablations in young monkeys. In these experiments, more than one type of visual problem was presented to the animals before surgery. The monkeys in the Orbach and Fantz study learned a red versus green discrimination, a light versus dark discrimination, and a diamond versus stripes problem in the preoperative period. The animals differed in terms of which problem was overtrained, and additional trials varied from 245 to 1000 in the two studies. In this investigation the overtraining trials came on one of the problems after all of the tasks were first learned, although in the Chow and Survis experiment, overtraining was instituted immediately after criterion was reached on one of the discriminations.

The findings in these two studies were comparable. The time between learning a problem and cortical surgery was not a determinant of retention, whereas which problem was overtrained clearly affected postoperative performance. In fact, the overtrained problem usually was retained perfectly, even though the other problems may have required more trials postoperatively than was needed for original learning in the preoperative period. The effects of overtraining thus appeared to be very beneficial, but at the same time very specific, with minimal carry-over to related but different visual discriminations. This can be seen in Table 10.2.

Table 10.2
Learning Scores on Visual Discriminations[a]

Task	Subjects	Number of trials		
		Initial learning	Preoperative retention and overtraining	Postoperative relearning
Color	1	40	0	0
	2	123	0	0
	3	210	—	91
	4	60	—	43
	5	71	—	31
	6	62	—	10
Brightness	1	216	—	48
	2	120	—	93
	3	70	18	0
	4	225	0	109
	5	156	—	60
	6	60	—	63
Pattern	1	73	—	66
	2	40	—	94
	3	46	—	245[b]
	4	41	—	245[b]
	5	93	16	2
	6	48	30	0

[a] From Orbach, J., and Fantz, R. L. *Differential effects of temporal neo-cortical resections on overtrained and non-overtrained visual habits in monkeys.* Journal of Comparative and Physiological Psychology 1958, 51, 126–129. *Copyright 1958 by the American Psychological Association. Reprinted/adapted by permission of the author.*

[b] Subjects 3 and 4 did not meet the criterion within the specified number of trials.

Another example of recovery of function following overtraining in brain-damaged animals can be found in an experiment conducted by some of us at Washington University (Weese, Neimand, and Finger, 1973). In this study, one group of rats was kept in their home cages until testing, whereas a second group was trained to criterion on a ridge-smooth tactile discrimination. A third group was trained to the same criterion and given 100% overtraining on that discrimination. After this, one half of the rats in each of the three groups then received large, but incomplete lesions of the somatosensory cortex (damage was centered in the first projection zone), whereas the remainder received sham operations. All of the animals were then tested to the same stringent criterion on the identical tactile stimuli that had been employed in the first part of the study (see Figure 10.8).

When no pretraining was given, the sham operated rats were much more successful in learning the task than those with cortical lesions. When the animals were trained to criterion, but not beyond, the sham group was still better, although lesion group scores improved. In contrast to these results, no lesion effect appeared among the overtrained groups where seven of the nine animals with ablations performed well within the control group range. Although the sham operated animals did not seem to improve any further with overtraining, the animals with lesions clearly did; in all but two cases, their deficits were no longer noticeable.

That the effects of overtraining may be specific to the overtrained task, and not to closely related problems, was mentioned previously in the context of the monkey studies on the temporal neocortex, and further support for this position was noted in an extension of the aforementioned investigation. Here, Weese, Neimand, and Finger went on to test the animals on a second, more difficult tactile problem that was not experienced before. Under these conditions, all of the groups with lesions performed worse than their respective control groups and no differently from each other, despite the fact that the animals had different amounts of experience on a related, but easier, tactile discrimination.

The ability of preoperative overtraining to attenuate some lesion effects is not restricted to instances of cortical damage. As a case in point, preoperative overtraining was found to facilitate postoperative retention of a visual pattern discrimination in rats that sustained brain-stem lesions in the pretectal region (Lukaszewska and Thompson, 1967). In addition, preoperative overtraining has been found to improve the active avoidance scores of dogs and rats with lesions of the amygdala (Fonberg, Brutkowski, and Mempel, 1962; Thatcher and Kimble, 1966). This can be seen in Table 10.3.

Just as with other brain lesion phenomena, failures to find overtraining effects also exist, most notably with brightness discrimination retention after visual cortex lesions. In 1921, Karl Lashley gave rats that required 100 or fewer trials to learn a brightness discrimination up to 1200 additional trials prior to surgery. Despite this massive amount of preoperative overtraining, his rats still performed poorly

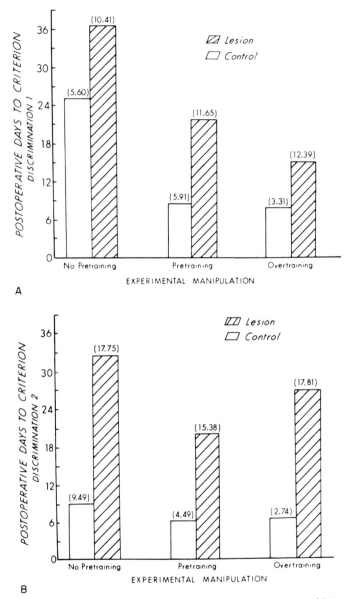

Figure 10.8. *Means and standard deviations for rats with somatosensory cortical lesions and sham operations on the tactile discrimination experienced by the animals given training before surgery (A), and then on a harder tactile discrimination not previously encountered (B). (From Weese, Neimand, and Finger, 1973.)*

Table 10.3

Percentage Savings on an Avoidance Task after Lesions of the Amygdala or Control Operations[a]

Amygdala	Operation controls	Normals
Nonovertrained subjects		
− 100	+ 78	+ 66
+ 91	+ 47	+ 100
+ 23	+ 65	− 15
+ 77	+ 30	+ 86
− 100	+ 39	+ 80
+ 41	+ 65	+ 40
− 100		
Overtrained subjects		
+ 100	+ 87	+ 90
+ 68	+ 86	+ 76
+ 96	+ 80	+ 89
+ 66		+ 91
+ 93		+ 93
+ 98		+ 100

[a] After Thatcher and Kimble, 1966.

[b] Savings = $\dfrac{\text{Trials to acquistion} - \text{trials to retention}}{\text{Trials to acquisition}}$

on the brightness discrimination after posterior cortical lesions. Lashley's finding has been confirmed a number of times (e.g., Glendenning, 1972), although later experiments have had fewer overtraining trials.

Whether the beneficial effects of overtraining seen in some animal experiments have an analogue in the human clinical literature is unclear at the present time. Norman Geschwind (1974), of the Harvard University Medical School, has tried to find parallels between impairments seen in animal experiments and speech defects after left hemispheric lesions in man. Although he does not distinguish between individuals who used little and much speech before brain damage, his position is that overtraining may be somewhat overplayed as a factor influencing performance after brain damage in man since patients may show severe and prolonged deficits in the ability to use language after lesions of the left hemispheric speech areas, even though "this may be the most overlearned skill they possess [p. 490]."

Whether Geschwind is correct in his assessment or not, the experimental data clearly show that overtraining can affect performance in brain-damaged subjects under certain conditions. As we noted earlier, overtraining represents only one of many specific training techniques that may account for variability in performance after brain lesions. When seen in this perspective and when the enrichment and nutritional literatures are considered, there can be little question but that the experiential history of the subject must be seriously considered in any attempt to understand the diversity of individual responses to brain injury.

Before leaving the topic of the training history of the subjects, one additional remark should be made about what these factors can show us in brain lesion studies. It is that although subjects may perform extremely poorly on a behavioral test after brain damage, it is often tenuous to conclude that the capacity for making the necessary discriminations has been lost. This is brought out in studies in which animals are first advanced through easy problems to tasks that would otherwise pose great difficulty for them.

Consider, for example, two serial lesion experiments that were conducted by one of us. In one experiment (Simons, Puretz, and Finger, 1975), rats given sequential unilateral lesions of the somatosensory cortex proved to be very poor in relearning a difficult ridge-smooth discrimination. In fact, these animals were as impaired as rats given one-stage lesions on this discrimination. But in another study, where the rats were slowly worked through a series of easier tactile discriminations prior to encountering the identical "difficult" problem, the animals with serial lesions were able to perform within the control group range, even though deficits still appeared among the one-stage subjects (Finger, Marshak, Cohen, Scheff, Trace, and Neimand, 1971).

This striking difference between animals slowly advanced to a difficult problem and those required to perform a difficult discrimination without prior learning does not appear to be an isolated case. We have noticed the same trend in some of our other experiments, with and without serial lesions, and we have even seen cases where naive rats without lesions could not master a problem with daily testing that has gone on for over 1 year; yet, when the same problem was preceded by a graded series of easier problems, the difficult discrimination was mastered in just a few days, and after less than 1 month of postoperative testing on all of the problems combined. Obviously the lesion did not *eliminate* the capacity for making the discrimination, although it did affect performance in other ways.[3,4]

---

[3] We have also found this principle helpful for teaching cats to learn to discriminate between two warm surfaces with their paws, something that other experimenters have been unable to accomplish at all (see Finger and Norrsell, 1974; Norrsell, 1978). In this case, months were spent trying to teach cats to distinguish between a surface 11°C above room temperature (22°C) and one 1°C above room temperature in a modified T-maze, but without any success. Other cats, however, proved adept in distinguishing between two cool surfaces with receptors located in or near their paws. Therefore, in a final attempt to establish a warm versus warm discrimination, a "fading out" technique was employed in which a warm stimulus (11°C above room temperature) was to be distinguished from a cool stimulus (−3°C relative to ambient temperature), with the temperature of the latter surface being slowly increased toward and then above the ambient temperature as successive criteria were met. The change in experimental procedure proved to be effective as the cats rapidly learned +11°C versus −3°C, and then recognized situations where the cold stimulus was decreased until it matched the ambient temperature. When the previously cold stimulus was moved into the warm range, the cats continued to perform well, now mastering the +11°C versus +1°C discrimination and situations

Throughout this chapter we have stressed the role of experience in learning and perceptual-learning situations. Before ending it, one final set of studies should be described because it clearly illustrates the point that experiential factors can also affect the appearance of symptoms that one might attribute to the integrity of more primitive parts of the brain—deficits and structures more closely associated with homeostasis than with learning per se.

T. L. Powley and Richard Keesey, of the University of Wisconsin, have devoted many hours to studying the effects of lateral hypothalamic lesions (LH) on eating and drinking. Typically, very large LH lesions result in a cessation of eating (aphagia) and drinking (adipsia) from which animals die if special interventions, such as force-feeding special liquid diets, are not attempted. With moderate or small lesions, survival rates improve as eating and drinking are more prone to recover.

In 1970, Powley and Keesey compared the effects of lateral hypothalamic lesions in animals of normal weight to those of animals that have been starved to 80% of their normal weight just prior to surgery. As expected, the normal animals with lesions of moderate size showed adipsia and aphagia and lost weight until stabilization occurred at 88% of the control group weight. A different pattern appeared among the starved animals. They had only a very brief period of anorexia and adipsia, and after a few days their *weights went up* from 80% of normal to 88% of normal.

When the same manipulation was attempted on animals with somewhat smaller lesions, the trend was even more dramatic. The starved animals now showed no anorexia or adipsia and actually ate more than the control group during the period immediately following the lesions. These animals stabilized at 93% of control group weight—the same level that the nonstarved animals declined to after surgery. These findings are presented in Figure 10.9.

The fact that under some conditions animals gain weight after LH lesions

---

with even less separation between the two warm stimuli. The most surprising finding of all was that the cats went on to show that they could discriminate between two warm stimuli that were only about 1°C apart. This behavioral technique thus revealed that the paw of the cat is remarkably sensitive to small differences in warm temperatures, rather than being insensitive to heat below noxious levels, as had been previously believed.

[4] A recent experiment conducted by Patricia Goldman (1976) also deserves mention. She noticed that if infant monkeys received lesions of the orbital frontal cortex, they did not recover spontaneously. Rather, performance at 2 years of age depended upon whether the animals operated upon in infancy had been postoperatively tested at 1 year of age. All of the brain-damaged monkeys that were tested at the end of year 1 were at first very debilitated. A year later, the preoperatively trained group showed complete recovery, while the animals that experienced no training at 1 year of age were very impaired. An interesting further observation is that the training does not always have to be specific to the task since testing on nonspatial problems also facilitates recovery on the delayed spatial alternation problem (Goldman and Mendelson, 1977). It may be that "as long as the animals are kept busy at something" after they are brain-damaged, they are more likely to do better than their counterparts kept from learning or some type of novel stimulation.

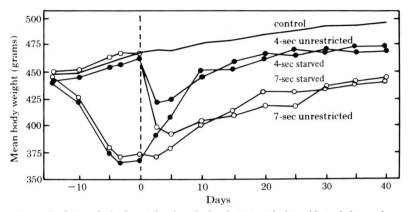

Figure 10.9. *Reducing the body weight of rats before lesioning the lateral hypothalamus shortens or eliminates the expected postlesion period of aphagia and anorexia. Two groups of rats receiving lesions of 4 seconds (n = 10) or 7 seconds (n = 13) duration showed aphagia and anorexia before regulating their body weights at a reduced level. Two other groups were given equivalent lesions after having been starved to 80% of their normal body weight. Of the starved groups, those receiving 7-second lesions (n = 17) showed only very brief periods of aphagia and anorexia; those receiving 4-second lesions (n = 10) showed no aphagia or anorexia, but instead became hyperphagic for the first week postlesion. (From Keesey and Powley, 1975. Reprinted by permission, American Scientist, Journal of Sigma Xi, The Scientific Research Society.)*

shows that the "centers" for eating and drinking are not being destroyed by the surgery as earlier investigators had postulated. Rather, the lesions appear to be lowering the "set point" for body weight regulation in a way that is still not clear (see Keesey and Powley, 1975). Although the new set point seems to be largely determined by the size of the lesion, whether the animals will starve in the presence of food or overeat clearly appears to be dependent upon prior experience.[5]

---

[5] Even presurgical manipulation of illumination seems to influence the outcome of brain injury in certain cases. Saul Balagura and his colleagues demonstrated that lesions of the lateral hypothalamus not only disrupt feeding, but also produce a syndrome consisting of hypokinesia, somnolence, and waxy flexibility (Coscena and Balagura, 1970). Balagura, Harrell, and DeCastro (1978) subsequently manipulated illumination levels by placing rats in continuous darkness or light for 5 days prior to LH surgery. In the rats kept in constant darkness prior to or after surgery, the motor impairments were much less severe despite the fact that the animals were aphagic and adipsic. Balagura and his colleagues attribute the limited sparing of function to the possibility that the illumination conditions altered the level of neurotransmitters at the time of, and after, surgery. This is a reasonable hypothesis that should be examined more systematically. It implies that presurgical manipulations (enrichment, general stimulation, etc.) could "set" circuitry in the central nervous system at different levels which, in turn, would then influence the outcome of brain damage. In this context, one might be tempted to ask whether pretreatment with tranquilizers prior to brain surgery would be more (or less) beneficial than pretreatment with neuroleptics. Questions such as these have hardly received any attention in the literature, although the answers could be germane to the treatment of patients suffering from cerebral traumas.

In summary, in this chapter we have tried to present an overview of some of the experiential factors that can play a role in recovery from brain damage. As we have seen, experience can be a significant variable in brain lesion studies with animals and people. Both specific learning experiences (e.g., training and overtraining) and nonspecific environmental enrichment are among the many factors that must be given serious consideration in this context. Still, much remains to be explored in this field. For example, the long-term effects of some experiential factors have not been given the attention that is needed to understand fully when and why they work, and many questions remain to be answered about the generality, applicability, and utility of some of these effects.

Why some, but not other, symptoms that follow brain damage can be attenuated by environmental interventions is indeed puzzling. Perhaps answers to important questions like this one will emerge when these studies are viewed from a new or different perspective. As seen developmentally, the effects of experience seem to be greatest when the brain is still in the process of growth. Yet, laboratory studies show that many experiential effects can still be observed well after the period of sexual maturity. As organisms grow old, the potential for experiential modification of brain lesion symptoms seems to diminish even more. At Clark University, for example, we have recently observed that neither pre- nor postoperative exposure to very complex environments seemed to facilitate recovery from bilateral frontal cortex lesions in 18-month-old rats who were tested on a spatial alternation task. (Rats are sexually mature well before they are 3 months old, and although not senile, are considered quite old when 18 months of age.) Why prolonged enrichment (more than 6 months in one case, and more than a year in another experiment) failed to help aged, brain-damaged rats remains a mystery ripe for investigation, especially since there are some data to show that people may still benefit from stimulating environments very late in life, at a time when there usually is massive brain cell attrition.

To be sure, the experimental literature on lesion–environment interaction effects is still in an embryonic state, thwarted perhaps by the notion that the mammalian central nervous system is predetermined in its connections, and subject to scant little modification after the earliest stages of infancy. Yet, even the few studies cited here seem to suggest some principles that should be considered in the context of therapy for brain damage in man. One might be to try to provide therapies as soon as possible after insult. Another would be to try to make sure that institutionalized and bedridden patients receive high-quality stimulation. The research literature also suggests that active participation in responding to the environment should be encouraged. In fact, self-initiated responding for satisfaction of needs might be the best therapy available, especially when combined with a relatively high level of sensory and psychological input, such as might be found in some behaviorally oriented rehabilitation programs. We will return to these points in Chapter 17.

Although we have not discussed the role of motivation in recovery from brain damage, it goes without saying that this factor can also play a major role in the patient's capacity to recover lost behavioral functions. This important variable has *not* received adequate attention in well-controlled studies, although it is probably one of the most important factors to consider in any setting where the ultimate goal is to achieve recovery of function.

References

Bakwin, H. Emotional deprivation in infants. *Journal of Pediatrics*, 1949, *35*, 512–519.

Balagura, S., Harrell, L. E., and DeCastro, J. M. Organismic states and their effect on recovery from neurosurgery: A new perspective with implications for a general theory. *Brain, Behavior and Evolution*, 1978, *15*, 19–40.

Beach, F. A., and Jaynes, J. Effects of early experience upon the behavior of animals. *Psychological Bulletin*, 1954, *51*, 239–263.

Bennett, E. L., Diamond, M. C., Krech, D., and Rosenzweig, M. R. Chemical and anatomical plasticity of the brain. *Science*, 1964, *146*, 610–619.

Bennett, E. L., Rosenzweig, M. R., and Diamond, M. C. Rat brain: Effects of environmental enrichment on wet and dry weights. *Science*, 1969, *163*, 825–826.

Bland, B. H., and Cooper, R. M. Posterior neodecortication in the rat: Age at operation and experience. *Journal of Comparative and Physiological Psychology*, 1969, 69, 345–354.

Bland, B. H., and Cooper, R. M. Experience and vision of the posterior neodecorticate rat. *Physiology and Behavior*, 1970, *5*, 211–214.

Chapin, H. D. A plea for accurate statistics in infants' institutions. *Transactions of the American Pediatrics Society*, 1915, *27*, 180–185.

Chow, K. L., and Survis, J. Retention of overlearned visual habits after temporal ablation in the monkey. *Archives of Neurology and Psychiatry*, 1958, 79, 640–646.

Coscena, D. V., and Balagura, S. Avoidance and escape behavior of rats with aphagia produced by basal diencephalic lesions. *Physiology and Behavior*, 1970, *5*, 641–657.

Denenberg, V. H., Woodcock, J. M., and Rosenberg, K. M. Long-term effects of preweaning and postweaning free-environment experience on rats' problem-solving behavior. *Journal of Comparative and Physiological Psychology*, 1968, *66*, 533–535.

Donaldson, H. H. Anatomical observations on the brain and several sense organs of the blind deaf mute, Laura Dewey Bridgeman. *American Journal of Psychology*, 1891, 248–294.

Donaldson, H. H. *The growth of the brain: A study of the nervous system in relation to education.* New York: Scribner's, 1895.

Donovick, P. J., Burright, R. G., and Swidler, M. A. Presurgical rearing environment alters exploration, fluid consumption, and learning of septal lesioned and control rats. *Physiology and Behavior*, 1973, *11*, 543–553.

Dru, D., Walker, J. P., and Walker, J. B. Self-produced locomotion restores visual capacity after striate lesion. *Science*, 1975, *187*, 265–266.

Ferchmin, P. A., Bennett, E. L., and Rosenzweig, M. R. Direct contact with enriched environment is required to alter cerebral weights in rats. *Journal of Comparative and Physiological Psychology*, 1975, *88*, 360–367.

Finger, S. Environmental attenuation of brain lesion symptoms. In S. Finger (Ed.), *Recovery from brain damage: Research and theory.* New York: Plenum, 1978, 297–329.

Finger, S., Marshak, R. A., Cohen, M., Scheff,S., Trace, R.,and Neimand,P. Effects of successive and simultaneous lesions of somatosensory cortex on tactile discrimination in the rat. *Journal of Comparative and Physiological Psychology*, 1971, 77, 221–227.

Finger, S., and Norrsell, U. Temperature sensitivity of the paw of the cat: A behavioural study. *Journal of Physiology*, 1974, *239*, 631–646.

Fonberg, E., Brutkowski, I., and Mempel, E. Defensive conditioned reflexes and neurotic motor reactions following amygdalectomy in dogs. *Acta Biologiae Experimentalis* (Warsaw), 1962, *22*, 51–57.

Forgays, D. B., and Forgays, J. W. The nature of free-environment experience in the rat. *Journal of Comparative and Physiological Psychology*, 1952, *45*, 322–328.

Fuller, J. L. Experiential deprivation and later behavior. *Science*, 1967, *158*, 1645–1652.

Geschwind, N. Late changes in the nervous system: An overview. In D. G. Stein, J. J. Rosen, and N. Butters (Eds.), *Plasticity and recovery of function in the central nervous system*. New York: Academic Press, 1974, Pp. 467–508.

Gilbert, J. G. Mental efficiency in senescence. *Archives of Psychology*, 1935, *27*(188).

Glendenning, K. L. Effects of training between two unilateral lesions of visual cortex upon ultimate retention of black–white discrimination habits by rats. *Journal of Comparative and Physiological Psychology*, 1972, *80*, 216–229.

Goldman, P. S. The role of experience in recovery of function following orbital prefrontal lesions in infant monkeys. *Neuropsychologia*, 1976, *14*, 401–412.

Goldman, P. S., and Mendelson, M. J. Salutary effects of early experience on deficits caused by lesions of frontal association cortex in rhesus monkeys. *Experimental Neurology*, 1977, *57*, 588–602.

Greenough, W. T. Experiential modification of the developing brain. *American Scientist*, 1975, *63*, 37–46.

Harlow, H. F. The formation of learning sets. *Psychological Review*, 1949, *56*, 51–65.

Hebb, D. O. *The organization of behavior*. New York: Wiley, 1949.

Hebb, D. O., and Williams, K. A. A method of rating animal intelligence. *Journal of General Psychology*, 1946, *34*, 59–65.

Hertzig, M. E., Birch, H. G., Richardson, S. A., and Tizard, J. Intellectual levels of school children severely malnourished during the first two years of life. *Pediatrics*, 1972, *49*, 814–823.

Hughes, K. R. Dorsal and ventral hippocampus lesions and maze learning: Influence of preoperative environment. *Canadian Journal of Psychology*, 1965, *19*, 325–332.

Keesey, R. E., and Powley, T. L. Hypothalamic regulation of body weight. *American Scientist*, 1975, *63*, 558–565.

Kelche, C. R., and Will, B. E. Effets de l'environnement sur la restauration fonctionnelle après lésions hippocampiques chez des rats adultes. *Physiology and Behavior*, 1978, *21*, 935–942.

Lashley, K. S. Studies of cerebral functioning in learning. II. The effects of long continued practice upon cerebral localization. *Journal of Comparative Psychology*, 1921, *1*, 453–468.

Levitsky, D. A., and Barnes, R. H. Nutrition and environmental interactions in the behavioral development of the rat: Long-term effects. *Science*, 1972, *176*, 68–71.

Lewis, M. E. *The influence of early experience on the effects of one- and two-stage hippocampal lesions in male rats*. Unpublished Master's thesis, Clark University (Worcester, Mass.), 1975.

Lukaszewska, I., and Thompson, R. Retention of an overtrained pattern discrimination following pretectal lesions in rats. *Psychonomic Science*, 1967, *8*, 121–122.

Mackintosh, N. J. *The psychology of animal learning*. London: Academic Press, 1974.

Meyer, D. R., Isaac, W., and Maher, B. The role of stimulation in spontaneous reorganization of visual habits. *Journal of Comparative and Physiological Psychology*, 1958, *51*, 546–548.

Norrsell, U. Testing procedures and the interpretation of behavioral data. In S. Finger (Ed.), *Recovery from brain damage: Research and theory*. New York: Plenum, 1978, Pp. 199–216.

Oppenheim, R. W. Laura Bridgeman's brain: An early consideration of functional adaptations in neural development. *Developmental Psychobiology*, 1979, *12*, 533–537.

Orbach, J., and Fantz, R. L. Differential effects of temporal neo-cortical resections on overtrained and non-overtrained visual habits in monkeys. *Journal of Comparative and Physiological Psychology*, 1958, *51*, 126–129.

Paul, C. Effects of overlearning upon single habit reversal in rats. *Psychological Bulletin*, 1965, *63*, 65–72.

Powley, T. L., and Keesey, R. E. Relationship of body weight to the lateral hypothalamic feeding syndrome. *Journal of Comparative and Physiological Psychology*, 1970, 70, 25–36.

Rabinovich, M. S., and Rosvold, H. E. A closed-field intelligence test for rats. *Journal of Psychology*, 1951, *5*, 122–128.

Richardson, S. A., Birch, H. G., and Herzig, M. E. School performance of children who were severely malnourished in infancy. *American Journal of Mental Deficiency*, 1973, 77, 623–632.

Rosenzweig, M. R. Effects of environment on development of brain and behavior. In E. Tobach, L. R. Aronson, and E. Shaw (Eds.), *The biopsychology of development*. New York: Academic Press, 1971, Pp. 303–342.

Rosenzweig, M. R., Bennett, E. L., and Diamond, M. C. Chemical and anatomical plasticity of the brain: Replications and extensions. In J. Gaito (Ed.), *Macromolecules and behavior*. New York: Appleton-Century-Crofts, 1972, Pp. 205–277.

Salz, R. Effects of part time "mothering" on IQ and SQ of young institutionalized children. *Child Development*, 1973, 9, 166–170.

Schwartz, S. Effect of neocortical lesions and early environmental factors on adult rat behavior. *Journal of Comparative and Physiological Psychology*, 1964, *57*, 72–77.

Simons, D., Puretz, J., and Finger, S. Effects of serial lesions of somatosensory cortex and further neodecortication on tactile retention in rats. *Experimental Brain Research*, 1975, *23*, 353–366.

Skeels, H. M. Adult status of children with contrasting early life experiences. *Monographs of the Society for Research in Child Development*, No. 31, 1966.

Smith, C. J. Mass action and early environment. *Journal of Comparative and Physiological Psychology*, 1959, *52*, 154–156.

Sperling, S. E. Reversal learning and resistence to extinction: A review of the rat literature. *Psychological Bulletin*, 1965, *63*, 281–297.

Stein, Z., Susser, M., Saenger, G., and Marolla, F. Nutrition and mental performance. *Science*, 1972, *178*, 708–713.

Stoch, M. B., and Smythe, P. M. Does undernutrition during infancy inhibit brain growth and subsequent intellectual development? *Archives of Diseases of Childhood*, 1963, *38*, 546–552.

Tanabe, G. Remediating maze deficiencies by the use of environmental enrichment. *Developmental Psychology*, 1972, 7, 224.

Thatcher, P. W., and Kimble, D. P. Effect of amygdaloid lesions on retention of an avoidance response in overtrained and non-overtrained rats. *Psychonomic Science*, 1966, *6*, 9–10.

Thompson, W. R., and Grusec, J. E. Studies on early experience. In P. H. Mussen (Ed.), *Carmichael's Manual of Child Psychology* (3rd ed.). New York: Wiley, 1970, Pp. 565–654.

Watson, J. B. *Behaviorism*. New York: W. W. Norton, 1925.

Weese, G. D., Neimand, D., and Finger, S. Cortical lesions and somesthesis in rats: Effects of training and overtraining prior to surgery. *Experimental Brain Research*, 1973, *16*, 542–550.

Weinstein, S., and Teuber, H.-L. The role of preinjury education and intelligence level in intellectual loss after brain injury. *Journal of Comparative and Physiological Psychology*, 1957, *50*, 535–539.

Wells, A. M., Geist, C. R., and Zimmermann, R. R. Influence of environmental and nutritional factors on problem solving in the rat. *Perceptual and Motor Skills*, 1972, *35*, 225–244.

West, R. W., and Greenough, W. T. Effect of environmental complexity on cortical synapses of rats: Preliminary results. *Behavioral Biology*, 1972, 7, 279–284.

White, B., and Held, R. Plasticity of sensorimotor development in the human infant. In J. Rosenblith and W. Allinsmith (Eds.), *The causes of behavior: Readings in child development in educational psychology*. Boston: Allyn and Bacon, 1966, Pp. 60–70.

Will, B. E., and Rosenzweig, M. R. Effets de l'environnement sur la récupération fonctionnelle après lésions cérébrales chez les rats adultes. *Biology of Behavior,* 1976, *1,* 5–16.

Will, B. E., Rosenzweig, M. R., Bennett, E. L., Herbert, M., and Morimoto, H. Relatively brief environmental enrichment aids recovery of learning capacity and alters brain measures after post-weaning brain lesions in rats. *Journal of Comparative and Physiological Psychology,* 1977, *91,* 33–50.

Winick, M. Nutrition and nerve cell growth. *Federation Proceedings,* 1970, *29,* 1510–1515.

Winick, M. *Malnutrition and brain development.* New York: Oxford University Press, 1976.

Winick, M., Meyer, K. K., and Harris, R. C. Malnutrition and environmental enrichment by early adoption. *Science,* 1975, *190,* 1173–1175.

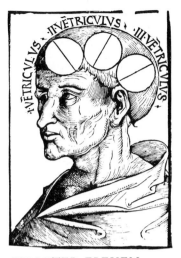

Drugs and Recovery:
Pyrogens and Hormones

Clinicians concerned with the physical therapy and general rehabilitation of persons with incapacitating brain lesions rarely make use of drugs to alter the course of the disease, and in general, the pharmacological management of these patients is only symptomatic [Brailowsky, 1980, p. 187].

CHAPTER ELEVEN

It is safe to say that most work in neuropsychology has been concerned with the identification of symptoms and deficits that follow traumatic central nervous system injury. There has been little emphasis on the derivation of "curative" or ameliorating treatments that can be applied to help the brain-damaged subject. Is there so little hope of success in trying to find the means to aid the recovery process, or are other factors partially responsible for this apparent gap in our knowledge?

Bernard Barber (1961), a sociologist at Columbia University, wrote an interesting monograph on the resistance of scientists to scientific discoveries. He pointed out that many factors limit the "open-mindedness" of scientists to new ideas or new discoveries. In some cases, the substantive concepts and theories held by scientists at a given time become a source of resistance to new ideas; the "paradigm" or system of beliefs concerning what constitutes a "fact" shapes attitudes about what will, or will not be, studied. According to Barber, the methodological conceptions scientists consider at any time constitute a second cultural source of resistance to scientific discovery and could be as important as substantive ideas in determining responses to innovation. Yet another source of resistance is the tendency of scientists to think in terms of established *models*—indeed to reject propositions outright because they cannot be put in the form of some model that is currently popular.

Perhaps because of these reasons, relatively few attempts have been made to manipulate recovery from brain damage by pharmacological intervention. As we have noted frequently in the preceding chapters, the prevailing view is that once damage to the central nervous system has occurred, there is little hope of functional recovery, or, on an anatomical level, of central nervous system regeneration. Until recently, beliefs about localization of function (a substantive concept in Barber's terms) and lack of appropriate techniques for facilitating or examining neuronal regeneration have kept neuroscientists from examining how damaged nerves repair themselves and whether the recovery process can be facilitated by drugs.

Both clinical and casual observations of patients with brain or spinal cord injuries seemed to support the view that nothing could be done, as did much of the work of the founding fathers of neurology (e.g., Paul Broca). Yet, as early as 1850, Brown-Séquard (1850a,b, 1851) had performed experiments on pigeons with complete transections of the spinal cord (see West, 1978). Brown-Séquard noted that at first the birds were very impaired, with only partial sensibility and limited voluntary movements. But by 15 months after the transection, the animals were almost normal in gait, balance, and use of their wings. Brown-Séquard's microscopic examinations of the spinal cord in the adult pigeons revealed that the two cut ends were reunited and that the grey and white matter *appeared* to be normal.

Today, at least limited neuronal regeneration in the spinal cord is an accepted fact (Chapter 4), but Brown-Séquard's work had to lay buried for more than 100 years before this idea could be accepted, perhaps because these observations were on birds and because the prevailing opinion was that similar phenomena would not be observed with mammals.

If, as we have seen, some regeneration can occur in mammals, how can it be enhanced and how can the functional efficiency of the "recovered" system be increased? We have already reviewed how experience can alter recovery from central nervous system injury (Chapter 10), but environmental manipulations require a lot of time, and basically such manipulations are well outside of the "medical" model, which contends that direct intervention in the form of pharmacologic agents is a more suitable (and dramatic) means to cure disability due to brain injury, if any cure is possible at all.

Although they were not the first to do research in this area, Sugar and Gerard (1940) broke the silence on the potential regenerative capacity of the spinal cord by showing that adult rats could recover effectively from complete cuts between sections T5 and T13 if extraordinary postoperative care was given to the animals. They argued that, in the past, spinal cord section rarely led to regeneration because the animals died as a result of bladder disturbance, edema, disrupted blood supply, and shock. Sugar and Gerard controlled for these factors and were able to demonstrate considerable recovery of movement (climbing, walking, hopping) in a few of their animals. They then correlated the behavioral recovery with the bridging of the *scar* by bundles of new axons "passing continuously between cord tracts on either side of the lesions" and noted that an adequate blood supply was critical for the regeneration to be seen (Sugar and Gerard, 1940, p. 16). However, other researchers have failed to note such dramatic recovery, or simply attributed any return of function to an incomplete disruption of the nerve fibers.

Although conflicting reports soon appeared in the literature, the stage was set to review the question of central nervous system recovery from injury more critically and to wonder about the possibility of manipulating the course of recovery by treatments that would reduce the scarring thought to block the successful regrowth of neurons. The studies emerging in this context were first concentrated on the spinal cord for several good reasons. In the first place, there were practical demands to deal with, such as the post–World War II cases of paraplegia due to combat-related injuries. Second, experimental manipulations in animals were more advanced for spinal cord research than for the brain itself. Third, it was believed that the major hurdle to functional regeneration after cord injury was the physical–mechanical barrier of scar tissue that prevented axons from bridging across the damaged zone. The thinking was that if this barrier could be surmounted, functional recovery might occur. In their 1940 paper, Sugar and Gerard prepared the groundwork for much subsequent research by concluding that:

> Spinal neurons with adequate blood supply start to regenerate cut processes. These fibers grow along structural pathways like peripheral nerve and using bands of glial nuclei *when possible,* but are mainly blocked by glia and scar tissue running transversely across the cord. When they successfully cross a scar, restoring anatomical continuity, nervous transmission across the lesion and coordinated function also return [p. 17].

To many investigators, the first step was to find a means to reduce the scarring and cyst formation that always seemed to occur after injury. One approach to the problem of providing a bridge or pathway across the scar was to ensure a good vascular bed as well as a "scaffolding" of muscle or nerve tissue. Sugar and Gerard accomplished this by transplanting bits of muscle or embryonic nerve tissue capable of liberating "neurotrophic" substances to stimulate growth. The transplantation of embryonic tissue that facilitates growth is interesting from experimental and theoretical perspectives, but insofar as practical (and ethical) applications go, such techniques are (and were in the 1940s) of limited value. Thus, it was thought more important to develop a *pharmacological* treatment to eliminate scarring; the idea being that injections of a "scar-dissolving agent" into the wound area would facilitate neuronal growth across the wound.

During the 1950s, William Windle and his students tried to expand upon Sugar and Gerard's ideas by performing many experiments to stimulate and enhance regeneration of nerve fibers across the cut spinal cords of adult cats and dogs. In one series of studies, they administered a pyrogenic substance derived from *Pseudomona* bacteria, which was called Piromen. In one case, Carmine Clemente and Windle (1954) examined recovery in 79 adult cats that had received complete spinal cord transections of the thoracic or upper lumbar regions. Postoperative care consisted of daily handling and manual stimulation of the bladder. Two experimental groups were formed. One received Piromen, the bacteria-derived polysaccharide, while the other group, with similar surgery, received nothing.

The drug was administered intravenously every other day for a 2-week period and gradually increased from 10 γ/kg to 125 γ/kg at the end of the period. The animals were given a 2-week rest period and then the drug was readministered. The 4-week "drug-no-drug" regimen was followed until the end of the project.

The cats were killed at different postoperative recovery periods and prepared for histology to examine the extent of healing and growth of axons across the glial barrier. During the first postoperative month, there was a clear difference in the healing of axons between the Piromen-treated and nontreated spinal animals. Clemente and Windle (1954) briefly stated, the pia-glial membrane, "which developed immediately over the cut ends of the spinal cord in non-treated cats failed to form in the Piromen-treated specimens [p. 717]." Clemente and Windle also noted that the treated animals also had more vascularization in the wound area and less collagenous connective tissue than the nontreated control cats. Sprouting of intraspinal neurons was the same in both groups; it began about 15 days after the injury. In the control group, the formation of the pial-glial barrier forced the regenerating neurons to "turn back," and ultimately their regenerative efforts ceased. In the drug-treated cats, "the neuron sprouts found no impenetrable barrier and made their way through the reticulum of loose connective tissue in the lesion site [p. 718]." These findings are shown in Figures 11.1 and 11.2.

Figure 11.1. *Four sections through the spinal cord transected 11.4 months previously, (Cat SP-36) showing reestablishment of a pathway of intraspinal nerve fibers (f) after Piromen therapy. The upper part of each figure is rostral. A constricting scar of fibrous connective tissue (ct) marks the site of the transection. Pyridine silver stain was used. × 35.*

(13) A longitudinal section at the site of the lesion taken midway ventrodorsally through the spinal cord. The rostral and caudal stumps are separated by the connective tissue scar, which is denser in sections ventral to the one pictured.

(14) A section 80 μ dorsal to that of (13). Regenerated nerve fibers begin to penetrate the connective tissue scar at this level, passing from the rostral to the caudal stump. A few fibers cross the lesion site.

(15) A section 160 μ dorsal to that shown in (13). Regenerated intraspinal fibers form a fascicle crossing the lesion site.

(16) A section 240 μ dorsal to the section shown in (13). This and (15) reveal the extent of regeneration achieved in this experiment. (From Clemente and Windle, 1954.)

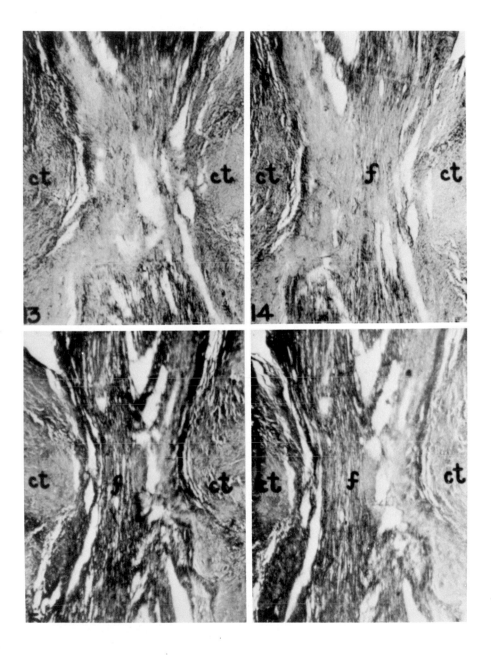

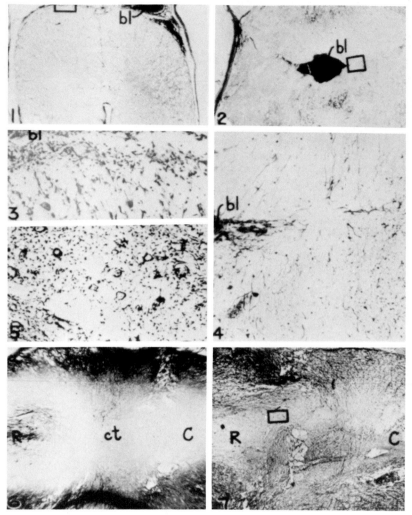

Figure 11.2. *(1) A longitudinal section of the caudal stump of the spinal cord transected 3 days previously: This is a nontreated control animal (Cat F-4). A membrane containing glial elements, and continuous laterally with the pia mater, covers the transected stump. Remnants of hemorrhage (bl) appear above this. For details of the portion enclosed by the square see (3). Silver protargol stain was used. × 11.25.*

(2) A longitudinal section of the spinal cord through the area of complete transection taken 3 days after the operation in a Piromen-treated animal (Cat F-3). No pia-glial membrane can be seen between the transected stumps of this spinal cord. For details of the portion enclosed by the square see (4). Silver protargol stain was used. × 11.25.

(3) A detail of the field designated in (1). This shows the earliest appearance of the pia-glial membrane, which grows over the cut ends of the spinal cord. Approximately × 99.

Despite their evidence for regeneration across the loose-knit glial scar in the Piromen-treated cats, Clemente and Windle did not examine the surviving cats for evidence of behavioral recovery, nor did they measure the pattern of gradual recovery (if indeed it existed) as the regenerating axons grew across the wound. Although the authors reported that, as time progressed, the regenerating fibers reestablished fascicles and tracts, their techniques did not permit them to determine whether the physiological properties of the new contacts were like those of the old contacts.

The attempts to replicate the findings of Windle and his students have met with only moderate success insofar as drug-treatments are concerned. In one very extensive follow-up experiment of Piromen effects, Robert McMasters (1962) performed spinal transections in more than 530 albino rats at the ages of 5, 6, or 7 days postnatally. He did observe their behavior for up to 4 months following surgery. Piromen was given to 376 of the animals while 58 received injections of sterile saline.

In brief, none of the 58 saline-treated rats showed any evidence of recovery of sensory or motor functions. The animals had urinary incontinence until they died (as did the majority of Piromen-treated rats) and this disorder accounted for almost all of the deaths. Of the 532 rats treated with Piromen, however, 22 showed a complete return of motor and sensory function, which began to be noticeable as early as 2–3 weeks after surgery.

Of the 216 rats operated on at 5 days of age, none showed any evidence of functional recovery when treated with Piromen. Obviously, these findings are not very indicative of a general effect after Piromen treatment, although McMasters did find some limited evidence of regeneration across the stump (i.e., some thin varicoselike neurons connecting the stumps) in some of the Piromen-treated

---

(4) A detail of the field designated in (2). A portion of the blood clot (bl) can be seen on the left. Absence of cellular overgrowth is evident. Approximately × 99.

(5) A photomicrograph showing the vascular matrix in the region of scar formation at the site of spinal cord transection in a Piromen-treated animal (Cat SP-45) 34 days after operation. This contrasts with relative avascularity of scars in nontreated control animals. Pyridine silver stain was used. Approximately × 99.

(6) A longitudinal section of the spinal cord of a nontreated control animal (Cat SP-57), showing the region of complete transection performed 62 days previously. Note the avascular, dense collagenous scar (ct) at the site of the lesion separating rostral (R) and caudal (C) stumps. Pyridine silver stain was used. × 13.5.

(7) A longitudinal section of the spinal cord at the transection site in a 4-month Piromen-treated animal (Cat LD-2). Note the regenerating fibers, shown at higher magnification in (8), which appear to come from the rostral stump, penetrating the connective tissue scar in the region of the lesion. Contrast the looseness of the scar tissue in the lesion area with that in the control shown in (6). Pyridine silver stain was used × 11.25. (From Clemente and Windle, 1954.)

rats.[1] There did appear to be less scarring in the rats treated with Piromen, but given the small numbers of animals actually showing behavioral recovery, it is difficult to conclude that the regeneration was due to the specific treatment itself, rather than spared fibers showing anomalous growth. Most important to note was that in some cases, the recovery that *was* observed was not always permanent. In these instances it persisted for only about a month after the treatments were discontinued, after which the animals regressed.

More recent attempts to find a "treatment" for spinal cord injuries have also been controversial and sometimes even discouraging. Often when one laboratory has reported significant evidence for spinal cord regeneration and behavioral recovery, a subsequent replication or slight modification made by another group has failed to produce the same positive results. As we mentioned previously, most attempts to facilitate spinal nerve regeneration have concentrated on developing techniques to help regenerating nerves cross the glial-pial scar that forms across the stumps of the damaged cord. Not all efforts have used tissue transplants or pharmacological interventions. In one experiment, for example, James Campbell and his associates (Campbell, Bassett, Husby, and Noback, 1957) used a mechanical scaffolding consisting of Millipore filters (nylon tubes impregnated with cellulose acetate) placed around the cut stumps of spinal cord in adult cats. The cellulose acetate filters at the third thoracic level of the cord permitted the fibers to develop "an orderly linear regeneration of axons in the gap without over-proliferation of glial tissue or of the pia-arachnoid complex [p. 929]," as can be seen in Figure 11.3. Unfortunately, as in many anatomical reports, no follow-ups of the animals' behavioral performance were made, so we do not know whether the technique was successful in promoting functional recovery.

Because of its limited or even questionable success, the use of pyrogenic agents to induce nerve regeneration has fallen out of favor with more contemporary investigators as they turned to other means to stimulate regeneration in the cord, such as hormone treatments. In one experiment, Joseph Harvey and Herbert Srebnik (1967) of the University of California, wanted to develop a model that resembled clinical cases of spinal cord injury. They reported that complete transection of the cord in humans is a relatively rare occurrence, although compression or laceration evokes symptoms that are very similar to those resulting from total transection of all fiber tracts.

These researchers studied the effects of thyroid hormone, which is essential for normal development of nerve tissue on regeneration of spinal nerves following acute compression of the cord. They compressed the cord for 1 minute at the 10th thoracic vertebra with a thumb forceps. During recovery, attempts were made to

---

[1] McMasters only performed histology on those rats that did recover. None of the animals that failed to recover were used in histological spinal cord evaluation, so we do not know if similar morphological changes might have occurred without functional recovery.

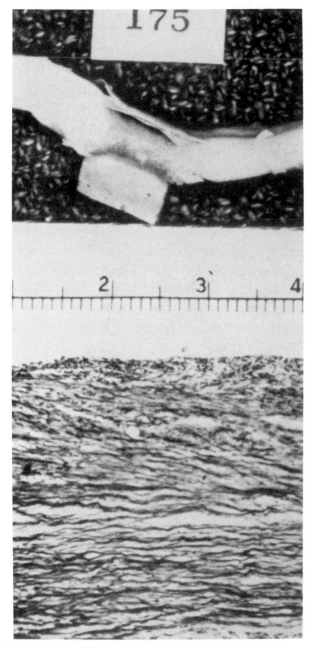

Figure 11.3. *(Top) Feline spinal cord 30 days after transection, Millipore tube opened (Formalin-fixed); (bottom) axons at the level of the transection, 30 days, Bodian (× 200). (From Cambell et al., 1957.)*

prevent urinary sepsis until the young adult rats regained bladder control. Of the 49 subjects used in the experiment, one group was given IP injections of L-thyroxine (4.5 µg) each day for 3 days *preceding* compression; one group received four injections of L-thyroxine (4.5 µg) *after* the cord was compressed; one group received 9.0 µg of the hormone postoperatively; and one group served as noninjected controls. All of the rats were tested from 10 to 180 days after the damage for locomotor functions of the hindlimbs.

In this experiment, all of the surviving rats showed some degree of recovery from the compression. This is shown in Figure 11.4. The untreated controls reached their maximum level of efficiency at about 30 days, but their motor performance was lower than any of the other groups. The rats that received thyroxine *prior* to injury were much better than these control animals by 120 days after the injuries were inflicted, and those given postoperative treatment of the hormone showed better motor control as well. Regardless of the treatments, the authors stressed that none of the rats with spinal compressions performed as well as normal animals; there *always* was a residual deficit.

To determine whether nerve fibers had actually regenerated across the damaged area, Harvey and Srebnik stimulated the cord *above* the site of the lesion with electric current and noted whether the animals showed hindlimb movements. Only rats given thyroxine treatments responded to the stimulation; none of the control rats were able to do so.

At the end of 6 months, the rats were killed for histology. The uninjected rats were observed to have scar tissue at the level of the compression, which consisted of neuroglia and connective tissue from the meninges. No regenerating fibers

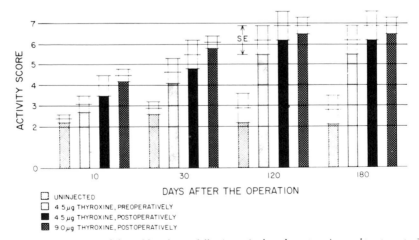

Figure 11.4. *Locomotor ability of female rats following spinal cord compression and treatment with L-thyroxine. See text for schedule of thryoxine injections. (From Harvey and Srebnick, 1967.)*

were seen crossing the scar in any of the noninjected animals. In the thyroxine-treated rats, in contrast, the scar tissue was thinner or absent, and fibers from the ventral or lateral columns of the cord could be seen growing across the crushed segments. This is shown in Figure 11.5.

The authors speculated that the thyroxine may have sustained the regrowth of nerve fibers by enhancing protein synthesis, inhibiting growth of scar tissue at the site of damage, and increasing vascularization of the same region—essentially, the correct physiological environment for the sustenance or growth of nerve fibers. Although this is speculative, and despite the fact that no animal showed complete recovery, the thyroxine obviously was able to facilitate the forward progress of the regenerating nerve fibers that usually is blocked by injury-induced scar tissue.

The most optimistic reports of recovery from spinal cord injury following enzyme "therapies" to break up scar tissue have come from the Soviet Union. L. A. Matinian and A. S. Adreasian (1973) have actively pursued research on spinal recovery for a number of years. They performed "total" chordotomies at the T-5 level in relatively young (6–7 weeks) rats and then examined locomotor and sensory functions of the hindlimbs for up to a year after surgery. As expected, there were severe impairments, and no sensory evoked potentials could be obtained in recordings taken from nerve fibers caudal to the transection when the cerebral cortex or fibers dorsal to the cut were stimulated. Experimental animals were then treated with various enzymes (lidase, trypsin, elastase, or hyaluronidase) to promote recovery of function. In general, the Soviet workers have claimed dramatic success; about 44% of the animals (total number used unknown) were said to show complete functional recovery with looser scar formation and better vascularization near the lesion zone. According to these researchers there was also an increased life span (of about 440 days) and 90% recovery of somatic functions in the drug-treated cases. Although these results are often cited, especially in the Russian literature, we have to stress caution in interpreting these data because no histology was presented. In addition, the statistical methods are questionable, and detailed experimental procedures were not made available.

As mentioned previously, others (see Guth, Albuquerque, Deshpande, Barrett, Donati, and Warnick, 1980) have been less successful in their attempts to obtain regeneration of nerve fibers across the transection. In fact, some authors have argued that the "apparent" growth across the scar is not growth at all, but rather the remnants of fibers that were missed during the attempt at a complete transection of the cord. Even those investigators reporting that enzyme therapy facilitates regeneration have noted that some return of motor function is possible after spinal shock has diminished if a few fibers are spared.

Recent attempts to replicate the Russian findings have not been encouraging. In one case, Earl Feringa and his colleagues (Feringa, Kowalski, Vahlsing, and

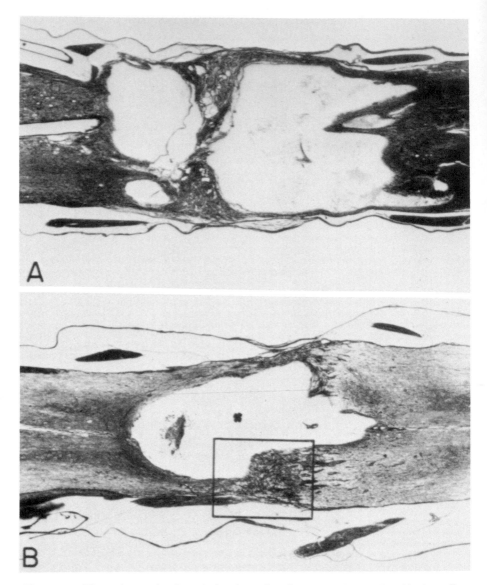

Figure 11.5. *Photomicrographs of rat spinal cord, 180 days after compression, sectioned horizontally about the level of the central canal. Cephalic end on the right. Bodian's protargol stain and aniline blue was used. (A) Section of spinal cord from uninjected rat. Note scar extending transversely across the cord, the large cysts on either side, and lack of nerve fibers traversing it; × 30. (B) Similar section from rat treated with L-thryoxine immediately after compression of the cord and for the following 3 days. Darkly staining and, presumably, regenerating fibers can be seen coursing through the scar tissue within the outlined rectangle; × 30. (C) Magnified view of rectangular area in (B). Note that many of the darkly staining fibers grow through the scar and toward the distal segments; × 110. (From Harvey and Srebnick, 1967.)*

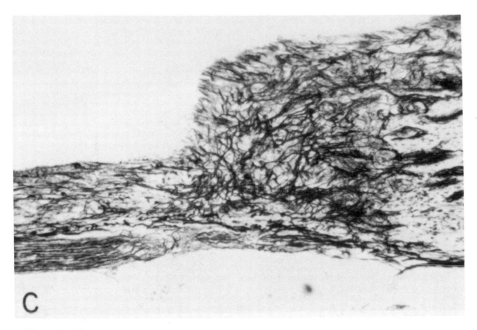

Figure 11.5C.

Frye, 1979) used pure hyalurondiase, trypsin, or trypsin plus elastase and examined female rats when the spinal cord was cut.[2] The enzymes were given for 15 days after the spinal cords were damaged. Feringa *et al.* found no recovery of function whatsoever. That is, no clinical differences were found between animals treated with enzymes thought to block scar formation and those that were untreated. There was also no return of cortical-evoked potentials when the cord caudal to the cut was stimulated.

Negative findings have also been reported by Guth and others (1980). They too attempted to repeat the findings of Matinian and Adreasian (1973) using the same "scar loosening" enzymes described earlier and were completely unsuccessful. Of 92 rats studied in Guth's experiments, not one showed any evidence of functional recovery following the treatments. Since some functional recovery was observed if there were sparing of neurons due to incomplete transections, Guth and his colleagues argued that whatever recovery was seen by the Russians must have been due to the incomplete nature of their lesions.

Based on the evidence at hand, and on work described in our earlier chapters, we have to conclude that the use of enzyme and pyrogenic treatments to promote functional recovery of the spinal cord cannot be given too much weight. At the

---

[2] Female rats were used to avoid or minimize some of the urinary tract complications often found after such surgery with male rats.

present time, whenever recovery *does* occur, and it often does, we should take into account the possibility that the transections were incomplete.[3] Nevertheless, because some functional restitution clearly is possible with only a few surviving fibers that are capable of sprouting into denervated regions of the cord, this phenomenon itself should be exploited in the treatment of paraplegia and related disorders. That is, although the cutting of specific, sensory projection systems or descending motor fibers may reduce the possibility of total recovery, this should not discourage us from attempting to promote rehabilitation by using spared fragments of a system whenever possible and developing agents that will keep these fragments healthy, even under adverse circumstances.

The concept of enhancing recovery with the use of pharmacological agents is not restricted to the spinal cord. The same paradigms can be applied to studies of higher order brain functions. Since some brain areas can be thought of as more "loosely coupled" than some specific sensory and motor projection systems, it might even be argued that drug treatments should be expected to be more successful at higher levels of the nervous system. For example, trophic hormones that stimulate growth could very well play an important role in facilitating recovery after brain injury. Despite the fact that enzyme therapy for spinal cord injuries has not been particularly successful or well viewed by scientists, the belief that any treatment for nervous injury might be worth pursuing has led at least a few investigators to examine whether hormone treatments could be used to enhance return of function after traumatic brain injury.

The initial studies on brain were practically direct extensions of experiments conducted with spinal cord preparations. About 30 years ago, for example, Windle, Clemente, and Chambers (1952) tried to get peripheral neurons, which have considerable regenerative capacity, to penetrate into the central nervous system in adult animals. They reasoned that such an attempt would serve as a model for understanding how the central nervous system might repair itself after injury. The logic was based upon their previous work showing that glial-pial scars after spinal cord transections block the growth of axons across the barrier. If it were possible to eliminate or reduce the glial barrier formed by astrocytes after lesions in the brain, perhaps regeneration at higher levels could occur.[4]

Accordingly, two adult cats served as subjects. With the animals under anesthesia, the temporal branch of their facial nerve was exposed as far as possible. A small opening was then made in the skull and the proximal stump of the cut nerve was inserted into the right temporal lobe to a depth of 3–4 mm. The cats were kept alive for 36 days and then killed for histological examination. One cat

---

[3] This argument would be weakened if investigators could show that the lesions were the same in both treated and untreated groups, with appropriate histological methods.

[4] This work was designed and conducted well before anomalous sprouting after central nervous system lesions had become a well-documented phenomenon—see Chapters 5 and 6.

was given pyromen (Piromen) intravenously for 28 days after the operation and the other received no medication. Silver and thionin stains were used to evaluate the penetration and regeneration of the cut facial nerve stumps.

In the nontreated cat, no blending of peripheral nerve with brain tissue was observed and there was a distinct glial scar at the wound site. Regenerating fibers were seen, but they did not enter into the brain. Instead, they grew along strands of connective tissue and membrane or were blocked by glia and turned back toward the center of the nerve—a phenomenon akin to that seen when spinal neurons were thwarted in their attempts to cross the transected stump of the cord.

According to Windle *et al.* (1952), the animal treated with pyromen showed a completely different picture. In this animal, the facial nerve merged with the brain tissue and there was no glial scar.

> The peripheral nerve implant in the Pyromen treated animal showed no sharp demarcation from the brain. The regenerating nerve fibers, neurolemma cells, connective tissue and blood vessels grew out in a radial manner to become indistinguishably blended with the brain [p. 361].

Windle and his students argued that the drug, pyromen, blocks scar formation and thus permits regenerating fibers to penetrate the brain. From this position, we can infer that the primary failure to obtain regeneration is due to a physical barrier that blocks the fibers from traversing the wound. Windle *et al.* (1952) suggest that pyrogens act to reduce scarring by stimulating the secretions of the adrenal gland.

> By this route and perhaps by direct action it (the adrenal) appears to alter certain connective tissue ground substances and cells. It exerts a powerful stimulating effect upon connection tissue cells of a low order of differentiation . . . and retards the proliferation of astrocytes which form glial scars. . . . We have recently produced a somewhat similar picture of spinal cord regeneration, in experiments substituting administration of ACTH for Pyromen (Clemente, 1951) [unpublished data], emphasizing the role of adrenal glands in this process [pp. 366–367].

The work of Windle and his students was extended, some 6 years later, by Clemente (1958). This author performed nerve implantation experiments in rats, cats, and rabbits in order to determine whether Windle's initial findings could generalize to other species, and also to respond to others who had failed in their attempts to obtain significant results. Basically, the new experiments were designed in the same way, except for the fact that wound healing after brain puncture *without* nerve implants was also examined. After surgery, some of the animals received either daily treatments with a pyrogen, ACTH, or cortisone, or they remained untreated until they were killed for histological examination from 1 to 180 days after surgery.

With respect to nerve regeneration in control animals, there was considerable activity, but the growing fibers did not penetrate into the substance of the brain itself. Clemente (1958) stated, "The fibers had grown to the outermost limits of the implanted nerve, but in control animals the fibers grew away from the brain substance, seeming to take the course of least resistance [p. 129]."

The results of the various drug treatments were mixed. In some of the animals, there were *no* beneficial consequences of the treatments, whereas others showed better wound healing, less scar formation, and blending of peripheral with central neurons following implantations. Why some animals provide a better matrix for repair than others had no simple explanation. In fact, the same phenomenon is often seen in clinical cases: Some patients show remarkable recovery after massive brain injury, whereas others with much less extensive damage remain permanently impaired. Unfortunately, these individual differences in response to brain damage are rarely given attention in the literature because the inductive method stresses *group* data and *averages,* rather than careful analyses of individual "exceptions" to the mean.

Experiments on implants of peripheral nerves into the material substance of the brain provide an interesting model for the study of regenerative phenomena. However, they say little about functional activity, nor do they directly answer the question of whether specific, pharmacological treatments can facilitate *behavioral* recovery from brain injuries. To answer these questions, we must turn to actual cases of brain damage and ask whether pharmacological agents can be effective in enhancing the reparative process following injury at the highest levels. For instance, if severed axons in the spinal cord could be made to regenerate by treatments with pyrogens, steroids, or enzymes designed to block glial scar formation, might not the same agents aid in healing cerebral wounds?

One of the first attempts to resolve this question was made by Clemente (1955). Pairs of young, but mature, rats of both sexes were first anesthetized and then given stab wounds of the cerebral cortex through a trephine hole made in the skull. One member of each pair was left untreated after the injury, whereas the other was given daily intramuscular injections of 5 mg / kg cortisone for a period of 3 weeks. The pairs of animals were then killed from 1 to 56 days after the injury and their brains examined for neuronal loss and connective scar infiltration in the area of the cortical wound. Clemente noted that the rats treated with cortisone showed a consistently smaller amount of connective tissue in the area of the lesion. There appeared to be less neuronal degeneration in the wound area as well.

A more detailed and systematic attempt to enhance central nervous system regeneration pharmacologically was made in 1971 by A. Fertig, J. A. Kiernan, and S. Sevan of Cambridge, England. The overall design of their experiment was quite similar to that described by Clemente (1955). Adult rats of both sexes were given stab wounds of the cortex and then were either left untreated or given chronic doses of corticotrophin (ACTH) or triiodothyronine (T3) a substance similar to thyroxine. In this study, the rats were killed 50 days after the stab wounds, so that their brains could be examined for fiber regeneration and the extent of scar tissue formation. Briefly stated, both ACTH and T3 appeared to produce beneficial consequences. Scars formed by connective tissue were less dense, and regenerating axons could be seen entering the gap caused by the stab wounds. Whereas all of the rats given chronic ACTH administration showed at least some evidence of axonal regrowth, only 5 of 24 control animals showed any evidence of regeneration in brain tissue adjacent to the wound area. Some of these findings are illustrated in Figures 11.6 and 11.7.

The specific drug actions that facilitate axonal growth and block excessive scar formation are still not well understood. Fertig and his colleagues speculate that ACTH limited the extent of collagen formation triggered by the stab wound. However, they point out that some connective tissue may be necessary to serve as a scaffold for regenerating axons trying to reestablish synaptic contacts with intact brain. A week of ACTH treatments seemed sufficient to produce the desired effects on collagen growth; more treatments actually seemed to inhibit the regeneration process. In contrast, T3, the thyroid hormone, was thought to facilitate nerve regeneration by a different mechanism. Instead of suppressing collagen, T3 was hypothesized to act by increasing protein synthesis in the affected axons. Such stimulation could assist the regenerating axons in competition with invading connective tissues, which could block the regenerative process.

Fertig's study is interesting because it was one of the first to demonstrate that pharmacological agents could modify cerebral anatomical response to injury. The changes, thought to be beneficial, were not merely due to the presence of spared neural elements, as might be the case after incomplete spinal cord transections. Unfortunately, Fertig's group did not collect any pre- or postoperative *behavioral* measures to determine if the stab wounds had any functional consequences and whether the treatment with ACTH or T3 restored behavior to preoperative levels of performance. Furthermore, one must consider the possibility that it may not even be the case that these agents are acting directly to facilitate regeneration. ACTH, for example, may simply reduce the edema that almost certainly follows traumatic manipulation of the brain. Fertig and colleagues noted that the steroid treatments were only effective during the first postoperative week—a time when edema is most prevalent. This is not to imply that the treatments are worthless, but rather that physiological processes thought to mediate axonal regeneration might be due to short-term mechanical events occurring in the wound area. It is also worth considering that ACTH and T3 might act to change the liquid milieu in the lesion zone—a factor which is often overlooked in the study of regenerative phenomena occurring in the central nervous system.

As we can see, there are a number of difficulties in using steroid hormones to facilitate recovery from brain damage, particularly as these substances have such widespread systemic effects. ACTH, for example, plays an important role in the

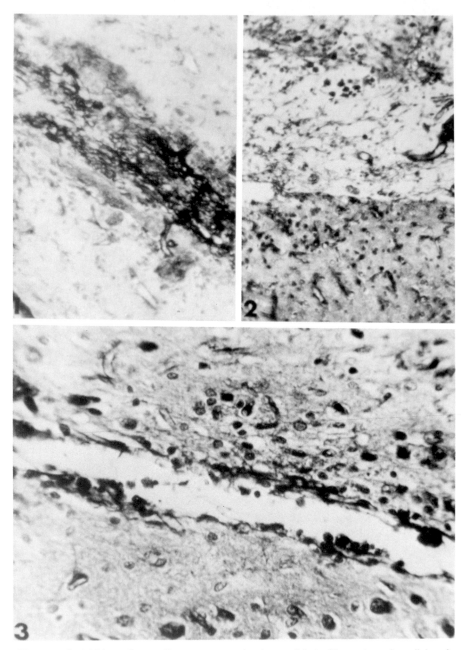

Figure 11.6. *(1) Shows dense collagenous connective tissue, with the fibers oriented parallel to the plane of the lesion, in a control animal. Azan.* × *40. (2) Shows loose connective tissue with fibers more or less randomly arranged. ACTH, short-term animal. Azan.* × *40. (3) Shows a lesion with hardly any connective tissue in the gap. ACTH, long-term animal. Azan.* × *200. (From Fertig et al., 1971.)*

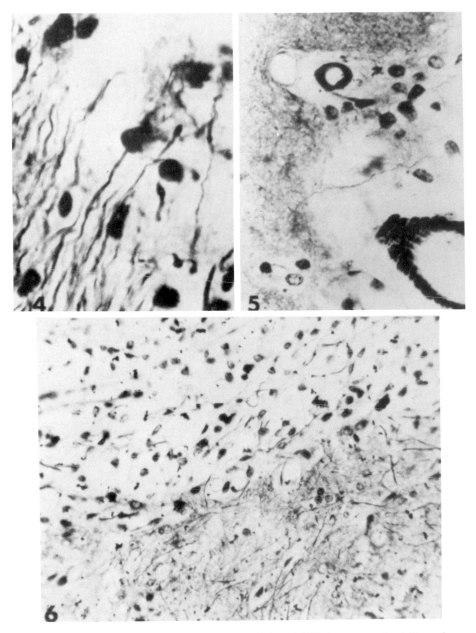

Figure 11.7. *(4) Shows regenerating axons entering lesion. ACTH, long-term animal. Urea-silver nitrate. × 300. (5) Shows a cortical axon regenerating for a considerable distance into the lesion of a rat in the ACTH, long-term group. Urea-silver nitrate. × 350. (6) Shows a wide lesion containing loose connective tissue into which many axons have regenerated. ACTH, short-term animal. Urea-silver nitrate × 200. (From Fertig* et al., *1971.)*

organism's response to stress, and certainly surgical trauma must be considered highly stressful. In addition, most experimental testing situations can also be considered stressful in that behavioral testing usually requires food or water deprivation, avoidance of painful stimuli, or sudden exposure to handling and novel stimulation. If focal brain damage does alter the output of the pituitary-adrenal axis, ACTH administration might "facilitate" behavioral recovery by increasing the animal's ability to respond to stressful situations. This is an alternative and simpler explanation for recovery than hypothesizing focal regenerative processes, especially if the recovery is very rapid.

Some indirect evidence to support this possibility comes from the work of Daniel Bush and his colleagues (Bush, Lovely, and Pagano, 1973). These investigators made bilateral lesions of the basolateral and basomedial amygdaloid nuclei in adult female rats and taught the animals to escape shock by running in a shuttle-box each time a tone was presented. In general, rats with lesions of the amygdaloid nuclei have difficulty in learning any aversively motivated tasks and, as expected, animals given placebo treatments before or after these lesions were very much impaired. Another group of brain-damaged rats received a subcutaneous injection of ACTH 1 hour prior to the initiation of training in the shuttlebox. These rats learned the task as well as control animals when both acquisition and extinction of the avoidance response were evaluated. Bush and his colleagues interpreted their data to indicate that the ACTH injection restored the animals' capacity to respond to stress and that this was the basis for their apparent "recovery" from brain damage. In this context, it would have been interesting to see if deficits would appear at a later time, once the effects of the hormone injection had worn off.

Despite the fact that hormones produce a broad spectrum of physiological effects (that make monolithic explanations of recovery very difficult), they do seem to enhance the organism's capacity to respond to brain injury. Not only has ACTH been examined, but more recently, some investigators have proposed that, under the appropriate circumstances, even insulin treatments could be beneficial in promoting recovery from brain damage.

In one experiment, John DeCastro and Saul Balagura (1976) created bilateral lesions of the dorsal hippocampus in adult rats after treating half the group with insulin (3 units) and the other half with saline injections. The brain-damaged rats were then compared to sham-operated controls in their ability to acquire an active avoidance response to electric shock. In this case, the conditioned stimulus was also a buzzer that preceded the onset of shock by about 10 seconds.

DeCastro and Balagura noted that the animals with hippocampal lesions were very impaired in learning the task and this included the group that had received the insulin treatment prior to surgery. However, the latter group performed significantly better than the group receiving saline injections, so there was some sparing produced by the insulin treatments. For the most part, the rats given

TABLE 11.1

Median and Range of Escape and Avoidance Latencies (Seconds) for the Four Groups[a]

Group	Median	Range	Median	Range
		Escape trials		
Insulin—sham	11.1	10.8–12.3	2.3	1.4–3.2
Saline—sham	11.0	10.9–11.3	1.6	1.1–2.8
Insulin—hippocampal	11.3	10.8–11.9	1.7	1.1–3.6
Saline—hippocampal	11.3	10.9–12.0	2.8	1.6–3.9

[a]*Reprinted with permission from DeCastro, J. and Balagura, S. Insulin pretreatment facilitates recovery after dorsal hippocampal lesions.* Physiology and Behavior. *Copyright 1976, Pergamon Press, Ltd.*

preoperative insulin took fewer sessions to learn to avoid, experienced fewer shocks during the learning process, and showed less emotionality (refusing to run and accepting painful shock—i.e., freezing) than saline-treated counterparts. This is shown in Table 11.1 and in Figures 11.8 and 11.9. Figure 11.10 shows a lesion representative of those sustained by the animals in this study.

We should note that the hypoglycemia produced by insulin treatment is a stressor and, as such, may have played a role in inducing the animals to run—an interpretation that would not be inconsistent with data described in the Bush *et*

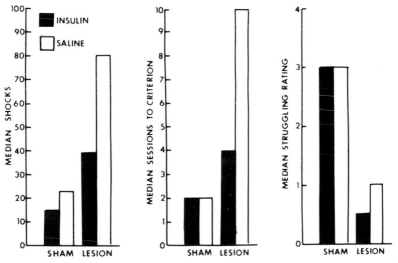

Figure 11.8. *The median number of shocks incurred (left) in the 10 sessions, the median number of sessions to attain criterion performance (center), and the median struggling ratings (right) for saline pretreated (white) and insulin pretreated (black) animals after either sham operation or dorsal hippocampal lesion. (Reprinted with permission from DeCastro, J. and Balagura, S. Insulin pretreatment facilitates recovery after dorsal hippocampal lesions.* Physiology and Behavior. *Copyright 1976, Pergamon Press, Ltd.)*

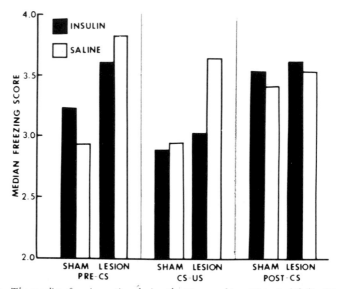

Figure 11.9. *The median freezing rating during the 10-second pre-CS period (left), CS-US interval (center), and post-CS period (right) for saline pretreated (white) and insulin pretreated (grey) animals after either sham operation or dorsal hippocampal lesion. The scores for the CS-US interval includes only those trials in which an escape response occurred. (Reprinted with permission from DeCastro, J. and Balagura, S. Insulin pretreatment facilitates recovery after dorsal hippocampal lesions.* Physiology and Behavior. *Copyright 1976, Pergamon Press, Ltd.)*

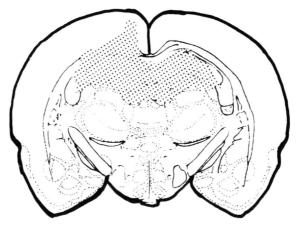

Figure 11.10. *Reconstruction of the maximum extent of the brain damage for a representative animal. (Reprinted with permission from DeCastro, J. and Balagura, S. Insulin pretreatment facilitates recovery after dorsal hippocampal lesions.* Physiology and Behavior. *Copyright 1976, Pergamon Press. Ltd.)*

al. (1973) experiment that we just discussed. In fact, there is very little evidence to suggest that insulin can have *direct* effects on neurons in the central nervous system, although it may affect the secretion of other hormones that could affect central nervous system functioning.

Again, the question of long-term, postoperative benefits of the insulin treatments were not examined, nor was there detailed anatomical analyses of sprouting or regeneration, so we do not know whether the reported "facilitation" was temporary and limited just to the specific test situation or whether the animals would have remained "recovered" on the series of tests long after treatments had been discontinued.

In general, treatments with hormones do indicate that the entire "internal milieu" of the animal may be changed by the hormone treatments such that the effects of focal lesions on behavior may not be the same. In previous chapters, we have seen how environmental manipulation can "tune" the central nervous system to respond to trauma in a way which would depend upon the kind of experience or life history that the organism has. This causes us to emphasize again that recovery—or the failure to observe it—in behavioral experiments is determined not just by the locus of the damage, but by other factors as well. The background matrix upon which the damage is inflicted may be the most important consideration in this regard.

References

Barber, B. Resistance by scientists to scientific discovery. *Science,* 1961, *134,* 596–602.

Brailowsky, S. Neuropharmacological aspects of brain plasticity. In P. Bach-y-Rita (Ed.), *Recovery of function: Theoretical considerations for brain injury rehabilitation.* Baltimore, Md.: University Park Press, 1980, Pp. 187–215.

Brown-Séquard, C. E. Experiences sur les plaies de la moelle épinière. *Comptes Rendus de la Societe de Biologie,* 1850, *1,* 17–18.(a)

Brown-Séquard, C. E. Régénération des tissus de la moelle épinière. *Comptes Rendus de la Societe de Biologie,* 1850, *2,* 3.(b)

Brown-Séquard, C. E. Sur plusiers cas ce citatrisation de plaies faites à la moelle épinière avec retour des fonctions perdues. *Comptes Rendus de la Societe de Biologie,* 1851, *3,* 77–79.

Bush, D., Lovely, R. H., and Pagano, R. R. Injection of ACTH induces recovery from shuttle-box avoidance deficits in rats with amygdaloid lesions. *Journal of Comparative Physiological Psychology,* 1973, *83,* 168–172.

Campbell, J. B., Bassett, C. A. L., Husby, J., and Noback, C. R. Regeneration of adult mammalian spinal cord. *Science,* 1957, *126,* 929.

Clemente, C. D. Structural regeneration in the mammalian central nervous system and the role of neuroglia and connective tissue. In W. F. Windle (Ed.), *Regeneration in the central nervous system.* Springfield, Ill.: Charles C Thomas, 1955, Pp. 147–161.

Clemente, C. D. The regeneration of peripheral nerves inserted into the cerebral cortex and the healing of cerebral lesions. *Journal of Comparative Neurology,* 1958, *109,* 123–151.

Clemente, C. D., and Windle, W. F. Regeneration of severed nerve fibers in the spinal cord of the adult cat. *Journal of Comparative Neurology*, 1954, *101*, 691–731.

DeCastro, J., and Balagura, S. Insulin pretreatment facilitates recovery after dorsal hippocampal lesions. *Physiology and Behavior*, 1976, *16*, 517–529.

Feringa, E., Kowalski, T. F., Vahlsing, H. L., and Frye, R. A. Enzyme treatment of spinal cord transected rats. *Annals of Neurology*, 1979, *5*, 203–206.

Fertig, A., Kiernan, J. A., and Sevan, S. S. A. S. Enhancement of axonal regeneration in the brain of the rat by corticotrophin and triiodothyronine. *Experimental Neurology*, 1971, *33*, 372–385.

Guth, L., Albuquerque, E. X., Deshpande, S. S., Barrett, C. P., Donati, E. J., and Warnick, J. E. Ineffectiveness of enzyme therapy on regeneration in the transected spinal cord of the rat. *Journal of Neurosurgery*, 1980, *52*, 73–86.

Harvey, J., and Srebnik, H. Locomotor activity and axon regeneration following spinal cord compression in rats treated with L-thyroxine. *Journal of Neuropathology and Experimental Neurology*, 1967, *26*, 666–668.

McMasters, R. E. Regeneration of the spinal cord in the rat: Positive influence of nerve growth factor. *Journal of Comparative Neurology*, 1962, *119*, 113–125.

Matinian, L. A., and Andreasian, A. S. Enzyme therapy in organic lesions of the spinal cord. *Brain Information Service*, UCLA, 1973, 162–169. (Translated from the Russian version).

Sugar, O., and Gerard, R. W. Spinal cord regeneration in the rat. *Journal of Neurophysiology*, 1940, *3*, 1–19.

West, J. R. Early history of mammalian nerve regeneration. *Neuroscience and Biobehavioral Reviews*, 1978, *2*, 27–32.

Windle, W. F., Clemente, C. D., and Chambers, W. W. Inhibition of formation of a glial barrier as a means of permitting a peripheral nerve to grow into the brain. *Journal of Comparative Neurology*, 1952, *96*, 359–370.

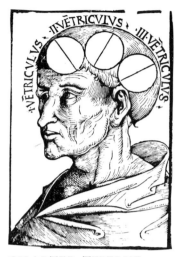

Drugs and Recovery: Nerve Growth Factor, Stimulants, and "De-blocking" Agents

Neodecorticate cats that have had a loss of visual and tactile placing of long standing usually exhibit these behaviors after treatment with amphetamines. Evidently, . . . recovery is possible in animals that lack those regions of the neocortex that have been considered to be completely indispensible [Meyer, Horel, and Meyer, 1963, p. 404].

CHAPTER TWELVE

Since the beginning of this century, embryologists have been trying to identify the growth factors responsible for the development, migration, and structural aggregation of neurons. One approach used by embryologists is to transplant bits of tissue (e.g., limb buds, spinal cord, ganglia) from one part of the developing neural tube to the other. Chick embryos are often used in such experiments because the patterns of innervation of the tissue transplants can easily be observed (Hamburger, 1980).

In 1948, a growth factor was accidently discovered when E. Beuker, working in Viktor Hamburger's laboratory at Washington University, decided to implant mouse sarcoma into the body cavity of chick embryos as a control for other kinds of tissue transplants. The tumor substance "took" and grew well in the body cavities of the embryos, but this was not the most impressive finding. The exciting result was that the tumor tissue was invaded by sensory and sympathetic fibers from the peripheral nervous system. Follow-up studies in Hamburger's laboratory revealed that the sensory and sympathetic ganglia in animals with tumor transplants were more than six times larger than normal. A potent neural growth factor seemed to be present in the sarcoma itself.

A short time after this discovery, Rita Levi-Montalcini, a well-known neurobiologist from the same univeristy, placed spinal and sympathetic ganglia isolated from embryos in solutions containing pieces of sarcoma. Even at a distance from the tumor tissue, the ganglia showed extensive growth, demonstrating that a diffusible trophic substance was responsible for the outgrowth. In 1953, Cohen and Hamburger identified the underlying stimulus as a protein, which they first called *nerve growth-promoting factor* (NGF) (Cohen, Levi-Montalcini, and Hamburger, 1954).

Since that time, many hundreds of studies have been performed on the biochemistry and physiology of NGF, partly because the protein has been viewed as an excellent tool for understanding neurotrophic principles.[1] Yet, despite this great interest in NGF and its obvious biological importance as a neurotrophic agent, there has been very little done to assess its effects on the central nervous system or on the behavior of intact or brain-damaged organisms. This may be due to the facts that first, until recently, questions existed over whether NGF could be found in the brain itself (see Walker Weichsel, Fisher, Guo, and Fisher, 1979); second, NGF was very difficult to produce in quantities sufficient for behavioral studies; and third, most investigators concerned with the biochemistry and physiology of the protein felt that it had little, if any, significance for central nervous system functions and probably nothing to do with behavior per se.[2]

The first attempts to explore the question of whether NGF had a *functional* role in the brain itself had to wait until 1972 when Anders Björklund and his associates in Lund, Sweden (Björklund and Stenevi, 1972; see also Bjerre, Björklund, and Stenevi, 1973) applied NGF to damaged, monoaminergic neurons in the medial forebrain bundle of rats. These workers were interested in the problem of regeneration of axons and, as we noted in Chapter 4, they developed a new way of studying the phenomenon. First, the Swedish workers transected the medial forebrain bundle and inserted a piece of iris taken from the eye of the same experimental animal. The iris is adrenergically innervated and the fibers of the medial forebrain bundle are also adrenergic, so they thought that the interposed tissue would serve as a "trophic target" if axons were to regenerate. This is shown schematically in Figure 12.1. Björklund and his colleagues used histofluorescence techniques to measure the extent and rate of regeneration. Under the right conditions, fibers containing monamines can be made to glow green or yellow-green when properly treated—the more catecholamine present, the more intense the reaction; and this is taken as an indication of regenerative activity.

Without any treatment there is some innervation of the transplanted iris,

[1] For recent reviews of NGF, the following can be consulted: Levi-Montalcini (1976), Levi-Montalcini and Calissano (1979), Bradshaw (1978), and Harper and Thoenen (1980).

[2] There is now some evidence that this protein, which appears to play a role in normal development, is taken up by retrograde axonal transport in adrenergic neurons where it affects an increase in tyrosine hydroxylase levels (Stoeckel and Thoenen, 1975) and lipid and protein synthesis (see review in Levi-Montalcini, Angeletti, and Angeletti, 1972). Varon (1975) cites data to suggest that NGF affects intracellular dopamine and tyrosine synthesis, and also plays a role in regulating RNA synthesis. Varon also mentions the possibility that NGF may alter membrane permeability and enhance the ability of neurons to adhere to glia, cells that are known to play an important role in guiding neurons to their appropriate target sites during development. Some of these data are presented in a recent review by Varon and Bunge (1978).

Figure 12.1. *Position of the iris transplant in the caudal diencephalon. The lesion produced by the transplantation (cross-hatched area) transects the two major ascending monoamine fiber systems; the dorsal catecholamine bundle (DCB), containing predominantly noradrenaline axons; and the medial forebrain bundle (MFB), containing indolamine axons (not represented in the diagram), dopamine axons (originating, inter alia, in the substantia nigra, SN), and also noradrenaline axons (originating in the ventral catecholamine bundle, VCB). In the specimens used for the present study, the transplant is in direct contact with the growing monoamine fibers in these two bundles. The magnitude of ingrowth into the transplant illustrated in the diagram is that observed in control specimens 7 days after the transplantation. Filled circles: dopamine-containing cell bodies; open circles: noradrenaline-containing cell bodies. Arrows indicate sites of injections. C, Close to the noradrenaline cell bodies in the locus coeruleus (LC); B, close to the noradrenaline axons in the DCB and, about 3 mm caudal to the site of the lesion; A, close to the DCB and is about 1 mm caudal to the lesion. When the transplant is placed in this position, fibers will grow into it from different locations: 1, the habenula region; 2, the DCB; 3, the MFB; 4, blood vessels (BV) at the base of the brain. Note: This is a schematic drawing of a transplant in a nonsympathectomized animal. The representation of the catecholamine bundles is that of Ungerstedt. (From Stenevi et al., 1974.)*

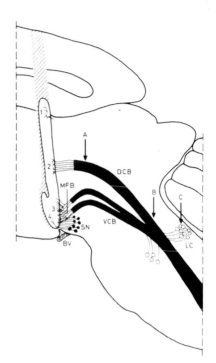

although it is at first rather sparse and thin (see Chapter 4). In contrast, when NGF was injected into the cerebral ventricles at the time of the iris transplant, the extent of the regeneration was considerable. There were abundant new nerve bundles growing into and around the iris, which showed intense fluorescence.

In later experiments, Björklund and his colleagues (Bjerre, Björklund, and Stenevi, 1974, Stenevi, Bjerre, Björklund, and Mobley, 1974) injected NGF in much smaller quantities directly into the area of the implant or into the area of the cell bodies that make up part of the medial forebrain bundle. Smaller doses of NGF in these regions were just as effective as larger amounts placed into the ventricles. However, in order to facilitate the regeneration, the NGF had to be given at the time of the transplants. Some of these findings are illustrated in Figures 12.2 and 12.3.

Although the studies by Björklund and his group were well executed and important in that they demonstrated that NGF can play a role in regeneration in the brain itself, they did not provide any evidence that such regeneration could have

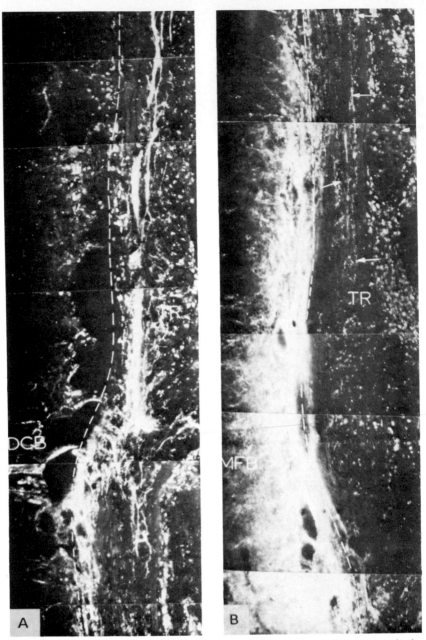

Figure 12.2. *(A) and (B): NGF-treated specimen given 200 B.U. of NGF, close to the locus coeruleus (Figure 12.1, injection site C) at the time of transplantation and killed 7 days later. (A) shows the upper half of the transplant (TR) extending from the DCB region up to the habenula region (cf. Figure 12.1). (B) shows the lower half of the same transplant reaching down to the MFB region (cf. Figure 12.1). In (A), extensive bundles and irregular networks of catecholamine fibers are seen growing into the transplant from the DCB. WIthin the transplant, these fiber formations extend dorsally up to the habenula region, and in (B) ventrally toward the MFB region (see arrows in B). Catecholamine fibers are seen in (B) on the caudal surface of the transplant, bordering the MFB, but practically no fibers are demonstrated within the transplant. The dashed lines indicate the caudal*

230

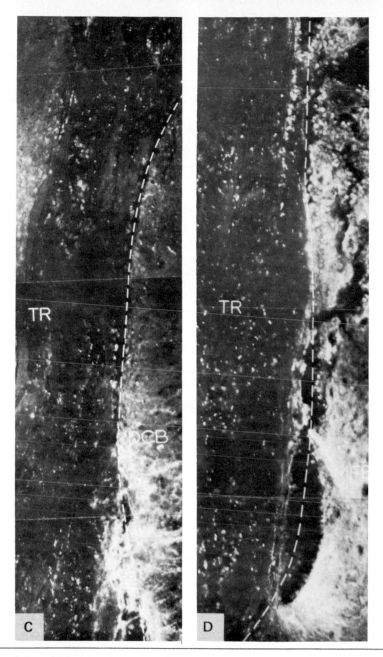

border of the transplant (× 130). (C) and (D); Control specimen given saline close to the locus coeruleus at the time of transplantation and killed 7 days later. (C) shows the upper half of the transplant (TR), as in (A) and (D); the lower half, as in (B). In (C), the catecholamine fibers growing from the DCB are restricted to the surface zone of the transplant facing the lesioned bundle (cf. the NGF-treated specimen shown in (A) and (B). (D): the very limited growth of fibers into the transplant from the MFB is similar to that of the NFG-treated specimen in (B). The dashed lines indicate the caudal border of the transplant (× 130). Abbreviations as in Figure 12.1. (From Stenevi et al., 1974.)

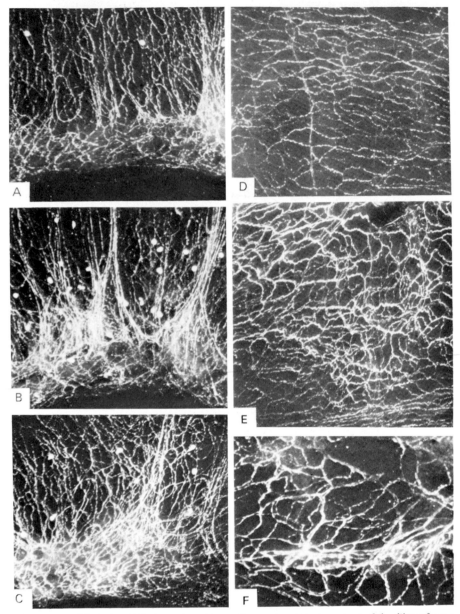

Figure 12.3. *Iris A, (× 130) shows the sphincter (bottom) and the inner part of the dilator from a 3-month-old mouse given saline (A); from a 4-week-old given NGF (B); and from a 3-month-old given NFG (C). All animals were killed 3 days after the last injection. Parts D and E (× 140) show the central part of the dilator from 3-month-old mice given saline (D) and NGF (C) and killed 3 days after the last injection. Part F (× 210) illustrated a hyperinnervated vessel in the dilator from a 3-month-old mouse given NGF and killed 3 days after the last injection. (From Bjerre et al., 1973.)*

functional or behavioral consequences. Even in the case of the innervation of the iris, it was not possible to tell whether the penetrating fibers were capable of adaptive physiological activity (i.e., neurotransmitter release and re-uptake). Might they have served to form aborted contacts or a kind of nonfunctional neuroma? This question was never approached. In fact, very little work has been done on the behavioral consequences of NGF treatments, whether they are applied to the central nervous system or to sympathetic ganglia.

Shortly after Björklund, Bjerre, and Stenevi published their papers, Barry Berger, C. David Wise, and Larry Stein (1973) did try to determine whether NGF could play a role in mediating functional recovery from brain lesions. Berger and his associates decided to give NGF injections to adult rats with lesions of the lateral hypothalamic area—a region of the brain considered critical for mediation of food intake and weight regulation. It is also an area rich in catecholaminergic neurons, which in turn are thought to be particularly sensitive to the effects of NGF.

Bilateral, single-stage lesions of the lateral hypothalamic area (LH) often produce severe aphagia and adipsia in well-fed animals and only careful handling and forced feeding can ensure the survival of affected animals. Berger et al. (1973) created LH lesions and at the same time administered 4 μg of NGF into the cerebral ventricles; another group with similar brain damage received a saline injection. In brief, the rats given NGF recovered faster than controls; the NGF-treated animals began to eat spontaneously and regained weight more rapidly.

Several months later, when both control and NGF-treated rats were regulating weight normally, the two groups were given injections of a neurotoxin, 6-OHDA, which destroys dopaminergic neurons. By itself, 6-OHDA can cause the "lateral hypothalamic syndrome," so it was not surprising that the deficits returned in both the experimental and control groups. However, the animals treated with NGF again showed much more rapid recovery of function than control animals.

Until recently, the Berger, Wise, and Stein report was the only one demonstrating behavioral effects of intracerebral administration of NGF in the mammal. That is, there were no attempts to extend their research any further. Because of this paucity of data and our interest in recovery of function, some of us at Clark University (Hart, Chaimas, Moore, and Stein, 1978) decided to examine the role of NGF in facilitating recovery of learned habits after lesions of the caudate-putamen complex. We chose to investigate the interaction between lesions of the caudate region and NGF administration because this complex is heavily populated by dopaminergic neurons, previously shown by Björklund and Stenevi (1972) to be sensitive to NGF, and because it had been shown (Shultze and Stein, 1975) that bilateral, single-stage lesions of caudate nucleus result in increased perseverative behavior (i.e., inability to "give-up" a previously learned habit) as well as severe deficits in active avoidance learning (i.e., running to escape footshock when a tone or other warning stimulus is presented). We also knew that caudate lesions can result in loss of capacity to regulate body weight. Overall, the caudate seemed like a good choice to begin our investigations.

In our first experiment, we used three groups of adult male rats as subjects. One group, given only sham operations, provided normal "baseline" performance data. Two other groups received bilateral, simultaneous damage to the caudate nucleus. Ten of these animals were given immediate bilateral injections of 2.5S NGF, while another ten received the same volume of the solution used as the vehicle for the NGF. All of the injections were made *directly* into the caudate, about 1 mm posterior to the electrode placement.

The rats were given a week to recover from the surgery and then began training on discriminative, active avoidance tasks. To avoid shock, the rats had to run to the initially nonpreferred side of a two-choice discrimination apparatus. Once they had learned to go to one side, the position of the "safe" box was reversed; what was correct became incorrect, and this reversal procedure was followed four times. We felt that this would be a good measure of performance after NGF treatments because, as we noted, rats with caudate lesions find it very difficult to reverse a previously learned habit.

Our results proved interesting. In the first place, with respect to spatial reversal performance, both groups of animals with brain damage were initially impaired. However, as the training continued, the rats given the single injection of NGF at the time of surgery began to perform as well as the sham-operated control animals. In contrast, the rats without NGF *continued* to show a learning deficit throughout their entire period of testing. This can be seen in Figure 12.4.

With respect to weight regulation and consummatory behaviors, the results were less dramatic. Still, the untreated rats tended to show a net loss in body weight following the lesions, whereas the animals given NGF all had exceeded their preoperative weights within 15 days after surgery. The rats treated with NGF also drank more water than control animals, but this may have been due to the fact that NGF is contaminated by renin—something we did not think about until later in our work.[3]

After behavioral testing was completed, the animals were killed for histo-

---

[3] It is now known that the increased drinking (polydipsia) seen after intracranial injection of NGF is due to the presence of isorenin bound to the 2.5S NGF molecule. Only additional purification steps can eliminate all renin-like activity (Levi-Montalcini, 1980). Recently, Avrith, Lewis, and Fitzsimmons (1980) showed that intracranial injection of angiotensin II or renin causes an immediate thirst and delayed sodium appetite; responses almost identical to those induced by 2.5S NGF injection. Because we were concerned that the learning facilitation that we observed in NGF-treated rats with caudate lesions could reflect this confounding, we (Sabel, Kardon, and Stein, unpublished) prepared animals with caudate lesions and treated them with intracerebral injections of renin alone. When tested using the procedures of Hart *et al.* (1978) these animals were impaired on the learning tasks. Thus, the effects of NGF and renin may be dissociated; renin may disrupt learning, whereas NGF seemed to be facilitory.

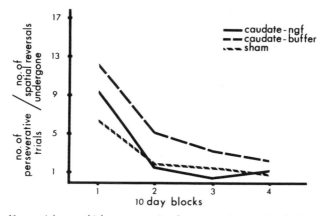

Figure 12.4. *Mean trials on which rats committed perseverative error(s) during spatial reversal testing. The dependent variable was generated by dividing number of perseverations in each 10-day block of trials by the number of spatial reversals. (From Hart et al., 1978.)*

logical analysis. We expected to find that the NGF treatments would spare more neurons in the damaged caudate nucleus, and so cell counts of intact neurons were compared to those found in the unoperated animals. Our analysis did *not* reveal any evidence of neuronal sparing; there were no differences in the number of healthy, intact neurons between those rats treated with NGF or those given only an injection of inert buffer. In fact, both operated groups had a similar net reduction in healthy caudate neurons. Figures 12.5 and 12.6 show brain sections from these animals.

What, then, could account for the behavioral sparing that we observed with the single intracerebral injection of NGF given at the time of surgery? In addition to counting intact neurons, we also examined the neuron to glia ratios and measured dopamine (DA) content in the caudate nucleus. There were no differences in DA content among the groups; steady-state levels of DA measured some 6 months after surgery were within the normal range, so long-standing differences in neurotransmitter levels could not explain our findings. We did observe that when the animals were killed for histology (6 months after surgery), there was a marked increase in the glia-to-neuron ratio for operated rats. However, the increase was significantly less in the animals given NGF than in their counterparts treated with buffer solution.

At the time, we though that the glia may have facilitated recovery of behavioral functions by assisting in the removal of debris, whereas the NGF treatments could then have played a role by suppressing astrocytic scar formation. Alternatively, we also speculated that the glia may have played a direct role in restoring function to remaining neurons, possibly by supplying nutriments to the

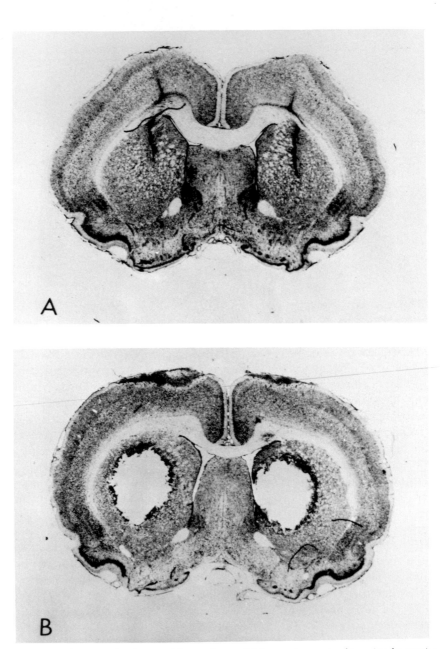

Figure 12.5. *Photomicrographs (× 28) for caudate nuclei damage in an animal permitted to survive 6 months postoperatively (Part A), and in a rat killed 5 days after the lesion was created by applying the same parameters (Part B). (From Hart et al., 1978.)*

remaining intact neurons of the caudate. In any case, although we could only guess at the mechanisms, it did appear that the administration of NGF directly into the brain facilitated morphological processes that correlated with functional recovery.

At first, we were surprised to find that NGF administration altered the glial reaction to injury, but a subsequent report by Ronald Lindsay led us to examine this question further. Lindsay (1979) first created an astrocyte reaction in the caudate nucleus of adult rats by injection of the neurotoxin, kainic acid, into that structure. The astrocytes were then cultured in vitro to provide a growth medium for sensory neurons taken from rat or chick embryos. As shown in Figure 12.7, the sensory neurons were able to survive and extend neurites in the medium containing the astrocytes, or in solutions of NGF itself. Sensory neurons placed in control media did not survive at all.

Lindsay thought his results indicated that glial cells actively support the growth of neurons and may secrete NGF under the appropriate conditions. He noted that application of anti-NGF sera to the medium blocked the growth-promoting effects of the astrocytes.

Lindsay's report encouraged us to perform an in vivo examination of the effects of intracerebral NGF administration on astrocyte activity in brain-damaged rats. We wanted to determine whether there was a time-dependent relationship between administration of NGF to a brain-damaged organism and reactive astrocytosis. In this study, we did not examine any postoperative behavior, preferring instead to use each experimental animal as its own histological control. Accordingly, we created bilateral lesions in the caudate nucleus of adult male rats and then injected NGF directly into the wound area on one side of the brain. The caudate nucleus in the opposite hemisphere was injected with an indentical volume of buffer control solution. Groups of animals were then allowed to survive from 8 hours to 60 days postoperatively. A comparable group of rats received injections of NGF on one side of the brain and buffer on the other, but were given no lesions. In this fashion, we could compare the number and size of reactive astrocytes on the NGF-treated side of the brain with the astrocytic reaction in the untreated damaged caudate. By using animals with no lesions as additional controls, we were able to examine whether the glial reaction to NGF would occur in brains that had received much less extensive injury (i.e., the opening of the skull and the inserting of the hypodermic needle into the brain tissue, as opposed to the creation of a large radiofrequency lesion). After the appropriate survival times, the animals were killed and their brains were sectioned and stained for reactive astrocytes.

Our analysis revealed that when postoperative survival was less than 30 days, NGF treatment did not alter reactive astrocytosis in the area of the lesion or in the tissue overlying the wound. In contrast, the rats that were allowed to survive from 30 to 60 days after surgery had more astrocytes on the side of the brain treated with

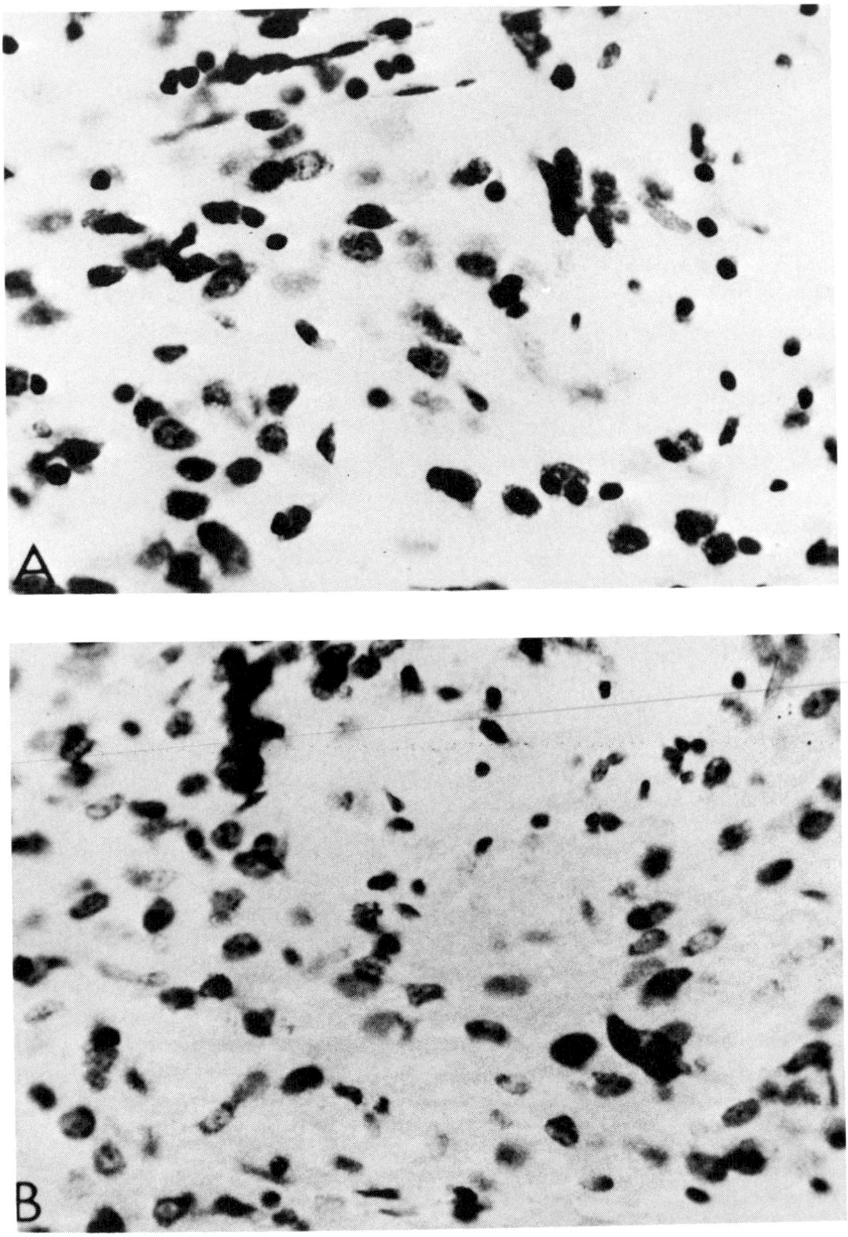

Figure 12.6. *Representative photomicrographs (× 126) of caudate nuclei in animals given lesions with NFG (A), lesions followed by inert buffer (B), or sham operation (C). See text for description. (From Hart* et al., *1978.)*

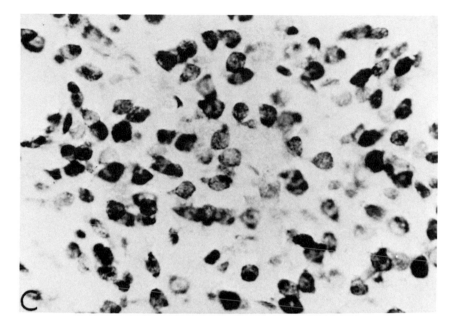

Figure 12.6C.

NGF than on the side treated with buffer solution.[4] At no point in time did the unoperated rats show an increased glial reaction due to NGF administration. Thus, there had to be a significant lesion before the effects of NGF on astrocytosis were manifested.

In observing the microscope slides, it seemed to us that the astrocytes began their development in the corpus callosum (where they may have lain dormant as interstitial cells) and swept down into the area of the lesion. Our observations also indicated that the largest and best defined astrocytes were found in the undamaged portions of the caudate nucleus *adjacent* to the lesions where they were interspersed with neurons. The borders of the lesions consisted of less dense-staining glial cells with smaller processes. We also noted that more than 66% of the rats surviving for 30–60 days had larger astrocytes on the NGF-treated side of the brain, whereas in the shorter survival times (0–20 days) there were no measurable effects of the NGF treatments.

A number of investigators have previously argued that NGF is not even present

[4] This finding does not contradict the data of Hart *et al.* (1978). In Hart's study, less gliosis was noted in the NGF group of brain-damaged animals than in the nondrug treated lesion group, but the animals were kept alive for 6 months after the surgery. In the present study, where more glial proliferation was noted in the NGF brain-damaged group than in the nondrug treated brain-damaged group, the observations were restricted to the first 2 postoperative months.

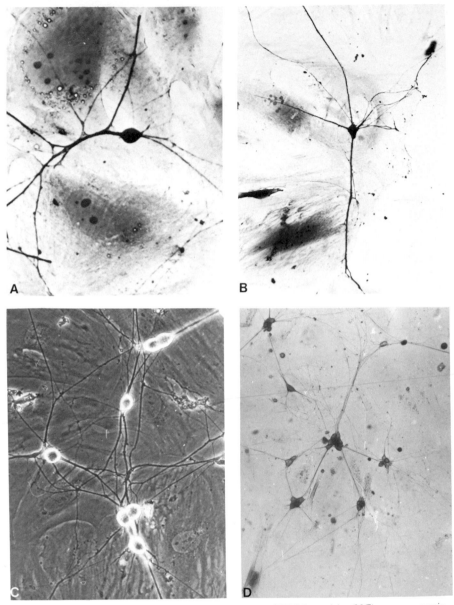

Figure 12.7. *Dissociated NFG-dependent (SCG, DRG) and NFG-insensitive (NG) neurones surviving indirect contact with adult rat brain astrocytes in the absence of exogenous NFG. Cultures were established as described in the text. A, Single rat SCG neurone straddling several RG18 cells, silver stained after 6 days in culture. B, Single chick embryo DRG neurone nuclei of two RG 18 cells, silver stained after 6 days in vitro. C, Network of rat embryo NG neurones on top of astrocyte monolayer, silver stained after 10 days in culture. D, Chick embryo NG neurones as seen by phase contrast, unstained preparation after 2 weeks in culture. Calibration bar, 100 μm. Similar observations are obtained when collagen gel is used, but the neuronal fibers extend in three dimensions, making photographic representation difficult. (From Lindsay, 1979. Reprinted by permission from Nature, 282, 80–82. Copyright © 1979, Macmillan Journals Limited.)*

in the brain of the adult mammal, a conclusion that we now believe was premature, although concentrations may be very low after infancy if the brain is intact (Walker *et al.*, 1979; see Figure 12.8). Also not everyone is convinced that NGF has a role to play in central nervous system functions. The latter view is held primarily because researchers have concentrated primarily on the effects of NGF on neurons per se, rather than upon the examination of satellite cells that may provide important trophic and sustaining roles in maintaining those neurons in a functional state when the system itself is damaged. Glia, if anything, are usually characterized as preventing neural regeneration or functional recovery by forming mechanical barriers to regenerative or collateral growth. Our research into this area is just beginning, so we can only speculate at present that glial cells may contribute positively to behavioral recovery (see Banker, 1980; Figure 12.9). It is difficult to imagine that the "filling" in of lesion zones by glia do nothing more than provide "bulk" in the formerly nectrotic zone, especially since glia are known to secrete NGF and other trophic substances as well as nutrients essential for neuronal metabolism (see Gaines, 1978, for a brief review).

The work of Björklund and his colleagues has demonstrated that NGF can play a role in facilitating the regeneration of catecholaminergic neurons in the brain, although the specific mechanism by which this process occurs is still unknown. It should be mentioned that James Turner and Kathleen A. Glaze (1978) have found similar effects of NGF treatments in the regenerating optic nerve of the newt, a much more primitive animal. A single injection of NGF near the

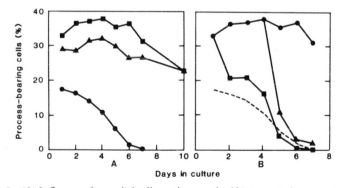

Figure 12.8. *(A) Influence of astroglial cells on the growth of hippocampal neurons. Neurons were cultured alone (circles), in the presence of astrocytes (triangles), or in medium conditioned by incubation with cultured astrocytes (squares). The number of neurons with one or more processes greater than two cell diameter in length was counted after various periods and expressed as a percentage of the number of those present 3 hours after plating. Neurons that had begun to degenerate were not included. (B) The effect of neuronal growth of withdrawing astrocyte-conditioned medium. Cultures of hippocampal neurons were established in conditioned medium. Some of the cultures (circles) were contained in that medium; others were transferred to control medium after 1 day (squares) or 4 days (triangles). The growth of cells established and maintained in control medium is shown for comparison. (From Banker, 1980. Copyright 1980 by the American Association for the Advancement of Science.)*

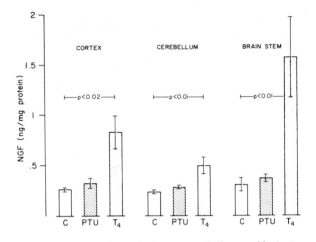

Figure 12.9. *NGF concentration in cerebral cortex, cerebellum, and brain stem of adult male mice. Bars indicate mean ± standard error (S.E.). The F ratios were highly significant for all three brain areas. Significance levels for the multiple comparisons by t tests, after logarithmic transformation of the data, were corrected for the number of tests performed (27). The p levels for the tissues when corrected in this manner were cortex, $p < .002$; cerebellum, $p < .003$; and brain stem, $p < .001$. (All levels of significance are for T_4-treated mice, compared to control mice.) No statistically significant differences were noted for PUT-treated mice, compared to control mice. (From Walker et al., 1979. Copyright 1979 by the American Association for the Advancement of Science.)*

transected nerve of the newt stimulated the rate of growth as well as the number of regenerating axons. Most interesting for us was their unexpected finding that the NGF treatments caused a significant increase in the astrocyte-like cells around the vicinity of the growing axons! These findings are presented in Figures 12.10–12.12.

Until the present time, all of our behavioral studies using NGF employed relatively young rats (90 days of age at the start of the studies). To determine whether NGF can facilitate recovery in old animals, we decided to test the use of highly purified renin-free NGF in rats that were 1½ years old. The experiment was essentially the same as that of Hart *et al.* (1978), but for the age differences of the animals. Our preliminary results were very encouraging. The aged brain-damaged rats treated with pure NGF learned the avoidance task in about the same number of trials as their intact counterparts. By comparison, the rats with caudate lesions without NGF did much worse. It is clear from these data that pure NGF can also facilitate recovery in aged brain-damaged subjects. In fact, the results from the present study suggest that the purified molecule may be even more potent than the 2.5S fraction previously used with younger animals.

In summary, when NGF is injected into the "intact brain," it seems to do very little and may actually disrupt normal behavioral performance and consum-

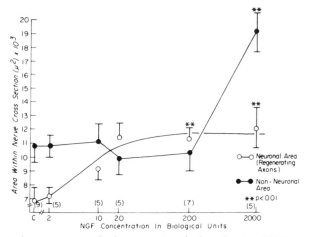

Figure 12.10. *A dose-response study demonstrating the log of various NGF concentrations, administered as single intraocular injections at the time of nerve transection, plotted against neuronal (regenerating axons) and nonneuronal (glial) areas within cross sections of regenerating nerves at 14 days after transection. Points represent mean values, with vertical lines indicating the standard errors. Values in parentheses indicate the numbers of nerves evaluated. (C) on the abcissa, represents the control value. (From Turner and Glaze, 1978.)*

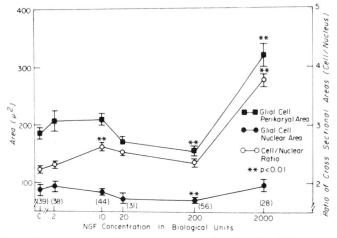

Figure 12.11. *A dose-response study demonstrating the log of various NFG concentrations, administered as single intraocular injections at the time of nerve transections, plotted against glial cell perikaryal and nuclear areas as well as the cell: nuclear ratios within regenerating nerve cross sections at 14 days after transection. Points represent mean values, with vertical lines indicating the standard errors. Values in parentheses indicate the numbers of cells analyzed at each NGF concentration. (C) on the abcissa, represents the control value. (From Turner and Glaze, 1978.)*

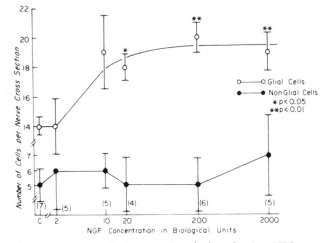

Figure 12.12. *A dose-response study demonstrating the log of various NFG concentrations, administered as single intraocular injections at the time of lesion, plotted against the number of glial and nonglial cells within regenerating nerve cross sections at 14 days postlesion. Points represent mean values, with vertical lines indicating the standard errors. Values in parentheses indicate the numbers of nerves evaluated. (C) on the abscissa, represents the control value. (From Turner and Glaze, 1978.)*

matory activity (Lewis, Brown, Brownstein, Hart, and Stein, 1979; Stein, Blake, and Wiener, 1980). Yet, when there is damage, its beneficial effects become more apparent. This is important because most studies done with NGF in the central nervous system have not first created lesions; the material is injected and then assays are performed on relatively intact tissue. This may be a reasonable strategy for biochemical assay work, but the results of such attempts may not provide any information whatsoever as to the actions of this protein in a disturbed neural system where the "rules of the game" might be very different. It is both curious and puzzling that so little work has been done on the behavioral effects of intracerebral NGF administration, given its tremendous importance to developmental neurobiology. Early work on NGF was carried out on the peripheral nerves because the neurons were directly accessible to study, but new techniques make this argument less valuable. Perhaps the day is coming when more attention to the central nervous effects of growth factor administration will be forthcoming because much more work in this area is certainly required. The principles of reorganization of function after injury probably have many factors in common with the processes that guide migration and organization of neurons in the developing nervous system. Studies with NGF administration in the central nervous system are an appropriate step toward applying developmental principles to an understanding of the mechanisms involved in functional recovery from brain lesions.

The use of trophic substances or enzymes that act upon neural or glial cells to enhance the possibility of recovery from brain damage represents but one of many approaches to the whole problem of understanding functional restitution after central nervous system injury. In one sense, the studies we have just described can be characterized by their attempts to manipulate directly the *growth* of nerve cells, either through the direct stimulation of neurons (e.g., NGF treatments) or by attempting to block the scar formation that is thought to abort anomalous neuronal growth.

Drugs that excite the central nervous system to higher levels of "activity" have also been used to facilitate recovery from brain damage. For example, in some very early experiments, Ward and Kennard (1942) came to the conclusion that certain stimulants (the cholinergic drug, Doryl; strychnine; and thiamin) can enhance the rate and degree of recovery from motor cortex damage in monkeys. Moreover, in a follow-up study, Kennard and Watson (1945) noted that the depressant, phenobarbital, could inhibit the recovery process and that Dilantin (diphenylhydantoin sodium) could prevent the recovery seen with Doryl (carbachol choline). In these studies, the issue of neural growth after the injury is not usually considered, and pharmacological rather than physiological doses are applied. Explanations of recovery, when given, tend to deal more with the drug's effects on neurotransmitter outputs, alterations in brain biochemistry, or changes in behavioral arousal levels, than with alterations in anatomy. The concept of *denervation supersensitivity,* to which we will devote an entire chapter, is a good example of a pharmacological "explanation" applied to recovery of function.

Actually, some very interesting experiments on the pharmacology of recovery were performed to determine what variables were involved in the behavioral changes seen after serial lesions of the cortex. For example, some time ago it had been demonstrated that rats with spaced ablations of the occipital cortex could learn to make a conditioned avoidance response to *light,* if the rats that served as subjects were kept under constant illumination during the interoperative interval. Rats kept entirely in the dark during the period could barely learn the task. It was assumed that "activity" produced by visual stimulation was necessary for "triggering" the serial lesion effect (Meyer, Isaac, and Maher, 1958). In the 1950s, the reticular activating system of the brain was considered essential for behavioral arousal, and arousal was required for "information processing." In this framework, it made sense to apply drugs to brain-damaged subjects that would "activate" the reticular system and thus facilitate the recovery of function that occurs after brain injuries (Rosner, 1974). As we will see, stimulant-induced recovery does not only occur in subjects with serial lesions (e.g., see Cole, Sullins, and Isaac, 1967); temporary elimination of symptoms can occur after drug administration, even when the damage is extensive and created bilaterally in a single stage.

In one study that can be used to characterize the approach, Patricia Meyer and her colleagues at Ohio State University (Meyer, Horel, and Meyer, 1963) removed the entire neocortex of adult cats and tested the animals for their placing responses. Essentially, a "placing response" requires the subjects to make visual-ly guided contact with the edge of a tabletop as they are moved toward it from some distance away. A sighted cat extends its paws as soon as the animal is within reaching distance of the table edge and then places its paws on the table in a smooth and organized fashion. Animals without the visual and / or motor cortices will make no attempt to extend their paws until they bump up against the edge of the table; such animals appear to be functionally blind.

Meyer *et al.* (1963) tested their decorticate animals for almost 1 year after surgery, and they found that during this time period, there was no recovery of placing. Six cats were then given intraperitoneal injections of 10 mg/kg dl-amphetamine sulphate and then were reexamined every 10 minutes until a response had appeared and subsequently disappeared.

The behavioral findings and histology are shown in Figures 12.13 and 12.14. In brief, Meyer *et al.* (1963) noticed an effect of the amphetamine within 10–20

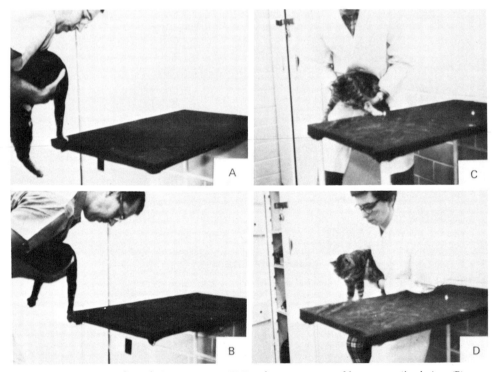

Figure 12.13. *Postdrug placing responses. (A) Postdrug appearance of forepaw tactile placing. (B), Postdrug disappearance of forepaw tactile placing. (C) Postdrug appearance of visual placing. (D) Postdrug disappearance of visual placing. (From Meyer, P. M., Horel, J. A., and Meyer, D. R. Effects of dl-amphetamine upon placing responses in neodecorticate cats.* Journal of Comparative and Physiological Psychology, 53, 402–404. *Copyright 1963 by the American Psychological Association. Reprinted by permission.)*

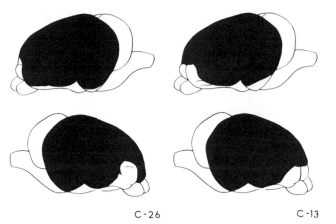

C-26   C-13

Figure 12.14. *Extent of neocortical damage in C-26 and C-13. (From Meyer, P. M., Horel, J. A., and Meyer, D. R. Effects of dl-amphetamine upon placing responses in neodecorticate cats.* Journal of Comparative and Physiological Psychology, 56, 402–404. *Copyright 1963 by the American Psychological Association. Reprinted by permission.)*

minutes after the injections. The effects included an increase in the rate and volume of respiration, piloerection of the fur on the animal's back and tail, retraction of the nictitating membranes, and other manifestations of arousal. Most important, the cats, under the influence of the amphetamine, showed a reappearance of the placing responses lost as a consequence of the decortication. Nevertheless, as the drug wore off, the visual deficits returned.

Although amphetamine injections do seem to restore some aspects of visual response, there is now more recent evidence to indicate that recovery of vision in decorticate preparations is not complete. In other words, the amphetamine does *not* restore animals to normal visual performance levels.

For example, to examine the visual capacity of cats with very large posterior lesions, Ritchie, Meyer, and Meyer (1976) trained adult cats on a series of complex visual tasks in which contours, contrast, and numerosity (number of objects on a visual panel) were manipulated. Normal cats can learn these discriminations even when contours and local differences in flux are equated. After removal of the visual cortex, the cats can still make the discriminations if the patterned stimuli are different with respect to *both* contour and numerosity. If both stimulus flux and contour are then equated, the animals show themselves to be form-blind and seem incapable of learning the discriminations. In addition to impairments in form vision, the decorticated cats fail to show placing responses, even with postoperative recovery periods of more than 1 year. But despite this handicap, a single injection of amphetamine restored visual placing for up to 3 weeks after the injections! In short, although the decorticated cats failed to learn form discriminations, they showed an ability, under the drug, to perform the placing response well.

There is no simple explanation for this interesting finding; certainly no alterations in anatomical pathways or anatomical growth could account for the temporary recovery followed by the return of deficit that occurs as the effects of the stimulant wear off. Donald Meyer (1972; Meyer and Meyer, 1977) has suggested that the lesions cause a suppression of retrieval of "engrams" that have been formed in the brain as a result of learning or experience. Thus, memory traces (engrams) are not destroyed by cortical lesions, but according to Meyer, access to them may be blocked. As a stimulant, amphetamine somehow allows the animals to overcome this block.

Meyer's concepts may be difficult to prove directly, but there is some indirect experimental support for his ideas from other laboratories. In one case Simone Faugier-Grimaud, Colette Frenois, and D. G. Stein (1978) examined the behavior of mature Java monkeys on visually guided placing reactions, before and after bilateral removals of the posterior parietal cortex (areas 5 and 7). The monkeys were tested daily, immediately after one- or two-stage removals of the cortical tissue, in order to determine if they demonstrated ataxia, abnormal reaching, and/or sensory neglect. In each case, it was noted that the unilateral ablation resulted in a contralateral deficit very similar to Balint's syndrome (Hécaen and DeAjuriaguerra, 1954) seen in humans following parietal lesions. The monkeys were unable to use the affected hand to reach for a small morsel of banana (about 2–3 mm^3) and place it in their mouths. As seen in Figures 12.15 and 12.16, they consistently misreached, or if they did obtain the banana, they missed putting it in their mouths. After a period of 10 days, recovery of the visually guided response was evident. (Each of the subjects was videotaped or filmed so that frame-by-frame inspection of their movements could be evaluated.) The movements became fluid, rapid, and accurate once more, and by no more than 2 weeks after surgery, the monkeys appeared to be completely normal. In some of the animals, a second lesion contralateral to the first, caused the deficit to reappear in the hand contralateral to the lesion (the previously unaffected side).

Once again, recovery took about 10 days to 2 weeks. Thereafter, the monkeys used the *initially* affected limb as if they had no lesions. All of the animals were tested daily on a series of visually guided discrimination problems, as part of another experiment, and then occasionally tested on the simple visual reaching task; they never showed any evidence of an impairment!

Almost 1 year after the surgery, the monkeys were given a very small dose of the drug used to induce anesthesia for surgery (ketamine, 5 mg). The dose administered was only 5% of that required for anesthesia. Under these conditions, Faugier-Grimaud *et al.* noted an immediate return of the deficit. If the lesions were only unilateral, the impairment was unilateral, but if the lesions were bilateral, then so was the impairment. As the drug effects wore off, normal visually guided reaching returned in the same motor sequence as had been observed during the recovery process that followed the surgery. Each time the drug was

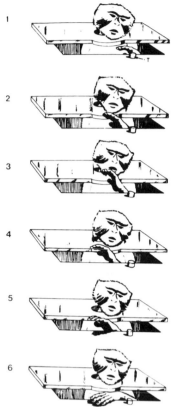

Figure 12.15. *Misreaching with the hand contralateral to the lesion. The monkey fixates the target (T), but misreaches several centimeters to the right of the target. Note that the hand approaches the target, wide open with the fingers fully extended. (Reprinted by permission from Faugier-Grimaud, S., Frenois, C., and Stein, D. G. Effects of posterior parietal lesions on visually guided behavior in monkeys.* Neuropsychologia, 16, 151–168. *Copyright 1978, Pergamon Press, Ltd.)*

readministered, the motor impairments returned only to disappear again as the ketamine effects wore off.

We think that these findings speak to the questions raised by Meyer concerning access to engrams in brain-damaged organisms. In the Faugier-Grimaud study, focal lesions produced a deficit which the animals were able to overcome in a short time. The movements utilized after recovery were virtually identical to those seen preoperatively—a case of restitution, rather than substitution of functions—at least at the behavioral level of analysis. Yet, despite the apparent recovery, the deficit in all of its manifestations seemed to lurk just below the "level of normal efficiency" accomplished by the animals. It would appear as if the level of arousal demanded by the test situation (i.e., motivation to obtain a piece of banana) was sufficient to permit "access" to the motor plan underlying visually guided behavior. When this level of arousal was diminished, perhaps access to the motor plan was now once again blocked!

Donald and Patricia Meyer (1977) hypothesize that the substrate for good per-

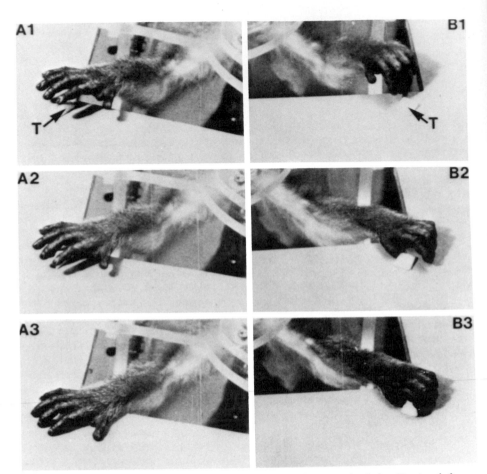

Figure 12.16. *Shaping of the affected hand arriving on target (T) in a monkey before (B$_{1-3}$) and after (A$_{1-3}$) lesion of area 7. (Reprinted with permission from Faugier-Grimaud, S. Frenois, C. and Stein, D. G. Effects of posterior parietal lesions on visually guided behavior in monkeys.* Neuropsychologia, *16, 151–168. Copyright 1978, Pergamon Press, Ltd.)*

formance in brain-damaged subjects can lie dormant, perhaps in adjacent areas of intact cortical or subcortical tissue. Thus, *therapy* should involve "a combination of treatments with an agent and behavioral procedures for the evocation of the memories to be reinstated [p. 72]." (Here memory should be taken in its broadest sense of response strategies, rather than as a collection of specific "items.") Thus, the goals of the treatments they envision would not be to help patients to recover by forming new habits but, instead, to permit them to make better use of the habits they already have available.

It is an interesting historical fact that Karl Lashley, in one of his last articles (1950), stated very much the same thing when he speculated that:

Amnesia from brain injury *rarely, if ever,* is due to the destruction of specific memory traces. Rather, the amnesias represent a lowered level of vigilance, a greater difficulty in activating the organized patterns of traces, or a disturbance of some *broader system of organized functions* [p. 472].

Despite Meyer's and Meyer's interesting proposals for "treatment" of the brain-damaged patient, there have been very few attempts to manipulate recovery in brain-damaged patients with drugs; the major thrust has always been on behavioral training and limited physical therapy, rather than direct intervention in the central nervous system.

The caution and conservatism is probably justified because successful pharmacological (hormonal–peptide, etc.) treatments have not been particularly well documented, and where experiments have been done, attempts at replication have often been equivocal. In addition, many experimental agents used in the laboratory often produce side effects that would be unacceptable in human subjects. In a stroke patient, administration of a stimulant might provoke higher blood pressure, which in turn could lead to additional damage. In other words, the drug might work in some cases, but the risk factor could be too great to warrant the treatment. Also, until very recently, prevailing concepts of brain function *precluded* the possibility of structural and neurochemical reorganization of function; theoretically, once damage occurred, the only possibility for rehabilitation was to train the patient to use alternative, but less effective, behavioral strategies. There was no real motivation to search for pharmacological agents to facilitate recovery because the popular belief systems concerning "plasticity" were basically negative. Yet, despite the prevailing pessimism concerning functional restitution by direct intervention, some work in humans has been done.

In particular, attempts have been made in the Soviet Union to facilitate recovery from brain damage in humans in pharmacological treatments. Consider the work of Alexander Luria and his colleagues who argue that focal brain lesions produce two types of functional disturbances (Luria, Naydin, Tretkova, and Vinarskaya, 1969). The first type is due to the actual death of neurons whose functions, of course, disappear completely. The second type of functional disruption results from the "inhibition" of intact neurons. Depending upon the type of injury, the relative proportions of these two components will vary from case to case. In the case of massive hemorrhage, destruction of active nerve cells will predominate, whereas in the case of concussion or lesions of the brain stem, there might be disturbances of the tonic influence of the reticular formation, which block the activation of the rest of the brain.

Luria and his colleagues hypothesize that:

> In cases where the role of inactivation assumes the foremost place in the disturbance
> of function, the main method of restoration of the disturbed function will be by
> deinhibition, or in other words, by the removal of the diaschisis, restoration of
> synaptic blocking, or, to use another term, by deblocking [p. 368].

Luria and his colleagues envision that such deblocking can be accomplished by drugs that modify synaptic transmission *as well as* by careful patient training "which can change the level at which a function takes place, and by involving the patient's residual powers in habitual forms of performance of activity [p. 369]." Thus, both training and drug treatments are often necessary to deinhibit the functions suppressed by brain injury. As we will see in the next chapter, Luria's notions are not entirely revolutionary. Constantin von Monakow (1914) talked about temporary disturbances in cerebral functions caused by shock-induced injuries many years earlier. He called this form of inhibition *diaschisis* and claimed that the shock could appear in regions of the brain far removed from the site of immediate damage. Luria and his colleagues see loss of behavioral and cognitive functions as sometimes being due to the "taking out" (i.e., *inhibition*) of systems or structures involved in the mediation of behaviors, rather than only being due to damage to a critical locus or center. If synaptic efficiency could be restored by the administration of a deblocking agent, and appropriate rehabilitation therapy given, the patient should at least partially recover.

Based on this logic, Luria and his staff at Moscow University administered drugs that block cholinesterase (the enzyme that "neutralizes" acetylcholine) in order to achieve higher levels of acetylcholine. They did this because they believed that pathologic processes such as hemorrhages liberate great quantities of cholinesterase so that normal neuronal activity in intact areas of the brain is suppressed.

Accordingly, the Russian investigators administered anticholinesterase drugs such as neostigmine, eserine, and galanthamine to brain-damaged patients. Luria reported that such treatments have remarkable, dramatic effects, often restoring lost functions immediately, even when the disease had lasted for years! Unfortunately, the primary findings are published in Russian and not easily available to Western researchers.

Luria himself stated that he injected neostigmine, in small doses, to patients (in the acute phase of brain injury) who suffered from paralyses; he argues that some recovery was noted because "temporarily inactive groups of neurons in a pathological focus or in the perifocal region *quickly return to work,* whereas the destroyed groups of neurons naturally remained inactive, thus sharply demarcating the "central" from the "secondary components of the disturbance [p. 372]."

In one experiment Luria administered neostimine to a patient with a nonpenetrating wound of the premotor area, which caused a disturbance of "delicate dynamic coordination." Luria recorded rhythmic tapping movements of this patient before and after neostigmine treatments and found evidence of restoration of dynamic coordination under the drug influence, even though prior training attempts had no effects. An important feature is that the observed improvement was stable and served as *the foundation* for later exercise therapy, which thereafter became much more effective.

Luria has also made claims that drug therapy can improve the rate of recovery from aphasia caused by gunshot wounds of the left hemisphere if the lesions are not localized in the "primary speech zones." The drug of choice in this situation is galanthamine, a Soviet-developed alkaloid now being tried in the United States as a means to treat cognitive deficits in senile dementia.

According to Luria, galanthamine is particularly effective in facilitating recovery of articulatory speech disturbances, but also is effective in aiding recovery from sensory defects important to speech. He claims that acoustic perception of sounds is improved, understanding of speech is better, and phonemic meaning is improved, to name a few of the derived benefits of galanthamine treatments. Luria does caution, however, that the treatments must be followed up with appropriate rehabilitation training based on individual needs of the patients.

In the Soviet experiments, it is possible that great success was obtained because the patients were carefully chosen. In other words, it would be important to know whether many of the subjects died of their injuries or were excluded from treatment for other reasons, and if only the hardiest or luckiest served in the experiments. This criticism notwithstanding, Luria's reports, based on a quarter-of-a-century of work with these drugs, are intriguing and certainly merit more attention than they have thus far been given in the West. Moreover, the animal experiments performed at Ohio State University (Meyer and Meyer, 1977) can be viewed as providing substantial confirmation of Luria's general concepts.

In closing this chapter we must emphasize that the most recent experimental reports with animals tested under highly controlled conditions are showing that pharmacological manipulation of damaged brains can occasionally be effective in reducing symptomatology. For example, Stanley Glick and Betty Zimmerberg (1978) have written extensively about pharmacologically induced recovery from frontal lesions in mice and rats (see Chapter 13 on denervation supersensitivity, for more details). Also, Edward Stricker and Michel Zigmond have used neurotoxic substances to create lesions in catecholamine-containing neurons in the brain stem that are implicated in feeding behavior (the LH syndrome). These investigators report that pre- and postoperative pharmacological treatments can affect synaptic mechanisms that lead to behavioral recovery in rats. For example, drugs that increase the sensitivity of remaining neurons to the available neurotransmitters seem to facilitate behavioral recovery. Thus, restoring levels of depleted neurotransmitters does seem to affect some behaviors (see Stricker and Zigmond, 1976).

In the case of human brain damage, no verdict can be rendered at the present time. Some risk-assessment studies should be attempted if for no other reason than to determine whether drug therapy is applicable in cases of severe brain damage. Clearly, the devastating consequences of brain damage to the patient and his family are sufficient to justify this attention, especially in instances where other approaches have failed.

References

Avrith, D. B., Lewis, M. E., and Fitzsimmons, J. T. Renin-like effects of NGF evaluated using renin-angiotensin antagonists. *Nature*, 1980, *285*, 248–250.

Banker, G. A. Trophic interactions between astroglial cells and hippocampal neurons in culture. *Science*, 1980, *209*, 809–810.

Berger, B. D., Wise, C. D., and Stein, L. Nerve growth factor: Enhanced recovery of feeding after hypothalamic damage. *Science*, 1973, *180*, 506–508.

Beuker, E. Implanation of tumors in the hindlimb field of the embryonic chick and the developmental response of the lumbro-scaral nervous system. *Anatomical Record*, 1948, *102*, 369–390.

Bjerre, B. A., Björklund, A., and Stenevi, U. Stimulation of growth of new axonal sprouts from lesioned monamine neurons in adult rat brain by nerve growth factor. *Brain Research*, 1973, *60*, 161–176.

Bjerre, B., Björklund, A., and Stenevi, U. Inhibition of the regenerative growth of central noradrenergic neurons by intracerebrally administered anti-NGF serum. *Brain Research*, 1974, *74*, 1–18.

Björklund, A., and Stenevi, U. Nerve growth factor: Stimulation of regenerative growth of central noradrenergic neurons. *Science*, 1972, *175*, 1251–1253.

Bradshaw, R. Nerve growth factor. *Annual Review of Biochemistry*, 1978, *47*, 191–216.

Cohen, S., Levi-Montalcini, R., and Hamburger, V. A nerve growth-stimulating factor isolated from sarcomas 37 and 180. *Proceedings of the National Academy of Sciences*, 1954, *40*, 1014–1018.

Cole, D. D., Sullins, W. R., and Isaac, W. Pharmacological modification of the effects of spaced occipital ablations. *Psychopharmacologia*, 1967, *11*, 311–316.

Faugier-Grimaud, S., Frenois, C., and Stein, D. C. Effects of posterior parietal lesions on visually guided behavior in monkeys. *Neuropsychologia*, 1978, *16*, 151–168.

Gaines, H. Intercellular transfer of proteins from glial cells to axons. *TINS* (Trends in Neurosciences, Elsevier-North Holland), October, 1978, 93–96.

Glick, S. D., and Zimmerberg, B. Pharmacological modification of brain lesion syndromes. In S. Finger (Ed.), *Recovery from brain damage: Research and theory*. New York: Plenum, 1978, Pp. 281–296.

Hamburger, V. Trophic interactions in neurogenesis: A personal historical account. *Annual Review of Neuroscience*, 1980, *3*, 269–378.

Harper, G. F., and Thoenen, H. Nerve growth factor: Biological significance, measurement and distribution. *Journal of Neurochemistry*, 1980, *34*, 5–16.

Hart, T., Chaimas, N., Moore, R. Y., and Stein, D. G. Effects of nerve growth factor on behavioral recovery following caudate nucleus lesions in rats. *Brain Research Bulletin*, 1978, *3*, 245–250.

Hécaen, H., and De Ajuriaguerra, J. Balint's syndrome (psychic paralysis of visual fixation) and its minor forms. *Brain*, 1954, *77*, 373–400.

Kennard, M. A., and Watson, C. W. The effect of anticonvulsant drugs on recovery of function following cerebral cortical lesions. *Journal of Neurophysiology*, 1945, *8*, 221–231.

Lashley, K. S. In search of the engram. *Symposium of the Society for Experimental Biology*, 1950, *4*, 454–482.

Levi-Montalcini, R. The nerve growth factor: Its role in growth, differentiation and function of the sympathetic adrenergic neuron. *Progress in Brain Research*, 1976, *45*, 235–358.

Levi-Montalcini, R. Polydipsia after intracerebral injections—A property of NGF or a contaminant? *Nature*, 1980, *284*, 577.

Levi-Montalcini, R., Angeletti, R. H., and Angeletti, P. U. The nerve growth factor. In G. H. Bourne (Ed.), *The structure and function of nervous tissue* (Vol. 5). New York: Academic Press, 1972, Pp. 1–38.

Levi-Montalcini, R., and Calissano, P. The nerve growth factor. *Scientific American*, 1979, *240*, 68–78.

Lewis, M. E., Brown, R. M., Brownstein, M. J., Hart, T., and Stein, D. G. Nerve growth factor: Effects on d-amphetamine induced activity and brain monoamines. *Brain Research*, 1979, *176*, 297–310.

Lindsay, R. M. Adult rat brain astrocytes support survival of both NGF-dependent and NGF-insensitive neurons. *Nature*, 1979, *282*, 80–82.

Luria, A. R., Naydin, V. L., Tretkova, L. S., and Vinarskaya, E. N. Restoration of higher cortical functions following local brain damage. In P. J. Vinken and G. W. Bruyn (Eds.), *Handbook of clinical neurology* (Vol. 3). Amsterdam: North Holland, 1969, Pp. 368–433.

Meyer, D. R. Access to engrams. *American Psychologist*, 1972, *27*, 124–133.

Meyer, D. R., Isaac, W., and Maher, B. The role of stimulation in spontaneous reorganization of visual habits. *Journal of Comparative and Physiological Psychology*, 1958, *51*, 546–548.

Meyer, D. R., and Meyer, P. M. Dynamics and bases of recoveries of functions after injuries to the cerebral cortex. *Physiological Psychology*, 1977, *5*, 72, 133–165.

Meyer, P. M., Horel, J. A., and Meyer, D. R. Effects of dl-amphetamine upon placing responses in neodecorticate cats. *Journal of Comparative and Physiological Psychology*, 1963, *56*, 402–404.

Ritchie, C. D., Meyer, P. M., and Meyer, D. R. Residual spatial vision of cats with lesions of the visual cortex. *Experimental Neurology*, 1976, *53*, 227–253.

Rosner, B. Recovery of function and localization of function in historical perspective. In D. G. Stein, J. J. Rosen, and N. Butters (Eds.), *Plasticity and recovery of function in the central nervous system*. New York: Academic Press, 1974, Pp. 1–29.

Sabel, B. A., Kardon, G. B., and Stein, D. G. Renin does not mediate behavioral recovery from caudate nucleus damaged rats, unpublished data.

Schultze, M., and Stein, D. G. Recovery of function in the albino rat following either simultaneous or seriatim lesions of the caudate nucleus. *Experimental Neurology*, 1975, *46*, 291–301.

Stein, D. G., Blake, C., and Weiner, H. Nerve growth factor disrupts metabolism and behavioral performance of intact rats but does not affect recovery from hypothalamic lesions. *Brain Research*, 1980, *190*, 278–284.

Stenevi, U., Bjerre, B., Björklund, A., and Mobley, W., Effects of localized intracerebral injections of nerve growth factor on the regenerative growth of lesioned central noradrenergic neurones. *Brain Research*, 1974, *69*, 217–234.

Stoeckel, K., and Thoenen, H. Retrograde axonal transport of nerve growth factor: Specificity and biological importance. *Brain Research*, 1975, *85*, 337–342.

Stricker, E., and Zigmond, M. Recovery of function after damage to central catecholamine-containing neurons: A neurochemical model for the lateral hypothalamic syndrome. In J. M. Sprague and A. N. Epstein (Eds.), *Progress in psychobiology and physiological psychology* (Vol. 6). New York: Academic Press, 1976, Pp. 121–172.

Turner, J. E., and Glaze, K. A. Glial reaction to nerve growth factor in the regenerating optic nerve of the newt (*Triturus viridescens*). *Experimental Neurology*, 1978, *59*, 190–201.

Varon, S. S. Nerve growth factor and its mode of action. *Experimental Neurology*, 1975, *48*, 75–92.

Varon, S. S., and Bunge, R. P. Trophic mechanisms in the peripheral nervous system. *Annual Review of Neuroscience,* 1978, *1,* 327–361.

von Monakow, C. *Die Lokalisation im grosshirn und der abbav der Funktion durch Kortikale Herde.* Wiesbaden: J. F. Bergmann, 1914. (Translated and excerpted by G. Harris. In K. H. Pribram, Ed., *Mood, states and mind.* London: Penguin, 1969, Pp. 27–37.)

Walker, P., Weichsel, M. E., Jr., Fisher, D. A., Guo, S. M., and Fisher, D. A. Thyroxine increases nerve growth factor concentration in adult mouse brain. *Science,* 1979, *204,* 427–428.

Ward, A. A., Jr., and Kennard, M. A. Effect of cholinergic drugs on recovery of function following lesions of the central nervous system. *Yale Journal of Biology and Medicine,* 1942, *15,* 189–228.

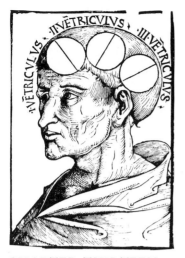

Diaschisis and
Neural Shock Models of
Recovery of Function

Immediately following an acute transverse lesion of the spinal cord there ensues a state known as spinal shock. Although not always recognized as such, an analogous situation can occur at more rostral levels, appearing, for example, subsequent to a rapidly developing lesion of a cerebral hemisphere [Kempinsky, 1958, p. 376].

CHAPTER THIRTEEN

In earlier chapters we were able to look at recent advances in anatomy and physiology, and, in a number of selected instances, we tried to show how phenomena such as "reactive synaptogenesis" and "silent synapses" could relate to recovery of function. It seems worthwhile to us at this point to reexamine some of the older theories of recovery, such as vicariation and substitution, to see how they have developed and fared over the years. We will also want to see how new data from anatomy, physiology, and the behavioral sciences can be incorporated into these theories.[1]

In discussing models of recovery of function, Hans-Lukas Teuber noted that as we cast about for explanations to account for what we observe, we sometimes stumble upon theories that were expressed many years earlier, but which seem to be largely ignored by contemporary investigators. He also felt that concepts that often seem to have little substantive explanatory value occasionally resurface because no reasonable alternatives have come along to replace them or because

---

[1] That there are a few general theories of recovery of function that keep appearing in one form or another is widely recognized and easily documented. However, just which theories constitute "acceptable" explanations and which do not represents an issue over which, to say the least, there has always been considerable disagreement. Much of the disagreement seems to originate more from certain predispositions about how the brain is, or should be, organized, rather than from specific instances of hypothesis testing. In fact, one can argue that whether laboratory experiments can be used to test some of the models and theoretical issues (e.g., vicariation) is in itself debatable. If localization of psychological functions, such as memory for places and problem-solving ability, in the normal brain is still being contested after years of experimental study, do we really have a solid premise from which to argue that "reorganization" is, or is not, taking place after brain injury?

verification must await the development of new techniques to test the proposed notions.

In particular, Teuber seemed intrigued with the concept of *neural shock,* about which all of the above statements might apply. Drawing upon his vast experiences in working with brain-damaged soldiers from World War II and the Korean conflict, he once described the case of a sailor, born and raised in the deep South, who was the victim of a massive left hemispheric brain injury (Teuber, 1974). The young man, who was rendered completely aphasic by the damage, was put in the care of a speech therapist from New England. One day the therapist came to Teuber to report that the patient was in fact "faking" his aphasia—that he had been malingering all along. She was upset because the sailor began to speak again, but in his old, heavy Southern drawl, rather than with the Connecticut accent of his tutor!

Teuber's story is interesting because it shows not only how the therapist was misled by her own ideas about how recovery should take place, but also because when speech did return to the sailor it was as if it had simply been lying dormant until the passage of time or the rehabilitation therapy "released" it from some uninjured part of the brain.[2] For cases like this one, the simplest explanation for recovery of function would just be that the structures originally mediating the behavior were never really destroyed by the lesions. Rather, they may have been put into a state of "shock" or "suppression" by the injury, which could, in fact, have destroyed tissue nearby or perhaps even some distance away.

Constantin von Monakow (1853–1930; see Figure 13.1), a Swiss neurologist of Russian extraction, is the person most frequently associated with the development of the concept of *suspension of function.* Von Monakow wanted to distinguish between the transient central nervous system disorders due to suppression of brain activity and the deficits that result from focal brain lesions that never seem to disappear. In the course of his investigations, von Monakow coined the term *diaschisis* to describe the relatively short-lived effects he believed were due to inhibition of activity in brain areas close to the initial site of damage. (He later also postulated a more resistant and protracted state of diaschisis.) According to von Monakow (1914; cited in Riese, 1950), diaschisis is an invariant feature of brain damage since "it goes without saying that after injury of such a delicate and intricate mechanism as the mammalian brain, far removed structures closely related morphologically or functionally to the region destroyed must be involved in one way or another [p. 101]."

Von Monakow began to emphasize the importance of remote lesion effects in the 1890s. This idea dominated his thinking by 1905, when the second edition of

[2] The apparent release of speech after brain injury can also be observed in cases of protracted aphasia. When placed under great stress, it is not unusual for a patient to suddenly utter one or two coherent statements or phrases, only to lapse back into garble and despair immediately afterward. This was something that Broca recognized when dealing with "Tan," his famous case of 1861.

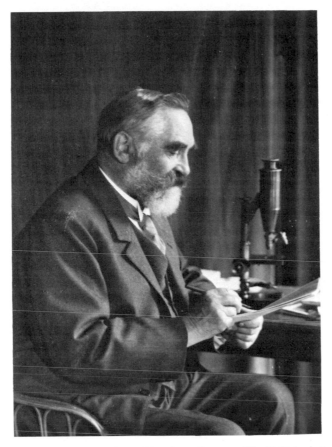

Figure 13.1. *Constantin van Monakow. (Courtesy of Paul I. Yakovlev)*

his *Gehirnpathologie* was published, and 1 year later he even spoke on ''Aphasia and Diaschisis'' to the Society of German Naturalists and Physicians. However, the concept of *remote lesion effects* can hardly be considered an entirely new idea. In ancient times, Galen contrasted the primary and secondary effects of disease in his *De Locis Affectis*. Moreover, von Monakow probably was familiar with the work of Edward Brown-Séquard (see Riese, 1950), who published his major thoughts during the 1870s and who argued that ''an alteration in any part of the nervous system . . . can, by producing an irritation, act on other parts, so as to produce the loss of function in those other parts [p. 97].'' Brown-Séquard (see Figure 13.2) even distinguished between inhibitory (influence d'arrêt) and excitatory (influence dynamique) distal reactions, and studied these remote effects experimentally in his laboratory.

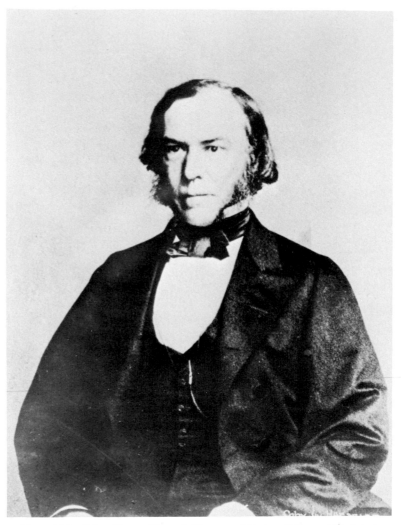

Figure 13.2. *Eduard Brown-Séguard. (Courtesy of National Library of Medicine)*

   Remote effects were often called *sympathetic effects* before von Monakow's popularization of the term *diaschisis*. The term *concensus partium* was also used to refer to them (see Riese, 1958). In 1840, Henle, who used the spinal cord as a model, even derived a set of neuroanatomical "rules" for the development of "sympathy." However, von Monakow developed his theory more fully than most of his predecessors, concerned himself to a greater degree with neuropathological experience, and was able to present his ideas at a time when neurology was just beginning to flourish and accept such concepts.

The key element in von Monakow's theory, as described in his massive work, *Die Lokalisationim im Grosshirn und der Abbau Funktion durch Kortikale Herde*[3] (1914), is that the inhibition of function will disappear over time without special training or drugs. When the inhibition does passively recede, the functions that are mediated by the traumatized, but undamaged structures, are able to reemerge. But while von Monakow used diaschisis to explain *transient symptoms,* he believed that his theory had little to say about remaining *residual symptoms.* In his mind, diaschisis neither accounted for the enduring losses that followed certain injuries, nor for any compensatory reactive strategies that may have developed as a result of such losses.

As conceived of by von Monakow, diaschisis is associated with concepts such as *abolition of excitability* and *functional standstill,* rather than with *irritation,* a term which appears in some of the earlier theories (e.g., Brown-Seguard), or *neural inhibition.* (Von Monakow did not believe in inhibitory synapses.) Furthermore, the mechanism underlying this abolition of excitability was considered to be selective in that some parts of the central nervous system seemed more sensitive to diaschisis-like effects than others. In one of his books, Walther Riese (1950) argued that the motor cortex is much more susceptible to transient shock effects than the sensory cortex. Furthermore, Riese states that functional distinctions have appeared within central nervous system areas. For example, distal motor functions (hand, foot) are supposedly more apt to be affected by remote lesions than are proximal motor functions (shoulders, hips). Diaschisis is also selective in terms of regional differences in the speed with which it dissipates. As von Monakow (1914; translated by Harris, 1969) stated

> The different rate in the regression of diaschisis is due to variations in the way individual neuron groups are linked, and in the type of excitability in different tectonic groups (everything else being equal, the groups that are more frequently used as a unit and are fortified by training will recover earlier than others) as well as to variations in the associated disorders of circulation, etc. [pp. 31–32].

We should stress that although the term *diaschisis* has been used in the contemporary literature to refer to a broad spectrum of actions at a distance from the actual site of damage, von Monakow (1914) himself only applied the term to a very restricted set of circumstances. In fact, he defined diaschisis very stringently as:

> an ''interruption of function'' appearing in most cases quite suddenly . . . and concerning widely ramified fields of function, which originates from a local lesion but has its points of impact not in the whole cortex (corona radiata, etc.) like apopletic shock but only at points where fibers coming from the injured area enter into

[3] Basic Translation: ''The Localization in the Cerebrum and the Loss of Function by Cortical Damage.''

primarily intact grey matter of the whole central nervous system. . . . Speaking
quite generally, the process of diaschisis may be regarded as being caused by abolition of excitability (functional standstill) due to local disruption of brain substance
within one neuron group, which is transmitted to neuron groups closely adjacent to
and directly related with the afflicted part of the brain [pp. 28–29].

The fact that the term *diaschisis* has been used to describe phenomena not included in von Monakow's own definition has led to some confusion and controversy in this field, with some writers employing the term only where originally
intended, others using it to describe a wide range of actions at a distance, and still
others utilizing more global terms such as *neural shock* (which Riese, 1950, clearly
distinguishes from *surgical shock*) and *reestablishment* to describe both cases that
seem to fit the original description of diaschisis and at least superficially related
phenomena. In any case, whether temporarily depressed states are always
mediated neurally or whether nearby or related areas are the only ones that may
show these phenomena, now seems to be of secondary importance to two facts.
The first is that lesions in one part of the nervous system can have profound effects
in other, sometimes distant, areas. The second is that some recovery of function
could be due to a resumption of normal functioning in areas that were only temporarily and indirectly affected by the lesions.

Transient suppressive events have received relatively little attention from
researchers in this country, in part because terms such as *diaschisis* have been
viewed as descriptive rather than explanatory, and because no one has really been
able to determine which of many factors actually are producing the inhibition.
Nevertheless, there have been direct attempts to study the physiological correlates of these distal events, and we are beginning to develop some understanding of how such processes can influence behavior after brain damage.

One frequently cited study was conducted in 1958 by Warren Kempinsky at
the Washington University School of Medicine. This investigator noted that in
cats, spontaneous and optically evoked potentials were temporarily depressed in
the intact hemisphere following a unilateral lesion of the opposite hemisphere.
However, a different pattern of electrical activity emerged in animals that had the
corpus callosum sectioned several weeks prior to unilateral cortical lesions
resulting from occlusion of the middle cerebral artery on one side of the brain.
These cats did not show evoked potential changes in the intact hemisphere, and
only half of the cats used in the study showed transient alterations in the electrocorticograms taken from the intact side. Kempinsky maintained that the distal
lesion effects that he observed under some conditions could not be accounted for
satisfactorily by direct disruption of the blood vessels feeding the affected areas
since depressed neural activity was observed in regions fed by different blood
vessels than those injured during the surgery. Instead, he concluded that the
transcortical effects were mediated neurally and that in severing the corpus

callosum, he had identified the pathway involved. In summarizing his results, Kempinsky (1958) proposed that:

> A unified concept of the conditions necessary for the development of either spinal or cerebral shock may now be proposed. Impulses from one aggregate of neurons constantly play upon the neurons of another, facilitating its activity. The first group is now destroyed; its function is suspended, or its fibers projecting to the second group are interrupted. The latter is thus deprived of one of its usual sources of facilitation. Consequently, it is less active during an interval immediately following the injury. There develops a wider expanse between its threshold and its maximal response to incoming stimuli, and its optimal preinjury performance may not be attainable. With time, the duration of which must depend upon the internal organization of the system and its other sources of afferent contributions, the second group of neurons assumes greater autonomy than before the injury and ultimately functions at a level more closely approximating that present initially [p. 388].

Kempinsky's model is consistant with the thinking of von Monakow and Walther Riese, an obvious follower of von Monakow, both of whom stressed neural, not vascular, bases for diaschisis effects.

That lesions in one hemisphere can have profound effects on the rate of blood flow in the opposite hemisphere, however, is now well known. This observation was made in man by Høedt-Rasmussen and Skinhøj (1964) and Skinhøj (1965). By injecting radioactive inert gas into the carotid artery and placing special detectors over each hemisphere, these investigators had little difficulty seeing dramatic bilateral reductions in blood flow after unilateral cerebral infarctions in their patients.

A more detailed study of cerebral blood flow, however, was conducted by Meyer, Shinohara, Kanda, Fukuuchi, Ericsson, and Kok in 1970. They studied the time course of the events that follow unilateral cerebral infarction and found that 3–16 days after a major accident, the hemispheric blood flow on the healthy side of the brain can be reduced almost as much as on the damaged side. The bilateral depression of circulation may only last a few weeks; within a month the blood flow gradually returns to normal on the intact side of the brain. Meyer and his colleagues showed that the same sequence of events can be observed after brain-stem lesions in man. They argued that changes in intracerebral pressure, generalized cerebral arteriosclerosis, severe hypertension, and hypotension are not factors that can account for this outcome.

The explanation proposed to explain such findings is that regional blood flow is determined by the CO_2 produced by the local brain metabolism (Lassen, 1959). This metabolic rate is low on the damaged side because of the loss of cells, and blood flow consequently is depressed. As a result of diaschisis, or a closely related neural process, there is also a suppression of neural activity on the opposite side of the brain. The blood flow on the intact side drops to reflect this change in neural activity and metabolism. Meyer *et al.* (1970) acknowledge that questions remain regarding the critical pathways involved in these events. They emphasize that the importance of the corpus callosum in producing bilateral reduction of metabolism, and hence blood flow, after a unilateral cortical lesion is clearly demonstrated in the experiments of Kempinsky (1958).

Whether this neurogenic theory of nonspecific neuronal depression is correct or not and whether vascular changes only follow or enhance, but do not in themselves create, diaschisis effects (as postulated by von Monakow, 1914) is still a matter of debate. What is clear is that regional cerebral physiology can be affected by focal events some distance away. This is apparent not only from experiments that have examined neurophysiological events, cerebral metabolism, and blood flow, but also from studies in which neurotransmitter levels have been analyzed in regions far from the site of physical damage. Robert Robinson and his colleagues (e.g., Robinson, Bloom, and Battenberg, 1977; Robinson, Shoemaker, Schlumpf, Volk, and Bloom, 1975) ligated the middle cerebral artery on one side of the brain in rats and reported that 5 days later there was a decrease in catecholamine content in the intact cortex, the cerebellum, and both ipsilateral and contralateral locus coeruleus—areas distant from the lesion and uninjured by the infarction. These transmitter levels returned to normal within 3 weeks and in some areas there was even an increase to a higher level after this time. Robinson and his co-workers hypothesize that these widespread changes to focal injury are capable of accounting for some of the poorly understood behavioral phenomena that often follow strokes. In many cases, poststroke depression and apathy have been difficult to understand solely in the context of focal destruction and frequently have been interpreted as being psychological reactions to pathology. When widespread biochemical changes resulting from stroke are viewed in a causal role, these behavioral states become more comprehensible. Structures comprising the limbic system, for instance, are not immune to the effects of distal cortical injury (Robinson and Bloom, 1978).

In this context, we should emphasize that physiological changes at a distance, like those discussed here, also bear on the validity and utility of some of the tests used to diagnose the presence and site of brain damage. Quite clearly, local reduction in regional cerebral blood flow, or depression of neurophysiological or biochemical activity, need not signify the presence of a nearby stroke, tumor, or injury. For that matter, such changes might not even be indicative of damage in the same hemisphere. This is why one has to be very careful when using behavioral tests to define the site of a brain lesion and why such tests should always be interpreted in terms of probabilities. Greater sensitivity, of course, would be achieved through the use of multiple tests that could be cross-correlated in terms of the symptoms that should (and should not) go together after particular lesions. Even when these techniques are used and the resulting profiles evaluated, errors in localization can still appear as a result of these remote lesion effects.

Some investigators have now attempted to correlate neurophysiologically depressed states, such as those reported by Kempinsky, with behavioral events. As mentioned in an earlier chapter, Robert Glassman (1971), of Lake Forest College, made small punctate lesions of the sensorimotor cortex in adult cats and was able to correlate the reappearance of normal sensory-evoked potentials in adjacent intact cortex with the animals' ability to perform a conditioned reaching response to obtain morsels of food. Glassman (1971) interpreted his results with reference to the concept of reestablishment, that is, to the capacity of suppressed but undamaged areas to resume their normal functions and again mediate the behaviors being investigated.

> It appears likely that the initial deficit as well as recovery were at least partly due to vegetative changes in the tissue near the lesion points. Such changes might include reduction of edema, reestablishment of blood supply, glial growth, or dissipation of toxic substances. The present data, then, appear to be in accord with the view presented by von Monakow . . . that the effects of brain damage are due not only to lost tissue, but also to some sort of temporary shock to regions adjacent or connected to the wound [p. 25].

More recently, Glassman reexamined the effects of lesions of the first somatic area (posterior sigmoid gyrus) and extended his efforts to the second somatic area (anterior ectosylvian gyrus) of the cat's cortex (Glassman and Malamut, 1976). Again, it was noted that evoked potentials in tissue near the small lesions exhibited a transient state of depression and that, for the most part, the observed recovery paralleled that found on a battery of neurological tests given to the cats. The EEG results in this study were characterized by a reduction in fast activity and more slowly activity, especially close to the site of the damage in the period immediately following the insult. Transient EEG effects like these are well known in man and occasionally are discussed in textbooks of clinical electroencephalography (see, for example, Kilch, McComas, and Osselton, 1972).

Irwin, Criswell, and Kakolewski (1973) have also collected data that bear on the reestablishment concept. They found that just by implanting electrodes into the brain-stems of rats, prolonged, nonlocalized, slow potential changes could be recorded across the cortex. Superimposed episodes of cortical spreading depression (Leao, 1944) accompanied these shifts and were associated with reduced nerve cell activity. The authors also examined rats subjected to small (3 mm), unilateral penetration wounds of the cortex. These animals displayed prolonged negative slow potentials in both hemispheres, although spreading depression was restricted to the damaged side. The electrophysiological changes tended to last about 5 days, and as the electrical activity returned to normal, so did motor activity.

One of the most recent attempts to test the concept of *diaschisis* in an experimental preparation failed to provide support for the model. James West, Sam Deadwyler, Carl Cotman, and Gary Lynch (1976) used the dentate gyrus of the hippocampus of the rat as a model system because its afferent projections are well known (see Chapter 6). As we have seen, the granule cells in the hippocampus receive projections from both entorhinal cortex and from the commissural system of the contralateral hippocampus. West and his colleagues hypothesized that if suppression of neuronal activity were produced by a lesion of the entorhinal cortex, the granule cells of the dentate gyrus should be less responsive to their remaining inputs. In the few animals studied, postoperative monosynaptic stimulation of the commissural pathway produced the same frequency, waveform, latency, and amplitude of dendritic potentials as that seen in the dentate gyrus preoperatively. This response pattern was observed from the first day of surgery until the experiment ended some 10 days later. This "test" of the diaschisis model has been subject to some criticism (see Markowitsch and Pritzel, 1978; West, 1978). Nevertheless, the data do serve as a reminder that diaschisis-like states might not always be found in sites to which damaged structures project and that the parameters governing these effects are still not well understood. (It might be noted that Kempinsky also reported two studies in which diaschisis was not observed. See Kempinsky, 1954, 1956.)

The extent to which the concept of diaschisis represents a valid *explanation* for behavioral recovery after lesions is not yet resolved. In fact, some theorists have argued that diaschisis is merely an a posteriori notion offering nothing more than a name for the observable remission of symptoms following injury to the central nervous system. Yet, despite the paucity of experimental confirmation of von Monakow's theory at the neuronal level, diaschisis still seems to be an appealing concept in both experimental and clinical neurology because certain behavioral phenomena seem to fit the notion of a time-dependent release from a suppressed level of functioning. For example, John Adametz (1959) suggested that cats with staged lesions of the rostral reticular formation show facilitated motor recovery and an absence of coma because serial lesions result in less neural shock than do one-stage lesions.

> While presumably destruction of the reticular activating system is a primary factor in the production of coma by mesial tegmental lesions, other considerations have importance also. The experiments herein establish a shock factor (diaschisis), more enduring in the instance of bilateral lesions produced in 1 sitting than in corresponding lesions produced in 2 stages [p. 25].

Explanations of this type also appear in the human clinical literature dealing with fast and slow growing lesions: Walther Riese (1948) has argued that signs of neural shock, which are obvious in such sudden lesions as brain injuries or apoplectic insults, and also in rapidly growing brain tumors, usually are absent in slowly growing neoplasms involving the same regions. He viewed the doctrine of neural shock as having far reaching implications for localizaing lesions in man and explaining unexpected symptoms after focal injuries.

We should note that Aaron Smith, Marion Walker, and Garth Myers (1978) also referred to the concept of *diaschisis* to explain some of the recovery that occurs after hemispherectomy in man. Their thinking is that pathologic influences radiating from the diseased hemisphere may inhibit or disrupt the functions of the opposite hemisphere and that this chronic depression potentiates the symptoms that patients show prior to surgery. However, distal effects dissipate soon after the diseased hemisphere is surgically removed. In theory, this "disinhibition" could account for some of the rapid improvements that these patients display on a variety of psychological and neurological tests administered shortly after hemispheric removals.

In the preceding chapter, we reviewed a number of studies that also relate to the concept of *diaschisis*. Specifically, in discussing pharmacological experiments, the point was made that lesions that at first appear to destroy certain "centers" in the brain may, in fact, only be suppressing neural functioning, as is evidenced by the rapid return of function following the administration of stimulants and other drugs. We pointed out that Patricia Meyer and her co-workers at Ohio State University found that neodecorticate cats that could not make placing responses under standard test conditions were able to show a rapid return of these reflexes under the effects of d-amphetamine, a central nervous system stimulant (Meyer, Horel, and Meyer, 1963). We also saw how "recovered" monkeys may exhibit a reemergence of deficits associated with parietal lobe insult after they are administered a low dose of a short-acting anesthetic (ketamine; Faugier-Grimaud, Frenois, and Stein, 1978). Studies such as these would also suggest that suppression of neuronal activity can account for some deficits seen after brain damage and that recovery of function can sometimes reflect the dissipation of an impaired state of functioning.

As noted in Chapter 12, clinical manipulation of neural shock or disinhibition following brain injury has thus far received the greatest attention in the Soviet Union, where attempts have already been made to treat lesion-induced disorders with pharmacological agents thought to unblock depressed central nervous system areas (Luria, Naydin, Tsvetkova, and Vinarskaya, 1969). The Soviet workers point out that disinhibition is the treatment of choice when "the role of inactivation assumes the foremost place in the disturbance of function [p. 368]," as in cases of concussion or other lesions, which disrupt tonic cortical activity.

Luria and his fellow investigators contend that states like diaschisis can be due to a loss of cholinergic transmission and that cerebral trauma (such as hemmorhage) can substantially increase levels of cholinesterase in nearby regions of the brain. The increased concentration of cholinesterase results in a "functional asynapsia," which is eliminated when levels of acetylcholine return to normal. To speed this process of functional recovery, the Luria group administers anticholinesterase drugs to their patients so that acetylcholine can again accumulate to levels where it can be used functionally.

The Russian investigators have described clinical cases in which single injections of eserine and neostigmine were able to restore motor function almost immediately after treatment (see Chapter 12). In particular, Luria and his colleagues claim that galanthamine, a potent alkaloid, can disinhibit previously lost gnostic, praxic, and speech functions in some patients (Pravdina-Vinarskaya and Rudaya, 1959). Behavioral restitution after galanthamine treatment is claimed to parallel the return of a normal-appearing EEG.[4]

In the Western clinical literature, there is some evidence to suggest that administration of cholinomimetic agents or choline itself can improve memory in senescent, demented patients (Drachman, 1977), but the data are not generally accepted as unequivocal. Clinical neuropsychologists and neurologists do occasionally report other phenomena that also can be related to the concept of *suppression*. For example, "recovered" aphasics often show a return of speech impediments when they are overly fatigued or when they have taken in too much alcohol.

In the context of findings such as these, it is not surprising that Teuber (1975) proposed that concepts such as *diaschisis* must be reexamined by contemporary neuroscientists. It seems appropriate to end this chapter with Teuber's words:

> Rather than postulating neuronal rearrangements, one should first consider a possibility advanced long ago by von Monakow, who spoke of hypothetical suppression and disruption of function . . . The concept has not fared well, having as yet no clear anatomic or physiologic counterparts. Nor did von Monakow help much by declaring that in some instances, diaschisis could be permanent. Yet, just such diaschisis-like processes will have to be identified, in our opinion, by appropriate histologic and histochemical means since the phenomena of recovery seem to demand it [p. 476].

References

Adametz, J. H. Role of recovery of functioning in cats with rostal reticular lesions. *Journal of Neurosurgery*, 1959, *16*, 85–98.

[4] In the West, these findings have been presented in chapters or in brief reports. Thus, some important questions can be asked about whether other drugs were used for comparison and whether control substances were given to still other patients with roughly comparable lesions. In addition, at the time that these studies were being conducted in the Soviet Union, very little was known about the roles of other neurotransmitters in the brain and perhaps how they might be affected by changes in the concentration of ACh. The study of central nervous system neurotransmitters, needless to say, has received much more attention in recent years, and it may be best to interpret these early reports with this in mind.

Drachman, D. A. Memory and cognitive function in man: Does the cholinergic system have a specific role? *Neurology*, 1977, *27*, 783–790.

Faugier-Grimaud, S., Frenois, C., and Stein, D. G. Effects of posterior parietal lesions on visually guided behavior in monkeys. *Neuropsychologia*, 1978, *16*, 151–168.

Glassman, R. B. Recovery following sensorimotor cortical damage: Evoked potentials, brain stimulation and motor control. *Experimental Neurology*, 1971, *33*, 16–29.

Glassman, R. B., and Malamut, D. L. Recovery from electroencephalographic slowing and reduced evoked potentials after somatosensory cortical damage in cats. *Behavioral Biology*, 1976, *17*, 333–354.

Henle, J. *Pathologische Untersuchungen*. Berlin: Verlag August Hirschwald, 1840.

Høedt-Rasmussen, K., and Skinhøj, E. Transneural depression of the cerebral hemispheric metabolism in man. *Acta Neurologica Scandinavica*, 1964, *40*, 41–46.

Irwin, D. A., Criswell, H. E., and Kakolewski, J. W. Spontaneous whole brain slow potential changes during recovery from neurosurgery. *Science*, 1973, *181*, 1176–1178.

Kempinsky, W. H. Steady potential gradients in experimental cerebral vascular occlusion. *Electroencephalography and Clinical Neurophysiology*, 1954, *6*, 375–388.

Kempinsky, W. H. Spatially remote effects of focal brain injury: Relation to diaschisis. *Transactions of the American Neurological Association*, 1956, *81*, 79–82.

Kempinsky, W. H. Experimental study of distal effects of acute focal injury. *Archives of Neurology and Psychiatry*, 1958, *79*, 376–389.

Kiloh, L. G., McComas, A. J., and Osselton, J. W. *Clinical electroencephalography* (3rd ed.). London: Butterworths, 1972.

Lassen, N. A. Cerebral blood flow and oxygen consumption in man. *Physiological Reviews*, 1959, *39*, 183–238.

Leao, A. A. P. Spreading depression of activity in the cerebral cortex. *Journal of Neurophysiology*, 1944, *7*, 359–390.

Luria, A. R., Naydin, V. L., Tsvetkova, L. S., and Vinarskaya, E. N. Restoration of higher cortical functions following local brain damage. In P. J. Vinken and G. W. Bruyn (Eds.), *Handbook of clinical neurology III*. Amsterdam: North Holland Publishing, 1969, Pp. 368–433.

Markowitsch, H. J., and Pritzel, M. Von Monakow's diaschisis concept: Comments on West et al. (1976). *Behavioral Biology*, 1978, *22*, 411–412.

Meyer, P. M., Horel, J. A., and Meyer, D. R. Effects of dl-amphetamine upon placing responses in neodecorticate cats. *Journal of Comparative and Physiological Psychology*, 1963, *56*, 402–404.

Meyer, J. S., Shinohara, M., Kanda, T., Fukuuchi, Y., Ericsson, A. D., and Kok, N. H. Diaschisis resulting from acute unilateral cerebral infarction. *Archives of Neurology*, 1970, *23*, 241–247.

Pravdina-Vinarskaya, E. N., and Rudaya, G. B. Reeducation of the gnostal, praxial and speech functions and disinhibition treatment with Galanthaminum (Russian). *Reports of the Academy of Pedagogical Sciences RSFSR*, 1959, *5*, 113–116.

Riese, W. Aphasia in brain tumors. *Confinia Neurologica*, 1948, *9*, 64–79.

Riese, W., *Principles of neurology in the light of history and their present use*. New York: Nervous and Mental Disease Monographs, 1950.

Riese, W. The principle of diaschisis. *International Record of Medicine*, 1958, *171*, 73–82.

Robinson, R. G., and Bloom, F. E. Changes in posterior hypothalamic self-stimulation following experimental cerebral infarction in the rat. *Journal of Comparative and Physiological Psychology*, 1978, *92*, 969–976.

Robinson, R. G., and Bloom, F. E., and Battenberg, E. L. F. A fluorescent histochemical study of changes in noradrenergic neurons following experimental cerebral infarction in the rat. *Brain Research*, 1977, *132*, 259–272.

Robinson, R. G., Shoemaker, W. J., Schlumpf, M., Volk, T., and Bloom, F. E. Effect of experimental cerebral infarction in rat brain on catecholamines and behavior. *Nature*, 1975, *255*, 332–334.

Skinhøj, E. Bilateral depression of CBF in unilateral cerebral diseases. *Acta Neurologica Scandinavica*, 1965, *41*(Suppl. 14), 161–163.

Smith, A., Walker, M. L., and Myers, G. *Hemispherectomy and diaschisis: Rapid improvement in cerebral functions after right hemispherectomy in a six-year-old child.* Paper presented at the 86th Annual Meeting of the American Psychological Association, Toronto, September 1978.

Teuber, H.-L. Recovery of function after lesions in the central nervous system: History and prospects. *Neuroscience Research Program Bulletin*, 1974, *12*, 197–209.

Teuber, H.-L. Recovery of function after brain injury in man. In *Outcome of severe damage to the central nervous system* (Ciba Foundation Symposium). Amsterdam: Elsevier, 1975, pp. 159–186, 476.

von Monakow, C. *Die Lokalisation im Grosshirn und der Abbau der Funktion durch Kortikale Herde.* Wiesbaden: J. F. Bergmann, 1914. (Translated and exerpted by G. Harris. In K. H. Pribram, Ed., *Mood, states and mind.* London: Penguin, 1969, pp. 27–37.)

West, J. R. The concept of diaschisis: A reply to Markowitsch and Pritzel. *Behavioral Biology*, 1978, *22*, 413–416.

West, J. R., Deadwyler, S. A., Cotman, C. W., and Lynch, G. S. An experimental test of diaschisis. *Behavioral Biology*, 1976, *18*, 419–425.

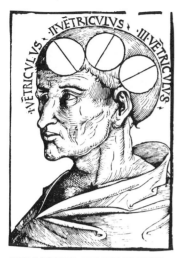

CHAPTER FOURTEEN

Supersensitivity as a Recovery Model

*The first effect of injury done to the nervous system
is a diminution of its functions; whilst the second or
ulterior effect is the augmentation of those functions*
[Hall, 1841, cited in Stavraky, 1961, p. 3].

If we accept the concept of *diaschisis* as a plausible explanation of functional recovery, we should be careful about falling into the trap of simply giving another name to the behavioral sparing that emerges as the time after injury increases. Assuming that neuronal activity *is* depressed by trauma, what, in fact, allows the synaptic dendritic and axonal potentials to return to levels capable of mediating behavior? Does it make sense to think that perhaps a post-traumatic state like diaschisis could serve as a stimulus for another series of physiological events that can subserve recovery?

In this context one should consider the possibility that diaschisis can sometimes be followed by a period of "supersensitivity," a state which permits remaining neurons to function effectively. In 1841, Marshall Hall anticipated modern thinking when he commented about injury to the central nervous system first diminishing functions and later augmenting them.

Increased sensitivity to chemical agents following partial deafferentation of postsynaptic elements is well known in some organ systems. This hypersensitivity has been demonstrated repeatedly for the glands, skeletal muscles, peripheral neurons of autonomic ganglia, and partially denervated spinal neurons (cf. Sharpless, 1964; Stavraky, 1961; Trendelenberg, 1963). For example, immediately after a muscle fiber is deprived of its normal inputs, smaller than normal contractions to acetylcholine are observed. However, the sensitivity to acetylcholine can rise substantially above normal base levels over a period of 1–2 weeks following the denervation. We know now that the supersensitive reaction is not due to greater release of acetylcholine from the remaining presynaptic terminals, but rather to an increase in the number of receptor sites at both the end-plate and extrajunctional regions. At peak levels, skeletal muscles may show a 1000–100,000 fold increase in sensitivity to acetylcholine following denervation than before it! Furthermore, the state of heightened sensitivity decreases as the muscle fibers become reinnervated.

Does the same kind of supersensitivity also occur in the central nervous system? In their well-known monograph, *The Supersensitivity of Denervated Structures: A Law of Denervation* (1949), Walter B. Cannon (see Figure 14.1), of the Harvard University Medical School, and Arturo Rosenblueth, of the Instituto Nacional de Cardíologia de México, extended the original "law of denervation" (Cannon, 1939) to hold that:

> When in a functional chain of neurons one of the elements is severed, the ensuing total or partial denervation of some of the subsequent elements in the chain causes a supersensitivity of all of the distal elements, including those not denervated, and effectors if present, to the excitatory or inhibitory action of chemical agents and nerve impulses; the supersensitivity is greater for the links which immediately follow the cut neurons and decreases progressively for more distal elements [p. 186].

The general concept of *denervation supersensitivity,* however, did not originate with Cannon and his associates. Budge (1855) described supersensitive phenomena after sympathetic denervation of the iris ("paradoxical pupillary dilation"), and in 1899, Lewandowsky reported that the response of the nic-

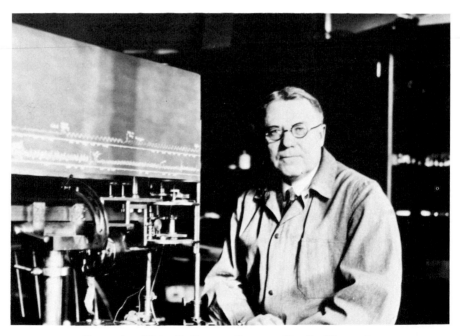

Figure 14.1. *Walter B. Cannon. (Courtesy of Bradford Cannon)*

titating membrane of the eye to intravenous injection of adrenal extracts was much greater in denervated than in intact tissue. According to Ullrich Trendelenberg (1963), Anderson (1904) carried out the first experimental analysis of denervation phenomena and showed them to be due to an increased sensitivity of the denervated muscle to epinephrine. More recent work on the nictitating membrane of the eye shows that chronic denervation increases sensitivity to norepinephrine, serotonin, and acetylcholine 125-, 50-, and 25-fold, respectively, over acute denervation levels.

Early descriptions of supersensitivity were not limited to the nictitating membrane or the eye. After destruction of the hypoglossal nerve, stimulation of a part of the facial nerve (the chorda tympani) produces a prolonged contraction of the tongue, but prior to any lesions, stimulation of the chorda tympani, which contains sensory, vasodilator, and secretory fibers, has no effect on the motor apparatus. This phenomenon is called the *Philipeaux-Vulpian effect,* after the investigators who first described it in 1863.

A related effect can be seen after the whole facial nerve is cut. Here there is an increase in sensitivity of the facial musculature to cervical sympathetic stimulation on the paralyzed side. This unusual finding was first observed in 1885 by Rogowicz. We now know that the basis of this effect, and that described by Philipeaux and Vulpian, lies in a dramatic increase in the sensitivity of the receptive organs to the action of acetylcholine from autonomic nerves (see Cannon and Rosenblueth, 1949). Phenomena such as these were encountered so frequently in the last century that Claude Bernard, one of the outstanding figures of the new physiology, wrote in his *Leçons de Pathologie Expérimentale* (1880) that the excitability of all tissues seems to increase when they are separated from the nervous influences which dominate them.

Although supersensitivity has been discussed thus far in relation to surgically denervating a structure, we should mention that any procedure that prevents neurohumors from being liberated by the nerve ending or from combining with the receptors on the effector organ can result in such sensitization. Thus, supersensitivity might also be seen after prolonged administration of pharmacological agents that block neuro-effector junctions (Emmelin, 1961) or following severe environmental deprivation conditions. The common element in all of these cases appears to be "disuse," and as contended by Seth Sharpless (1964), supersensitivity should not be viewed as a "pathological curiosity, [but rather as] a wide-spread physiological mode to adjustment in nervous junctions [p. 362]." [1]

---

[1] The concept of *supersensitivity* can make a certain amount of sense if one thinks in terms of design principles. Neural structures can be thought of as "modules" that have a greater capacity than would ordinarily be needed. When normally innervated, this excess capacity will go unnoticed. Following the loss of innervation, whether due to a lesion or to the normal loss of cells over a lifetime, this excess capacity may be called upon to maintain a relatively normal level of functioning of the modules.

In contrast to the extensive literature on supersensitivity in the peripheral nervous system, these effects are only now beginning to be directly studied in the brain itself. In one recent study (Creese, Burt, and Snyder, 1977), unilateral lesions of the nigrostriatal dopamine pathway were made in rats by injecting this pathway on one side of the brain with neurotoxin, 6-hydroxydopamine. Two to seven months later, the rats were given apomorphine, a dopaminergic agonist. Most of the animals responded to the apomorphine by repeatedly turning in a direction opposite to the side of lesion—a behavior that signified that the damaged side of the brain had become supersensitive (see Ungerstedt, 1971; Ungerstedt and Arbuthnott, 1970). One to ten weeks later, the experimenters examined the binding of (^{3}H)haloperidol, a dopamine antagonist, to rat striatal dopamine receptors and found it to be much greater on the damaged side of the brain, but only in those rats that displayed the turning indicative of supersensitivity. Additional assays revealed a 40% increase in the number of binding sites in the damaged striata, thus providing a clear mechanism for the observed supersensitivity. Some of these data are presented in Figure 14.2.

Ian Creese and his co-workers at the Johns Hopkins University School of Medicine think that their demonstration has significant clinical implications since indications of behavioral supersensitivity can also be observed in animals subjected to long-term treatments with neuroleptic drugs. Such rats provide an animal model for tardive dyskinesia, a state of heightened, abnormal motor activity that often is seen in human patients that have been treated for long periods of time with neuroleptic agents (Moore and Thornburg, 1975; Tarsy and Baldessarini, 1974). The behavioral supersensitivity observed in the animals treated with neuroleptics is also associated with enhanced (^{3}H)haloperidol binding to dopamine receptors, again reflecting an abnormally high number of binding sites (Creese, Burt, and Snyder, 1977).

In a related experiment combining physiological and behavioral measures, Lars-Göran Nygren, Kjell Fuxe, Gösta Jonsson, and Lars Olson (1974), of the Karolinska Institute, gave adult rats injections of another neurotoxin, 5,6-dihydroxytryptamine, in the lateral ventricle. Fluorescence histochemistry performed on the brain tissues 8, 12, and 14 days later revealed a complete or almost complete disappearance of 5-hydroxytrypamine (5-HT) terminals in the gray matter of the spinal cord. The Swedish scientists then examined hindlimb extensor reflexes after injections of nialmide and L-tryptophan and noticed a clearcut behavioral supersensitivity (no supersensitivity had been apparent 2 days postlesion). One to three months after the lesion, 5-HT terminals began to increase and 5-HT uptake began to recover, although incompletely. These events were paralleled by a normalization of the reflex to the drugs. These data, shown in Figures 14.3 and 14.4, were interpreted to suggest that the disappearance of 5-HT terminals caused a 5-HT receptor supersensitivity and that this supersensitivity diminished as new terminals grew out to normalize the functions of the 5-HT synapses.

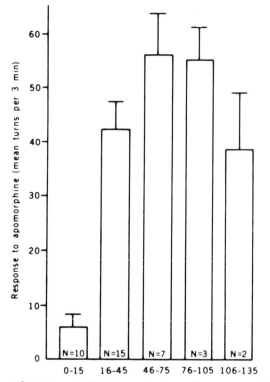

Figure 14.2. *Increased (^{3}H)haloperidol binding in the lesioned striatum and behavioral supersensitivity to apomorphine in rats with unilateral nigrostriatal lesions induced by 6-hydroxydopamine. Rotational behavior in response to subcutaneous injection of apomorphine (.25 mg/kg) was measured 2-7 months after the lesions were made. The binding of (^{3}H)haloperidol was assayed in the lesioned and control striatum of each rat separately 1–10 weeks later and is expressed as the percentage increase in radioactivity (counts per minute) of specific (^{3}H)haloperidol bound in the lesioned striatum compared with the control striatum at four concentrations of (^{3}H)haloperidol (.4–4.0 nM). (From Creese, Burt, and Snyder, 1977. Copyright 1977 by the American Association for the Advancement of Science.)*

Prior to the appearance of reports such as these, supersensitivity in the central nervous system was only studied indirectly or inferred from the way brain-damaged subjects responded to certain drugs. George Stavraky, of the University of Western Ontario, provides a number of interesting examples of this in his book, *Supersensitivity following Lesions of the Nervous System* (1961).

One case involved a patient who had an area of the left frontal lobe undercut and isolated on three sides. Ten months later, in preparation for a frontal lobotomy, both frontal lobes were exposed and electrocorticograms were recorded. A high voltage, rhythmic spike discharge appeared only on the damaged side when the cortex was irrigated with an acetylcholine solution. The discharge became so severe that the patient had to be put under pentobarbital anesthesia.

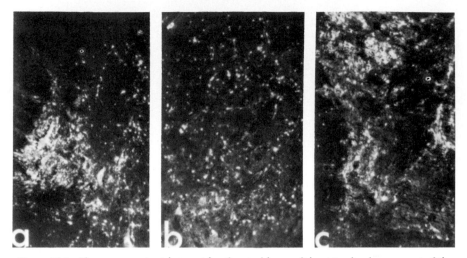

Figure 14.3. *Fluorescence microphotographs of ventral horns of the upper lumbar segment of the spinal cord. Transverse sections (× 105). (a) saline treated rat, 12 days. Dense pattern of CA and 5–HT nerve terminals. (b) 5,6–HT treated rat, 12 days. The sparse distribution of terminals seen depends on a complete absence of 5–HT and a slight decrease in number of CA terminals. (c) 5,6–HT treated rat, 3 months. The 5–HT terminals have reappeared as a dense, somewhat diffuse pattern of yellow fluorescent, small varicosities, partly masking the more distinct CA varicosities seen in (b). (From Nygren et al., 1974.)*

In the opinion of Echlin and McDonald (1954), findings like this provide clear evidence that denervated or partially denervated cerebral cortex can become supersensitive to certain types of stimuli.[2]

As an explanation for recovery of function, the concept of *denervation supersensitivity,* when used by itself, may be limited. This is because it depends on damage to a given neural system or subsystem being incomplete, so that a minimal amount of neurotransmitter would be left to activate postsynaptic elements. In addition, since afferent inputs may be greatly diminished, the model would best apply to those systems where the exact pattern or number of presynaptic neurons activated would not be a critical factor in information transmission.

In their own conception of the role of supersensitivity in recovery of function, Walter B. Cannon and Arturo Rosenblueth (1949) placed great emphasis on the importance of remaining, normally unused pathways and synapses. They sug-

[2] The exaggerated response of the cerebral cortex to pharmacological agents can be seen not only with drugs, but also with direct electrical stimulation. Obrador (1947) noted this in dogs that sustained lesions that partially isolated the motor cortex 2 months earlier. This was also seen by Bard (1933) in an experiment in which the electrical threshold for movement was lower on the damaged side of the brain than on the intact side in cats with cortical lesions.

gested that "devious neural connections" not used in the healthy state could become functional as a result of the supersensitivity that develops after the normal pathway to an area is inactivated. Cannon and Rosenblueth hypothesized that once used, such connections may remain functional, even after the supersensitivity subsides.

Hence, supersensitivity, which may under some conditions only involve spared elements of an incompletely damaged neural pathway, but which under other circumstances may involve the conversion of unusual "subliminal" connections into a functional pathway, can be viewed as one type of a reorganizational theory. As Cannon and Rosenblueth (1949) themselves stated

> Since spinal semisection has been shown to lead to the supersensitivity of partially denervated neurons to the influence of impinging nerve impulses, it appears likely that this supersensitivity is one of the important mechanisms for the opening of vicarious pathways indicated by the restoration of function in the chronically semisected animals, i.e., that it is an important factor in so-called reorganization of the central nervous system after injuries [p. 214].

We thus find that *reorganization* to Cannon and Rosenblueth, at least as defined in their discussion of the spinal cord, does not mean the establishment of new connections, but rather only the use of pathways and synapses that are already present, but which presumably do not play a major role in the particular function in the normal state. (We discussed the idea of unused pathways in Chapter 7, in the context of Patrick Wall's notion of *latent synapses*.) In the absence of spared routes to a supposedly critical structure, recovery, in their opinion, could not take place.[3]

Although denervation may result in both supersensitivity and, as we noted in earlier chapters, axonal sprouting, the emphasis placed by Cannon and Rosenblueth on established neural structures would rule out a place for sprouting in their limited, supersensitivity recovery model. This would be consistent with the work of McCouch, Austin, Liu, and Liu (1958). They observed sprouting 2–3 weeks after semisection of the rat spinal cord, but found that reflexive responses indicative of supersensitivity became exaggerated on the side of the injury considerably earlier. Stavraky (1961), who acknowledged the work of McCouch *et al.*, hypothesized that, if anything, sprouting may function as an important component in the later phases of functional compensation in the nervous system. Indeed, it seems plausible to view sprouting as a possible response to supersensitivity, but incorrect to view supersensitivity as a by-product of sprouting; in fact,

---

[3] One of the more interesting questions that can be asked is why these devious connections are present to begin with. One possibility is that they are the remnants of a system that was important long before the brain reached its present state of development. As new, more efficient systems emerged, these older systems were not necessarily eliminated, but perhaps simply bypassed.

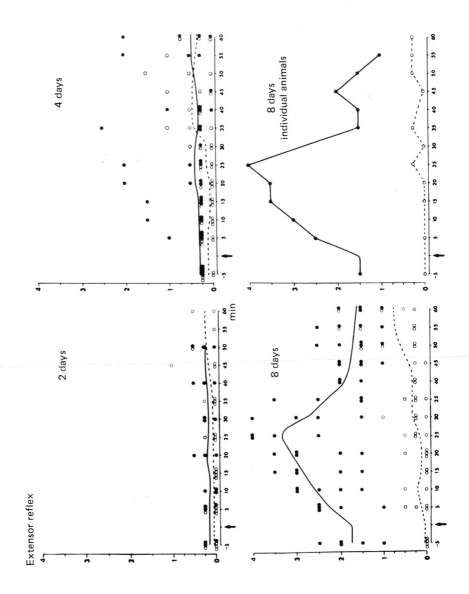

Extensor reflex

4 days

2 days

8 days
individual animals

8 days

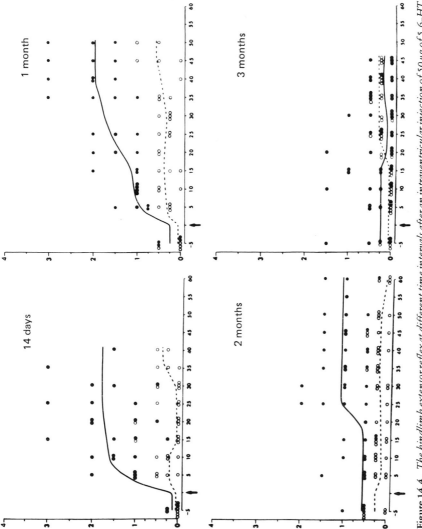
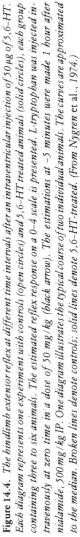

Figure 14.4. *The hindlimb extensor reflex at different time intervals after an intraventricular injection of 50 μg of 5,6-HT. Each diagram represents one experiment with controls (open circles) and 5,6-HT treated animals (solid circles), each group containing three to six animals. The estimated reflex response on a 0–4 scale is presented. L-tryptophan was injected intravenously at zero time in a dose of 50 mg/kg (black arrow). The estimations at –5 minutes were made 1 hour after nialamide, 500 mg/kg IP. One diagram illustrates the typical course of two individual animals. The curves are approximated to the median. Broken lines denote controls; solid lines denote 5,6-HT-treated. (From Nygren et al., 1974.)*

sprouting should eliminate supersensitivity by reestablishing a more normal complement of presynaptic terminals.

On the basis of what is known about supersensitivity, we can hypothesize that recovery of function might be facilitated by first inflicting damage elsewhere in the central nervous system that would partially denervate the brain area under study, or by administering a drug that reduces the release of a neurotransmitter in that area prior to subtotal physical insult. Stanley Glick and Stuart Greenstein (1972) tested the first idea indirectly by making lesions of the frontal cortex in rats to eliminate some of the catecholaminergic inputs to the lateral hypothalamic region. They damaged the lateral hypothalamus 30 days later to determine whether the expected "supersensitive" state permitted remaining lateral hypothalamic neurons to mediate weight regulation. Glick and Greenstein showed that these animals were able to regulate body weight, but that rats receiving lateral hypothalamic and frontal cortex lesions at the same time, or only 10 days apart, did not eat and drink (Table 14.1).

In a test of the second prediction, Stanley Glick, Stuart Greenstein, and Betty Zimmerberg (1972) administered α-methyl-paratyrosine to block the synthesis of dopamine and norepinephrine, neurotransmitters believed to be important in the regulation of eating and drinking. Some rats were given the drug for 3 days prior to *subtotal* lateral hypothalamic lesions with the expectation that it would

TABLE 14.1

Mean Postoperative Weight Changes (Percentage of Preoperative Weight) following Lateral Hypothalamic Lesions [a]

Days after LH surgery	Groups [b]				
	LH	SFC–LH	10-day FC–LH	30-day FC–LH	Sham
1	87.7	87.1	89.8	89.9	99.2
2	81.3	80.9	85.9	87.7	101.8
3	75.4	76.3	82.5 [c]	85.7	103.8
4	70.8	72.5	78.7 [c]	85.8	105.6
5	65.8	68.2	74.7 [c]	86.2	108.1
6		64.8	70.5 [c]	88.9	110.0
7			66.4	90.4	111.3
8				93.8	111.2
9				94.7	111.8
10				96.1	114.1

[a] From Glick and Greenstein (1972). (*Reprinted by permission from* Nature, 239, 187–188. *Copyright* © 1972, *Macmillan Journals Limited.*)

[b] LH = lateral hypothalamus; SFC = simultaneous frontal cortical; group means computed only for days on which all rats of a group still surviving.

[c] Significantly greater than LH or SFC–LH at $p < .05$ (*t* test); all 30-day FC–LH rats recovered; one 10-day FC–LH rat recovered, but is not included in data in table.

make the lateral hypothalamic circuitry supersensitive. As shown in Table 14.2, with adequate dosages of the drug, these animals satisfactorily regulated body weight following the hypothalamic lesions. In contrast, animals receiving the same drug after surgery, thus further depleting neurotransmitter levels, lost considerable weight and died.

Glick and his colleagues at the Mount Sinai School of Medicine have extended their experiments on supersensitivity after brain lesions to include dependent measures other than feeding and weight regulation. In one set of studies they examined spontaneous and drug-induced rotation after unilateral lesions of the nigrostriatal tract (which is believed to result primarily from an imbalance in dopaminergic transmission). Amphetamine, which stimulates release of dopamine from presynaptic terminals, increases circling toward the side of the lesion by acting primarily on the intact side of the brain (Ungerstedt, 1971). In contrast, apomorphine, a direct dopamine receptor antagonist, had little effect on this circling immediately after unilateral nigrostrial lesions. However, as time passed, the apomorphine caused increases in rotation toward the side opposite the lesion. Glick and his colleagues attributed the increased contralateral turning behavior to the development of supersensitivity on the denervated side of the brain (Glick, Jerussi, and Fleisher, 1976).

George Stavraky (1961) provides a number of examples to show that the time period between lesion production and the development of measurable supersensitivity can vary tremendously with experimental conditions. The duration of the supersensitive state also seems highly variable. In some cases, it may appear within a week and last for only a matter of days, but in other cases, the picture may be quite different. The point is made in a study in which cats had the corpus

TABLE 14.2
Mean Weight Changes (Percentage of Weight Prior to Surgery) after Lateral Hypothalamic Lesions [a]

Days after surgery	Lesions (saline)	Lesions αMT (10 mg/kg)	Lesions αMT (75 mg/kg)	Lesions αMT (100 mg/kg)	Sham-operated
1	86.8	86.2	89.3	87.5	99.2
2	80.9	80.4	87.3	85.2	101.8
3	75.0	74.6	85.9	83.6	103.8
4	70.1	69.7	83.6	84.1	105.6
5	65.2	65.0	81.8	88.7	108.1
6	61.4	61.6	79.8	90.5	110.0
7	—	58.6	80.1	92.2	111.3
8	—	—	82.3	95.3	111.2
9	—	—	84.4	95.6	111.8
10	—	—	85.9	96.0	114.1

[a] From Glick, Greenstein, and Zimmerberg (1972). (*Copyright 1972 by the American Association for the Advancement of Science.*)

callosum divided and then were tested to see how sensitive they were to convulsions when pharmacologic agents were administered (Teasdall, 1950; Teasdall and Stavraky, 1950). No differences appeared between the corpus callosum and control groups during the first 8–9 months that followed the surgery. The cats with lesions then became progressively more sensitive to the drug, penthylenetetrazol. Their seizures became so severe and prolonged that some even died during the stage of status epilepticus. The animals with lesions that did not succumb continued to show extreme sensitivity to the convulsant drug for more than a year after the supersensitivity was first noticed.[4]

In a related study, Hoefer and Pool (1943) found that sensitivity to convultions in cats and monkeys with corpus callosum transections may be *reduced* before it is heightened. Although this effect may have been due to anesthesia, we can also view these findings as suggesting that the supersensitivity was influenced by a diaschisis-like state, which appeared in the first few weeks after the lesions were made, a possibility discussed at the start of this chapter.

As a model, supersensitivity has been useful in providing a theoretical framework for some serial lesion effects (Glick and Zimmerberg, 1972). For example, it can be argued that animals with staged lesions do not show symptoms of brain damage as readily as their one-stage counterparts because the initial operation produces a state of supersensitivity in critical loci, such as in target tissue opposite to that which is initially damaged. A large, but incomplete second lesion, in such a case, may allow an animal to use a spared fragment of tissue that might not be used by an animal sustaining comparable lesions on both sides of the brain at the same time. Conceivably, the development of supersensitivity at other loci might also account for some of these instances of recovery.

Although neuronal supersensitivity has the potential to facilitate recovery of function, we must consider the possibility that a state of heightened sensitivity could also be maladaptive under some conditions. If a structure normally receives afferents from two distinct sources, one of which is damaged, supersensitivity to inputs from the remaining source would be expected to develop. If these circuits are normally antagonistic to the ones damaged, marked deficits and exaggerated reactions could develop. Stavraky (1961) contends that this effect underlies the clinical syndrome of sensory ataxia (an inability to regulate voluntary movements as a result of posterior column or dorsal root injury). He argues that sensory ataxia

---

[4] The possibility that this finding may also reflect a related state called *kindling* should be acknowledged. Kindling refers to the fact that repeated brain stimulation can induce the development of behavioral and electrical seizures and a state of supersensitivity to pharmacological agents. With more and more stimulation, these reactions intensify as each stimulation induces more neural excitability. Kindling can be long lasting and possibly even permanent. The interested reader should see Birchfiel, Duchowny, and Duffy (1979) for an analysis of kindling and for additional references about this phenomenon.

is not just due to the loss of inputs, but is the result of a composite functional alteration in which lack of sensibility and increased excitability together affect symptomatology. This can be seen in postural reflexes, some being absent and some being exaggerated, and in the way the limbs may "overshoot" the target in response to certain stimuli.

Stavraky also points out that unusual sensations and pain reactions (paresthesias, dyesthesias, and hyperesthesias, such as thalamic pain and causalgia) also appear to be associated with partial denervation of certain areas of the central nervous system.

> Such a supersensitive state would account well for the paroxysms of bizarre, poorly localized, but exaggerated and therefore intolerable, pain that is felt when these areas of the central nervous system are activated through their remaining connections. The effect of sensitization is shown particularly clearly in mesencephalic tractotomy which abolishes the original pain for which it is done, but leads to a gradual development of an insufferable dyesthesia [p. 92].

In terms of adaptation, it is important to consider the point that animals with focal brain lesions probably have very short survival times in the wild and that in the absence of modern medicine, the same can probably be said for people. If this is the case, one can legitimately ask why supersensitivity evolved and if its relationship to recovery of function after a lesion is anything more than a chance affair. This is a difficult question to answer, but some clues may be found when the nervous system is viewed in a developmental perspective.

We might speculate that early in life there may be more postsynaptic receptor sites than fibers that grow toward them. This would increase the probability that at least some synapses will be formed and enhance the chances that those that are formed will be effective in driving the postsynaptic cell. At maturity, if cells are lost or the system is injured, there may be a throwback to this earlier developmental phase of increased receptor sites, and supersensitivity would occur.

Whether the supersensitivity is beneficial or deleterious may depend on whether the system remains in a state of balance or whether it is thrown out of balance following cell loss. As cells are depleted with advancing age, for example, there may be an increase in the sensitivity of the remaining connections in the brain, which allows the system to function at a reasonable level of efficiency. In this case, the increased sensitivity would be beneficial. This is because it would not be confined to just one brain area or input where it could result in exaggerated responses that would disrupt the normal balance of excitation and inhibition needed to mediate adaptive behavior.

With a focal lesion, the picture may be different. In this case the supersensitivity that follows will also represent a return to an earlier developmental phase, but its adaptive significance may be questionable. Since the supersensitive reaction probably did not evolve for recovery, the effect may or may not be beneficial. In the final analysis, the nature of the inputs remaining to the denervated structure may prove to be the critical factor. If it is just a question of fewer inputs from a homogeneous population, the effects could be beneficial, whereas if one of two types of inputs is lost, the supersensitive reaction would exaggerate the influence of the remaining, unbalanced input even more, and this could well be deleterious, as evidenced in some of the examples presented by Stavraky.

Although supersensitivity can account nicely for some phenomena, we should mention that another of several problems that must eventually be addressed is that of defining the sites in the central nervous system that have become supersensitive and which might account for some cases of behavioral recovery. In drug studies, it would be presumptuous to conclude that pharmacological agents such as α-methyl-paratyrosine are acting only upon the structures that are later subjected to damage since catecholamine-containing neurons can be found throughout the brain. Thus, changes such as supersensitivity can be taking place in sites far removed from the actual locus of the injury, and far removed even from the particular circuitry that is under investigation. Even when the most detailed anatomical and physiological analyses accompany the behavioral data, effects at a distance may raise interpretive problems, a point acknowledged by some investigators (e.g., Creese, Burt, and Snyder, 1977).

Finally, it is important to realize that the theory of supersensitivity, as an explanation for recovery of function, often must be considered in the context of other processes that can determine the outcome of brain injury. For example, vicarious functioning, multiple control, and behavioral compensation must also be viewed as possible explanations when all of a structure, or specific parts of a very highly organized area, are severely damaged. Some recovery of function, for instance, may be observed following total ablation of the precentral motor regions. Especially if there are no spared fragments, supersensitivity *by itself* could not account for the restitution; however, supersensitivity may still play some role in mediating the recovery that is witnessed. In particular, the somatosensory cortex is known to have some motor units and many connections to and from the motor cortex. It may be that the motor cortex lesions altered the sensitivity of the motor circuitry in the somatosensory cortex such that this small population of motor units might now be capable of effective functioning. Hence, the recovery could reflect some sort of multiple control or "vicarious functioning" (see Chapter 15), but this, in turn, may be dependent upon the lesion-induced supersensitivity. Of course, such ideas are speculative, but the more we know about restitution, the more apparent it is becoming that all of our theories and notions about recovery could be intertwined and that it is extremely improbable that any one theory will be able to explain all of the data that fall under the heading of "recovery of function."

References

Anderson, H. K. The paralysis of involuntary muscle, with special reference to the occurrence of paradoxical contraction. Part 1. Paradoxical pupil dilation and other ocular phenomena caused by lesions of the cervical sympathetic tract. *Journal of Physiology*, 1904, *30*, 290–310.

Bard, P. Studies on the cerebral cortex. *Archives of Neurology and Psychiatry*, 1933, *30*, 40-74.

Bernard, C. *Leçons de Pathologie Expérimentale* (2nd ed.). Paris: Ballière, 1880.

Birchfiel, J. L., Duchowny, M. S., and Duffy, F. H. Neuronal supersensitivity to acetylcholine induced by kindling in the rat hippocampus. *Science*, 1979, *204*, 1096-1098.

Budge, J. L. *Über die Bewegung der Iris, für Physiologen und Ärzte*. Braunschweig: Vieweg, 1855.

Cannon, W. B. A law of denervation. *American Journal of Medical Science*, 1939, *198*, 186, 737–750.

Cannon, W. B., and Rosenblueth, A. *The supersensitivity of denervated structures*. New York: Macmillan, 1949.

Creese, I., Burt, D., and Snyder, S. Dopamine receptor binding enhancement accompanies lesion-induced behavioral supersensitivity. *Science*, 1977, *197*, 596–598.

Echlin, F. A., and McDonald, J. The supersensitivity of chronically isolated and partially isolated cerebral cortex as a mechanism in focal cortical epilepsy. *Transactions of the American Neurological Association*, 1954, *79*, 75–79.

Emmelin, N. Supersensitivity following pharmacological denervation. *Pharmacological Review*, 1961, *13*, 17–37.

Glick, S. D., and Greenstein, S. Facilitation of recovery after lateral hypothalamic damage by prior ablation of frontal cortex. *Nature New Biology*, 1972, *239*, 187–188.

Glick, S. D., Greenstein, S., and Zimmerberg, B. Facilitation of recovery by α-methyl-p-tyrosine after lateral hypothalamic damage. *Science*, 1972, *177*, 534–535.

Glick, S. D., Jerussi, T. P., and Fleisher, L. N. Turning in circles: The neuropharmacology of rotation. *Life Sciences*, 1976, *18*, 889–896.

Glick, S. D., and Zimmerberg, B. Comparative recovery following simultaneous and successive-stage frontal brain damage in mice. *Journal of Comparative and Pysiological Psychology*, 1972, *79*, 481–487.

Hall, M. *On the diseases and derangements of the nervous system*. London: H. Bailliere, 1841.

Hoefer, R. F. A., and Pool, J. L. Conduction of cortical impulses and motor management of convulsive seizures. *Archives of Neurology and Psychiatry*, 1943, *50*, 381–400.

Lewandowsky, M. Über die Wirkung des Nebennierenextractes auf die glatten Muskeln, im Besonderen des Auges. *Archiv für Anatomie und Physiologie*, 1899, 360–366.

McCouch, G. P., Austin, G. M., Liu, C. N., and Liu, C. Y. Sprouting as a cause of spasticity. *Journal of Neurophysiology*, 1958, *21*, 205–216.

Moore, K. E., and Thornburg, J. E. Drug-induced dopamine supersensitivity. *Advances in Neurology*, 1975, *9*, 93–104.

Nygren, L.-G., Fuxe, K., Jonsson, G., and Olson, L. Functional regeneration of 5-hydroxytryptamine nerve terminals in the rat spinal cord following 5,6-dihydroxytryptamine induced degeneration. *Brain Research*, 1974, *78*, 377–394.

Obrador, A. S. Hiperexcitabilidad de neurones motoras producida par aislamiento parcial de areas de la corteza cerebral. *Revista Clínca Española*, 1947, *25*, 171–174.

Philipeaux, J. M., and Vulpian, A. Note sur une modification physiologique qui se produit dans le nerf lingual par suite de l'abolition temporaire de la matricité dans le nerf hypoglosse du même coté. *Comptes Rendus des Academie Science Paris*, 1863, *56*, 1009–1011.

Rogowicz, N. Über pseudomotorische Einwirkung der Ansa Vieussenii auf die Gesichtmuskeln. *Pflüger's Archiv für die gesamte Physiologie*, 1885, 1–12.

Sharpless, S. K. Reorganization of function in the nervous system—use and disuse. *Annual Review of Physiology*, 1964, *26*, 357–388.

Stavraky, G. W. *Supersensitivity following lesions of the nervous system*. Toronto: University of Toronto Press, 1961.

Tarsy, D., and Baldessarini, R. J. Behavioural supersensitivity to apomorphine following chronic treatment with drugs which interfere with the synaptic functions by catecholamines. *Neuropharmacology*, 1974, *13*, 927–940.

Teasdall, R. D. *A study of the response of partially denervated (deafferented) neurones of the central nervous system to pyramidal impulses and to reflex and chemical stimulation*. Unpublished doctoral dissertation, University of Western Ontario, London, Canada, 1950.

Teasdall, R. D., and Stavraky, G. W. Effect of section of the corpus callosum on experimental convulsions. *Federation Proceedings*, 1950, *9*, 124–125.

Trendelenberg, U. Supersensitivity and subsensitivity to sympathomimetic amines. *Pharmacological Review*, 1963, *15*, 225–276.

Ungerstedt, U. Striatal dopamine release after amphetamine or nerve degeneration revealed by rotational behavior. *Acta Physiologica Scandinavica*, 1971, Suppl. 367, Pp. 49–68.

Ungerstedt, U., and Arbuthnott, G. W. Quantitative recording of rotational behavior in rats after 6-hydroxydopamine lesions of the negrostriatal dopamine system. *Brain Research*, 1970, *24*, 485–493.

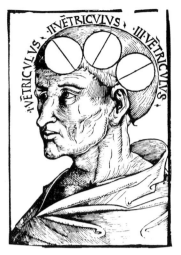

Vicariation Theory and Radical Reorganization of Function

That reorganization takes place within remaining portions of the cortex has been shown previously, since removal of such regions as the prefrontal areas or the postcentral gyrus greatly augments motor deficit when areas 4 and 6 have been previously extirpated in infancy, whereas ablation of the prefrontal or postcentral area from a normal cortex has no effect on skilled motor acts [Kennard, 1942, p. 238].

CHAPTER FIFTEEN

In 1886, David Ferrier wrote to dismiss, in no uncertain terms, a concept of recovery based on the idea that parts of the brain that are intact after focal injury can take over the functions of the damaged zone. He stated

> It has been assumed . . . that apparent recovery of voluntary control over the limbs . . . justifies the hypothesis of Flourens and his followers that a process of compensation is effected by other parts of the hemispheres taking up and performing the functions of the centres which have been destroyed. [This] hypothesis is altogether inconsistent with the *theory* of specific localization of function. If we were to suppose it possible that the functions of the leg centres could be taken up by the neighboring occipito-angular region, we should have the very remarkable substitution of a motor by a sensory centre. Such a mode of interpretation is no more justifiable than the supposition that the organ of vision may take up the functions of the organ of hearing . . . or perform both functions at once [pp. 368–369].

Ferrier clearly stood in opposition to Flourens and his followers, and through a series of experiments on dogs, monkeys, and other animals (see Chapter 3), set the stage for the thousands of brain ablations and stimulation experiments that eventually led to more contemporary theories of brain function. Despite Ferrier's strident argument against vicariation, brain researchers have not abandoned the concept altogether, and it usually appears under such terms as vicarious function, substitution, spontaneous reorganization, and the like (see Laurence and Stein, 1978, for further elaboration). The fact is that organisms *do* recover, even after bilateral injuries that destroy structures almost entirely. Given this observation, and in keeping with the doctrine of assigning specific functions to specific loci rather than to diffuse operations of remaining tissue, investigators should at least consider the possibility of a "take-over" of function by other brain regions following injury (see Spear, 1979, and Scheff and Wright, 1977, for recent approaches to the problem).

The theory of vicariation, like diaschisis and denervation supersensitivity, has had its well-known advocates. Hermann Munk (1839–1912; see Figure 15.1), who was working in Berlin more than 100 years ago, is often cited as an early proponent of vicariation theory (see Rosner, 1974). In a particularly important study, reported in 1877, he ablated a part of the occipital lobe in some dogs and a large segment of the temporal lobe in others. His observations led him to conclude that these animals suffered a "mind blindness" (loss of memory for visual images) in the former case, and a "psychic deafness" (loss of memory for auditory images) in the latter. Over a period of 1–2 months, however, the animals seemed to recover completely, and in a way which led Munk to postulate that the animals were relearning material exactly as it had been learned in their earliest years. In his opinion, this was because neighboring tissue had taken over the function originally controlled by the cerebral mass that he had damaged. In support of this hypothesis, Munk reported that if he spared the area that produced "mind blindness," but damaged surrounding tissue, little or no effect on visual functioning could be found. But when he damaged the same neighboring tissue (see Figure 15.2) in completely recovered animals (who had been rendered mind-blind as a result of an initial lesion in the occipital area), the newly relearned memories were lost once again, and the dogs no longer walked without stumbling or avoiding obstacles. Munk called them "cortically blind."[1]

It is both interesting and important to note that the basic paradigm used by Munk more than 100 years ago has been, and still is, the most popular method for "demonstrating" or "proving" vicariation, in spite of the fact that it clearly is based on a number of very shaky and questionable assumptions. The paradigm involves showing that damage to area 1 impairs performance on some behavioral measure, but that there is at least partial recovery over time or with therapy. It also requires showing that lesions of area 2 do not produce this deficit when the rest of the brain is healthy, or at least when area 1 is intact. If these two conditions can be met, it is assumed that area 2 takes over for area 1 if damage to area 2 reinstates the deficit in subjects who had recovered from area 1 lesions.

But how infallible is this logic? One point that is sometimes overlooked is that the absence of a lesion effect does not constitute proof that an area is not playing

---

[1] A discussion of Peter Spear's (1979) work on lesions of the visual cortex was presented in Chapter 7. Some of his data can also be interpreted in terms of nearby areas taking over the functions of a damaged visual cortex. Spear tested cats on pattern discriminations and used the same general paradigm employed by Munk. His two main findings were (a) that lesions of the neighboring suprasylvian gyrus (excluding Brodmann area 19) had no effect on visual pattern discrimination when the visual cortex was intact; but (b) that the integrity of the suprasylvian gyrus was very important for this behavior after the visual cortex (areas 17, 18, and 19) was ablated.

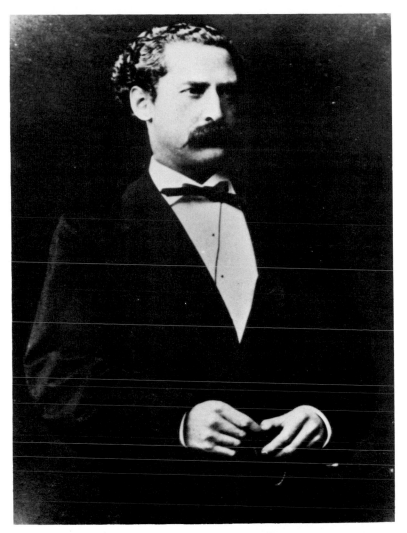

Figure 15.1. *Hermann Munk. (Courtesy of Mary Brazier)*

an important role in a function in the organism without brain damage. In our example, it certainly seems possible that area 2 was involved from the beginning, but that area 1 has the capability to mediate the function in the absence of area 2. Furthermore, we have described data which show that the presence of a behavioral deficit cannot be regarded as proof that an area is solely, or even directly, concerned with a function in the healthy brain. Area 1 lesions, for example, may produce deficits because they not only involve the loss of some cells, but

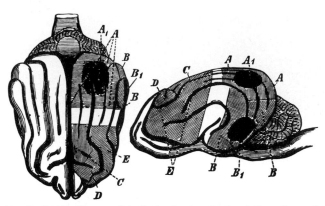

Figure 15.2. *Munk's (1881) diagram of the brain of a dog. A, visual; B, auditory; C, D, E, touch. Bilateral removal of A_1 results in psychic blindness; bilateral removal of B_1 results in psychic deafness.*

also because they temporarily suppress the activity in other parts of the brain (e.g., area 2). Therefore, lesions of areas 1 and 2, alone or together, can yield results like those reported by Munk, but for entirely different reasons than those postulated by him.

The concept of vicariation, which has waxed and waned in popularity over the years, seems to have been especially popular after World War I. Foerster (1930) and Bethe and Fischer (1931), for example, were advocates of the idea that functions could be taken over by structures not previously concerned with them, and even Pavlov argued for a large "safety factor" in the nervous system, in the sense that there probably are always potential pathways (roundabout associative connections) for the establishment of conditioned reflexes that are never normally used by the subject. In that indirect connections probably exist from every part of the brain to every other part, such a position would not seem to be as radical as it is often made out to be, provided that receptors and effectors and some of their projection areas are left intact.

Rather than just concern themselves with whether vicariation can or cannot take place, many of the investigators at the turn of this century attempted to study cases suggesting vicariation in sufficient detail to permit them to define the conditions that must be met for its occurrence. Otfrid Foerster (1930) and Shepherd Franz (1923), for instance, concentrated on the role of active learning and reeducation in the vicariation process.

Some support for the active learning position can be found in an experiment conducted by Robert Ogden and Shepherd Franz in 1917. They made unilateral motor cortex lesions in four monkeys and then gave each animal a different postoperative treatment, which for one animal included massaging the paralyzed segments, for another, forced usage of the paralyzed limb, and for a third, both therapeutic procedures. They found little recovery of motor function in the one monkey that was left to its own devices. However, they did report that:

> The method of treatment recommended by neurologists, general massage, does produce a slight amount of improvement but not to an extent to enable the animal to use the arm and hand properly for such ordinary operations as feeding and climbing, although these activities may be carried out after such treatment in an awkward manner. When, however, efforts are directed to the special nerves and muscles, and when the sound side of the animal is restrained so that movements of climbing and feeding must be made, if at all, by the use of the paralyzed segments the improvement is rapid and the recovery is practically complete [p. 45].

Another of the important issues that has sparked considerable debate concerns the question of which structures are actually substituting for those that are damaged. Karl Lashley (1938) stated that Shepherd Franz, who had published many papers with him, took the extremist position that almost any part of the brain might take over for another part, and that structure sets virtually no limits on the potential for recovery. After examining the evidence in favor of such a view, Lashley came to a different conclusion: He argued that successful reeducation depends upon the preservation of some part of a system that normally is concerned in the same function. Lashley (1938; see Figure 15.3) took the position that there is not an unlimited capacity for vicarious function, "but a limitation to the system which is more or less directly concerned with the same function under normal circumstances [p. 741]."

Whether or not one agrees with this position, it is quite clear that three basic interpretations have appeared within the framework of vicariation theory:

Hypothesis 1: The function is taken up by the homologous area on the opposite side of the brain. (This hypothesis, of course, is only applicable to unilateral lesions and to asymmetrical bilateral lesions.)

Hypothesis 2: The function is taken up by uninjured areas on the same side of the brain.

Hypothesis 3: The function is now being mediated by a center located at another level of anatomical organization.

Each of these hypotheses has been examined in cases of recovery from motor cortex lesions. As we have seen, after the period of infancy and in absence of special therapies, one-stage lesions of the motor areas typically result in paralyses of the contralateral limbs in man and primates, after which there usually is at least some recovery. In dogs, there is often considerable recovery within a matter of days or weeks, and the recovery process seems to be even more rapid in rabbits and rats, although more subtle motor deficiencies may persist for long periods of time.

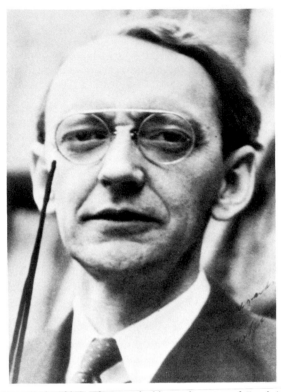

Figure 15.3. *Karl Lashley. (Photographed by, and courtesy of, Frank A. Beach)*

Hypothesis 1, which contends that the intact hemisphere takes over for the damaged one, has been "tested" in a number of instances with the multiple lesion paradigm. However, there has been very little evidence emerging to support this hypothesis, especially if the damage is inflicted upon adults. Lashley (1938) notes that Fritsch and Hitzig themselves were unable to support the hypothesis of takeover by the nondamaged hemisphere, and their negative results were upheld in an important early study by Carville and Duret (1875). The latter observed a dog who had recovered from left hemiplegia due to removal of the motor areas of the right cerebral cortex. The investigators noted that a subsequent lesion in the corresponding area of the left hemisphere was not followed by a reappearance of the left side paralysis, although as expected, a right hemiplegia appeared. In other dogs with lesions placed simultaneously in both hemispheres, almost complete recovery of motor functions ultimately was noted. Carville and Duret concluded that the corresponding areas on the intact side of the brain contributed very little to the recovery process.

This general conclusion has been supported in other experiments on dogs (e.g., Franck, 1887; Ogden and Franz, 1917). In addition, Leyton and Sherrington examined a monkey who had shown considerable motor recovery after a lesion of the left cortical arm area and found no worsening of the residual deficit when the right arm area was ablated 60 days after the first operation.

The best support for Hypothesis 1 comes from research on newborn animals and humans. Dodds (1887–1888), in an early review of localization theory, states that Soltmann ablated the whole prefrontal lobe and part of the postfrontal lobe of the left side in a 4-day-old dog. Three months later, stimulation of the paw area of the right hemisphere elicited movements of both the right and left forepaws.

In people, the finding that the right hemisphere appears to take charge of language functions after early left hemispheric damage (Chapter 8) might also be construed as evidence for the position that one side of the brain can take over the functions of the other side, especially early in life. In such cases, barbiturate injections into the arteries feeding the hemispheres have revealed a pattern of speech representation on the right side of the brain that is rarely encountered among healthy subjects. But here, and perhaps in other cases as well, there is an important theoretical dilemma, and it concerns whether significant right hemispheric mediation of speech *normally* takes place very early in life, before a period of specialization. For instance, there are data showing that right hemispheric damage may be more likely to at least temporarily arrest speech in children than in adults (see Hécaen and Albert, 1978), and this may mean that there is considerable right hemispheric involvement in this function early in life. If this interpretation is correct, the application of vicariation theory to the speech data would be questionable since vicariation usually means that the function is taken over by a structure not directly involved with it (or, as held by some authors, only minimally or indirectly involved with) prior to insult. In these cases, recovery might represent only the continued and uninhibited development of a right hemispheric function that is present at the time of left hemispheric damage, and not an instance of one hemisphere taking over a function that is new or foreign to it.

Hypothesis 2, which holds that there are areas on the same side of the brain that take over for the damaged region, probably has attracted the greatest number of adherents, in part because it can be invoked to account for bilateral as well as unilateral lesion data. Carville and Duret (1875) favored this position, and they contended that new "functional" centers are formed in the vicinity of the damaged ones.

Some support for Hypothesis 2 can also be found in the experiments of Margaret Kennard (1936, 1938) on young monkeys. As we pointed out in Chapter 8, she examined postural and locomotor abilities after lesions of Brodmann areas 4 and 6 and found that considerable motor sparing could be observed if the lesions were made early in life (or in stages). Kennard postulated that by some unidentified process, the nearby frontal association cortex and the postcentral gyrus (somatic cortex) took over the motor functions from areas 4 and 6. She used Munk's paradigm to arrive at these conclusions:

1. Lesions of the frontal association areas, or the parietal lobe, did not affect motor performance when the motor zones were left intact.
2. Motor cortex lesions were followed by considerable recovery when the damage was inflicted early in life.
3. After recovery from motor cortex damage, removal of one or both of these nonmotor cortical areas on the same side of the brain reinstated and potentiated the original deficits.

Support for Hypothesis 2 has not been consistent, especially where animals past the period of infancy have been studied. Lussana and Memoigne, contemporaries of Carville and Duret, for instance, failed to support the hypothesis in two tests of it (cf. Dodds, 1877–1878). First, after signs of paresis had disappeared, stimulation of the tissue surrounding the motor cortex wound did not produce movement. And second, removal of this neighboring gray matter did not reinstate the original paralysis.

These early negative findings were replicated by Leyton and Sherrington (1917) in an analysis of the events that follow motor cortex lesions in the monkey. These investigators studied monkeys that had the arm region of the motor cortex damaged and who showed signs of recovery. They found that additional ablations around the previous arm area did not reinstate the deficits. In addition, electrical stimulation of the elbow and shoulder areas of the motor cortex had no effect on arm movements. The possibility that the sensory cortex (postcentral gyrus) was mediating the recovery was also examined with both lesion and electrical stimulation techniques; again with no evidence of a new motor area for the arm being present.

In retrospect, it is somewhat surprising that Sherrington and others were unable to obtain motor movements when they stimulated the somatic areas (postcentral gyrus) in their subjects. Some years after Kennard formulated her vicariation hypothesis to account for motor recovery, Kennard herself presented data that showed that stimulation of the postcentral gyrus could elicit movements in animals sustaining motor cortex lesions in infancy (Kennard and McCulloch, 1943). Woolsey and his co-workers have since been able to replicate Kennard's observation with adult-operated monkeys—a significant finding that could provide a basis for the recovery witnessed after therapy (Ogden and Franz, 1917) or serial lesions (Travis and Woolsey, 1956) in mature subjects. These data and related anatomical and physiological observations are reviewed by Woolsey (1958) in a way that clearly shows that there are well organized motor pathways from the postcentral gyrus to the periphery, in spite of the fact that Sherrington's opposing viewpoint (that motor areas have no sensory functions, and vice versa) has sometimes dominated thinking in this area. The motor representation on the postcentral gyrus is shown in Figure 15.4.

The last hypothesis, that a function can be taken over by a center at another level, has received very little experimental attention relative to the other theories, although it is possible that some recovery of motor function could be due to subcortical extrapyramidal efferents that are now playing a broader role in behavior.

With Hypothesis 3, even with subcortical damage, it is almost automatically assumed that the recovery will have its basis in structure located *lower* in the system. Still, it is possible to argue from lesion data that higher centers can take over for lower ones, at least in an indirect way. This can be exemplified by a series of experiments carried out by Philip Teitelbaum and Jerzy Cytawa (1965; see also Cytawa and Teitelbaum, 1967). These investigators made lesions of the lateral hypothalamus in rats and observed adipsia and aphagia. In time, the animals went through the specific stages of recovery that were outlined previously, (see also Chapter 18) and eventually approximated normal animals in their patterns of

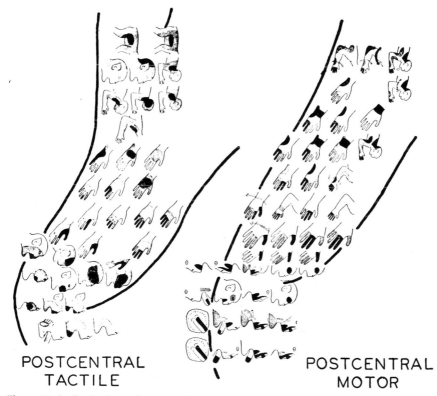

POSTCENTRAL
TACTILE

POSTCENTRAL
MOTOR

Figure 15.4. *Comparison of postcentral tactile localization pattern with the postcentral motor localization pattern of* Macaca mulatta. *(From Woolsey, 1958.)*

food intake. Once the rats had recovered, the authors applied potassium chloride to the frontal cortex to cause spreading depression, (a transient state of abnormal electrical activity). As a result of this, the lateral hypothalamic syndrome was reinstated, even though frontal cortex lesions alone did not reproduce the syndrome in other animals. These data could thus be used to argue that the frontal cortex took over the functions of the hypothalamus, much as Kennard argued that the parietal lobe took over the functions of the frontal lobe when motor function was at issue.

It is again worth remembering that these findings, like all findings using this paradigm, are subject to multiple interpretations. In the present case, one which appears to have considerable merit is that frontal and lateral hypothalamic lesions are producing a common disruption of function, which in turn contributes to the lateral hypothalamic syndrome. As Robert Dawson (1973) points out, both cortical spreading depression and lesions of the lateral hypothalamic area have been shown to affect forebrain norepinephrine concentrations. Therefore, it is conceivable that cortical spreading depression in a normal animal would fail to deplete norepinephrine to a "critical level," whereas the same manipulation in a subject already suffering sharply lower norepinephrine levels would be expected to have much more dramatic results.

The question of which part of the brain is taking over for another part that is damaged still remains unanswered. In fact, it is conceivable that which area will take over for another may be determined by more than just the site of the lesion itself. One of us (Finger and Simons, 1976; Simons, Puretz, and Finger, 1975) recently found that after recovery from somatosensory cortical lesions in rats, damage anterior and posterior to the lesion sites reinstated the deficits. As can be seen in Figure 15.5, these deficits were less severe in subjects who had originally experienced staged somatosensory cortex lesions than in animals who first had simultaneous lesions of the same areas. The additional lesions had virtually no effect on animals with the somatosensory cortex intact. These findings can be interpreted to mean that there may be different neural substrates mediating recovery after one-stage and staged lesions—a possibility that has also received some support from experiments showing that "recovered" one-stage and serial animals may respond in very different ways to pharmacological agents (e.g., Glick and Zimmerberg, 1972).[2]

[2]In this study, mice received one-stage or two-stage lesions of the frontal cortex and were tested for passive avoidance learning. Following recovery on the task, the groups were given 5mg/kg d-amphetamine. The group with serial frontal cortex lesions showed an eight-fold increase in latency to the drug. The one-stage recovered animals, however, showed mean latencies that increased from under 8 seconds to over 4 minutes. These data are suggestive of different substrates underlying the recovery. Nevertheless, an alternative explanation is that the substrates are the same and that only the time course of the recovery process is different. Glick and Zimmerberg (1972) themselves prefer the latter explanation and argue that denervation supersensitivity occurs much more rapidly in one case than in the other.

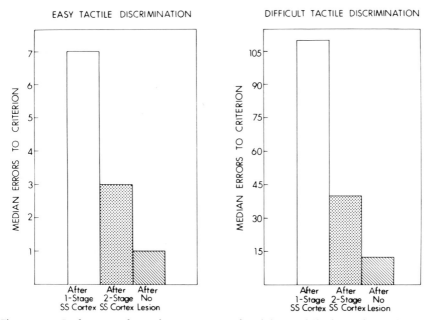

Figure 15.5. *Performance of animals on an easy (graph on left) on a difficult (graph on right) tactile discrimination following large lesions of the cortex anterior and posterior to the somatosensory areas. All animals previously had relearned the identical discrimination after either one-stage lesions of the somatosensory cortex, two-stage lesions of the somatosensory cortex, or sham operations. (Data of Finger and Simons, 1976, and Simons et al., 1975. From Finger, 1978.)*

As the theory of vicariation presently stands, it is possible to envision infinite backtracking since each time recovery is observed, in that one could always claim, after the fact, that another structure has taken over the function of the damaged region.

Had he lived to the present, this state of affairs would not have surprised Walther Riese. More than 30 years ago he realized the difficulties involved in testing the three hypotheses we have reviewed. In a manner that shows the profound influence that his remarkable predecessor, John Hughlings Jackson, had upon him, Riese (1950) wrote the following:

> Much experimental and clinical effort has been devoted to the solution of the problem to which regions of the brain substitutional and compensatory acts should be related. As mentioned above, preference has been given to the adjacent and to the symmetrical regions. The critical question involved is, whether structures not used before for the same purpose, can "take over" the endangered function. We stressed the fact that the problem of specificity of nervous structure and that of its plasticity is here involved. But most of the difficulties and controversies implied in the subject resulted from the ambitious but vain effort, to make conclusive statements as to the processes going on in the intact brain or its healthy and spared parts. Again, localiza-

tion of function (and not that of symptoms) is at the source of these difficulties [p. 112].

Whether there is really a good test of the theory of vicariation at the present time represents a good question in itself. If multiple lesions do not provide the rigorous test that is demanded by some individuals, what then can be used in its place? Although the technology is still developing, one possibility is that positron emission tomography (''pet scans'') will be of some help in this endeavor. These procedures can be used to measure brain metabolism while specific tasks such as reading and perceptual learning are being performed. In particular, when adapted to laboratory animals, these scans may allow us to see whether metabolic patterns change as a result of focal lesions and whether such changes do in fact correlate with the time course for recovery of function. However, interpreting such data may not be easy. It would still be necessary to determine whether the observed metabolic changes represent a true takeover of a new and unusual function by another brain area (i.e., vicariation), or only a change in strategy when addressing a problem. A strategy change that would allow the subject to use other brain areas exactly as they had been used in the past (e.g., a change from rote memory to visual imagery when given a mathematical problem), of course, would not be vicariation, but rather ''compensation,'' a response mode to injury that we will discuss in more detail in the next chapter.

Another issue that is only now beginning to be examined in the context of vicariation theory is how anatomical and physiological changes might relate to it. As we have seen, Ivan Pavlov and his students have described ''roundabout connections'' being present from the start, and their writings seem to imply that no special modifications are required of these connections for them to become functional pathways. Another position is that existing pathways may only become functional under special physiological conditions. One example of this type of thinking was described in the last chapter where Walter Cannon and Arturo Rosenblueth (1949) talked about ''devious neural connections'' becoming functional as a result of denervation supersensitivity.

Recently, attention has turned to sprouting, rerouted, and anomalous connections as possible substrates for vicarious functioning. The basic premise is that if intact neurons give off new terminals to fill vacated sites, and if such processes can be correlated with restitution, one can argue that the new projections have come to mediate the lost functions and that the role of the area receiving the new projections is no longer the same (see Loesche and Steward, 1977). This idea has been developed by Donald Meyer (1973), who utilized data from two reports; one by Horel, Bettinger, Royce, and Meyer (1966); and the other by Goodman and Horel (1966), to illustrate this possibility.

Like Karl Lashley (1929, 1935), James Horel and his co-workers (1966) noted that a learned black–white discrimination would be lost following large, posterior neocortical lesions in rats, but that a brain-damaged animal could relearn the problem in about as many trials as it would take a naive rat. Horel and his colleagues observed that intact naive rats performed more poorly during the early learning trials than did the brain-damaged animals. On the basis of these data, it was suggested that brightness discrimination in the rat could be mediated by at least two different structures. Donald Goodman and James Horel (1966) then showed that unilateral ablation of the occipital cortex produced sprouting from the optic tract to two subcortical visual areas ipsilateral to the lesion. From this, Donald Meyer (1973) proposed that brightness discrimination is normally mediated by the visual cortex, but that under conditions of marked anatomical reorganization, subcortical areas can take over for a damaged cortex.

The work of Patricia Goldman and Thelma Galkin that we described in Chapter 5 is also relevant to this issue. As we noted, Goldman and Galkin (1978) examined the anatomical and behavioral effects of *prenatal* damage to the dorsolateral frontal cortex. Rhesus monkey fetuses were subjected to unilateral or bilateral cortical insult at different embryonic stages, replaced in utero, and delivered at the end of their term of gestation. When examined years later, the brains of these monkeys showed several unexpected features. There were gross abnormalities of cortical fissurization even at sites distant from the lesions. Neurons in the dorsomedial thalamus were well preserved despite the fact that degeneration in this area normally is a reliable sequel to dorsolateral cortex damage. These anatomical results were more pronounced the earlier the prenatal lesions were performed. In addition, long-term behavioral testing of one monkey with a bilateral prenatal lesion revealed no impairment whatsoever on tasks usually sensitive to dorsolateral frontal cortex insult; that is, delayed deficits did not appear even when the animal was tested 2 years after surgery. These findings prompted Goldman and Galkin to offer several possible explanations to account for the behavioral results that they obtained, two of which are directly related to vicariation theory. One is that the behavioral sparing could be the result of other structures in the basal ganglia or thalamus taking over some of the functions of the damaged prefrontal cortex. The other holds that the sparing of cognitive function may have been due to young neurons in the process of migration toward the dorsal part of the frontal lobe, becoming rerouted to take up final positions in areas different from those where they were originally destined.

If sprouting and rerouted connections can be related to vicariation, as suggested by the research described earlier, the recent findings of Stephen Scheff and his co-workers might account for the observation that serial lesions usually result in faster and more complete recovery than one-stage lesions. Scheff, Bernardo, and Cotman (1977) reported that serial lesions of the entorhinal cortex resulted in more rapid (2 days) and denser collateral sprouting than that seen after one-stage damage (4–7 days). They suggested that the initial, small lesion could "prime" the relevant axons to sprout into the denervated areas. Scheff has also described

visual evoked potentials in cortex contiguous to the visual areas in serially damaged rats that had recovered the ability to master a black–white discrimination
problem (Scheff and Wright, 1977). These potentials were less prominent in rats
that failed to recover, suggesting that the new activity is a correlate of the recovery
process.

Even should anatomical changes like sprouting be found to underlie some instances where vicariation is suspected, there would be little reason to believe that
sprouting underlies all instances of vicariation. Indeed, as we have pointed out,
vicariation might also be initiated and sustained by a state of supersensitivity
(which should decrease as vacated terminals are occupied by new sprouts), or, as
in the case of some conditioned reflexes, it could conceivably occur in the absence
of these types of changes. Yet, under any of these conditions, the possibility that
vicariation might also have its deleterious effects should also be considered. That
is, if one functional area can acquire the ability to substitute for an injured one,
then the functions of the former might themselves be affected. As mentioned
earlier, Brenda Milner (1974) argued that this can, in fact, be seen when the right
hemisphere becomes dominant for speech in children who have sustained
diseases and injuries in the left hemisphere. Milner describes deficits on a variety
of tasks in these patients and suggests that some of the impairments could well be
the result of "crowding" too many functions into one part of the brain. Unfortunately, not enough experimental work has been conducted on this possibility,
so despite the fact that the hypothesis makes intuitive sense, its validity remains to
be determined.

In closing this chapter, we can say that although some *indirect* support for
vicariation theory can be found after injury in adults, more support for one brain
area taking over another's function probably can be found after lesions sustained
early in life. In a way this would bring us back to Hermann Munk, who believed
that vicariation could only occur if the substitute areas were "unoccupied" (not
functionally committed) at the time of trauma. While the role of age in vicariation still remains to be explored fully, it is interesting that Alf Brodal (1973),
more than 100 years after Munk presented his ideas, reflected on some of the same
developmental considerations when considering his own stroke. As an anatomist,
he not only deliberated about whether a "committed" structure could take on a
new function, but raised the related question: How could the brain's "great
reserve capacity" (dormant cells) escape disuse atrophy over the course of a
lifetime?

Questions and philosophical issues such as these and those raised by Walter
Riese merit considerably more attention than they have been given thus far,
especially as they bear on vicariation theory. Until they can be fully addressed and
until new experiments can be conducted with less invasive techniques, it would
seem premature to accept or reject the concept of *vicariation* outright.

References

Bethe, A., and Fischer, E. Die Anpassungs fähigkeit (Plastizität) des Nervensystems. *Handbuch der normalen und pathologischen Physiologie*, 1931, *15*, 1045–1130.

Brodal, A. Self-observation and neuro-anatomical considerations after a stroke. *Brain*, 1973, *96*, 675–694.

Cannon, W. B., and Rosenblueth, A. *The supersensitivity of denervated structures: A law of denervation*. New York: Macmillan, 1949.

Carville, C., and Duret, H. Sur le fonction des hémisphères cérébraux. *Archiv der Physiologie*, 1875, *7*, 352–490.

Cytawa, J., and Teitelbaum, P. Spreading depression and recovery of subcortical functions. *Acta Biologica Experamentalis*, 1967, *27*, 345–353.

Dawson, R. G. Recovery of function: Implications for theories of the brain function. *Behavioral Biology*, 1973, *8*, 439–460.

Dodds, W. J. On the localisation of the functions of the brain. *Journal of Anatomy and Physiology*, 1877–1878, *12*, 340–363; 454–494; 636–660.

Ferrier, D. *The functions of the brain*. London: Smith, Elder & Co., 1886.

Finger, S. Lesion momentum and behavior. In S. Finger (Ed.), *Recovery from brain damage: Research and theory*. New York: Plenum, 1978, Pp. 135–164.

Finger, S., and Simons, D. Effects of serial lesions of somatosensory cortex and further neodecortication on retention of a rough–smooth discrimination in rats. *Experimental Brain Research*, 1976, *25*, 183–197.

Foerster, O. I. Restitution der Motilität. II. Restitution der Sensibilität. *Deutsch Zeitschrif für Nerven*, 1930, *115*, 248–314.

Franck, F. *Fonctions Motrices du Cerveau*. Paris, 1887.

Franz, S. I. *Nervous and mental reeducation*. New York: Mcmillan, 1923.

Glick, S. D., and Zimmerberg, B. Comparative recovery following simultaneous and successive-stage frontal brain damage in mice. *Journal of Comparative and Physiological Psychology*, 1972, *79*, 481–487.

Goldman, P. S., and Galkin, T. W. Prenatal removal of frontal association cortex in the fetal rhesus monkey: Anatomical and functional consequences in postnatal life. *Brain Research*, 1978, *152*, 451–485.

Goodman, D. C., and Horel, J. A. Sprouting of optic tract projections in the brain stem of the rat. *Journal of Comparative Neurology*, 1966, *127*, 71–88.

Hécaen, H., and Albert, M. L. *Human neuropsychology*. New York: Wiley, 1978.

Horel, J. A., Bettinger, L. A., Royce, G. J., and Meyer, D. R. Role of neocortex in the learning and relearning of two visual habits by the rat. *Journal of Comparative and Physiological Psychology*, 1966, *61*, 66–78.

Kennard, M. A. Age and other factors in motor recovery from precentral lesions in monkeys. *American Journal of Physiology*, 1936, *115*, 138–146.

Kennard, M. A. Reorganization of motor function in the cerebral cortex of monkeys deprived of motor and premotor areas in infancy. *Journal of Neurophysiology*, 1938, *1*, 477–497.

Kennard, M. A. Cortical Reorganization of motor functions. *Archives of Neurology and Psychiatry*, 1942, *48*, 227–240.

Kennard, M. A., and McCulloch, W. S. Motor responses to stimulation of cerebral cortex in absence of areas 4 and 6 (*Macaca mulatta*). *Journal of Neurophysiology*, 1943, *6*, 181–189.

Lashley, K. S. *Brain mechanism and intelligence*. Chicago: University of Chicago Press, 1929.

Lashley, K. S. The mechanism of vision. XII. Nervous structures concerned in habits based on reactions to light. *Comparative Psychology Monographs*, 1935, *11*, 43–79.

Lashley, K. S. Factors limiting recovery after central nervous lesions. *Journal of Nervous and Mental Disease,* 1938, *88,* 733–755,.

Laurence, S., and Stein, D. G. Recovery from brain damage and the concept of localization of function. In S. Finger (Ed.), *Recovery from brain damage: Research and theory.* New York: Plenum, 1978, Pp. 369–407.

Leyton, A. S. F., and Sherrington, C. S. Observations on the excitable cortex of the chimpanzee, orangutan, and gorilla. *Quarterly Journal of Experimental Physiology,* 1917, *11,* 135–222.

Loesche, J., and Steward, O. Behavioral correlates of denervation and reinnervation of the hippocampal formation of the rat: Recovery of alternation performances following unilateral entorhinal cortex lesions. *Brain Research Bulletin,* 1977, *2,* 31–39.

Meyer, P. M. Recovery from neocortical damage. In G. M. French (Ed.), *Cortical functioning in behavior.* Glenview, Ill.: Scott Foresman, 1973, Pp. 115–129.

Milner, B. Hemispheric specialization: Scope and limits. In F. O. Schmitt and F. G. Worden (Eds.), *The neurosciences: Third study program.* Cambridge, Mass.: M.I.T. Press, 1974, Pp. 75–89.

Munk, H. Zur Physiologie der Grosshirnrinde. *Berliner Klinische Wochenschrift,* 1877, *14,* 505–506.

Ogden, R., and Franz, S. I. On cerebral motor control: The recovery from experimentally produced hemiplegia. *Psychobiology,* 1917, *1,* 33–49.

Riese, W. *Principles of neurology in the light of history and their present use.* New York: Nervous and Mental Disease Monographs, 1950.

Rosner, B. Recovery of function and localization of function in historical perspective. In D. G. Stein, J. J. Rosen, and N. Butters (Eds.), *Plasticity and recovery of function in the central nervous system.* New York: Academic Press, 1974, Pp. 1–29.

Scheff, S., Bernardo, L., and Cotman, C. Progressive brain damage accelerates axon sprouting in the adult rat. *Science,* 1977, *197,* 795–797.

Scheff, S. W., and Wright, D. C. Behavioral and electrophysiological evidence for cortical reorganization of function with serial lesions of the visual cortex. *Physiological Psychology,* 1977, *5,* 103–107.

Simons, D., Puretz, J., and Finger, S. Effects of serial lesions on somatosensory cortex and further neodecortication on tactile retention in rats. *Experimental Brain Research,* 1975, *23,* 353–366.

Spear, P. D. Behavioral and neurophysiological consequences of visual cortex damage: Mechanisms of recovery. In J. M. Sprague and A. N. Epstein (Eds.), *Progress in psychobiology and physiological psychology* (Vol. 8). New York: Academic Press, 1979, Pp. 45–83.

Teitelbaum, P., and Cytawa, J. Spreading depression and recovery from lateral hypothalamic damage. *Science,* 1965, *147,* 61–63.

Travis, A. M., and Woolsey, C. N. Motor performance of monkeys after bilateral partial and total cerebral decortications. *American Journal of Physical Medicine,* 1956, *35,* 273–280.

Woolsey, C. N. Organization of somatic sensory and motor areas of the cerebral cortex. In H. G. Harlow and C. N. Woolsey (Eds.), *Biological and biochemical bases of behavior.* Madison: University of Wisconsin Press, 1958, Pp. 63–81.

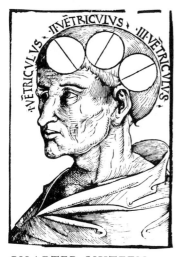

Behavioral Compensation and Response and Cue Substitution Theories

In example after example from the clinic, one can point to alternative behavioral strategies that seem to be active in covering for a neurological deficit. These clinical examples serve up fair warning that the improvement in function following neurological insult may not reflect recovery of function in a neurological sense. They may reflect the ingenious ability of the organisms to maintain a behavioral status quo by using other mental and behavioral resources [Gazzaniga, 1978, p. 413].

CHAPTER SIXTEEN

In observing people with handicaps, we are often surprised to see how effective many individuals are in their ability to overcome severe physical disabilities. For example, there are many cases of patients who, for one reason or another, are deprived of the use of their arms, but nonetheless manage to feed themselves, type, paint, and drive to work, using their feet to substitute for the loss of their hands. Whether or not the *means* are the same, these people achieve the goals that many of us aspire to, or in the case of driving or getting dressed, take completely for granted. In all of these cases, the handicapped individuals demonstrate functional compensation through the development of alternate behavioral strategies. To be sure, the alternative approaches may not be as efficient or as effective as other goal-directed behaviors used by people who have no afflictions, but a degree of independence and personal achievement is permitted.

In trying to understand how organisms with brain damage recover function, some investigators have suggested that it is more important to determine specifically *how* a goal is attained, rather than merely whether it is reached or not (Laurence and Stein, 1978). In more formal terms, the study of how a goal is reached supposes a careful analysis of response strategies; in animals, this would mean, for example, an examination of the postoperative changes in the pattern of movements used to run a maze ("a means analysis"). Contrast this approach to an "ends" analysis where the lowered IQ score, latency of response, number of errors made, number of perseverations, and so on, are used to assess the extent of a deficit. No attempt is made to determine *how* the organism attempts to cope with its altered perceptions and newly limited motor capacities.

Understanding the specific changes in response strategies after central nervous system injuries is very important for defining what we mean by "functional recovery." In the strictest sense, we could argue that there really is no true restitution of function if, by recovery, we mean a return to the identical behaviors seen prior to the injury (Dawson, 1973; LeVere, 1975). Instead, there may only be compensation: a state which may be characterized by the use of different stimulus cues, new groups of muscles, different cognitive strategies, and even various "tricks" that allow brain-damaged organisms to give the superficial impression that full recovery has occurred.

The compensation hypothesis of functional recovery has a certain simplicity to it because it would seem that no radical changes in the neural substrate are required to explain the observed behaviors; where long-term recovery is noted, you hypothesize, essentially, that the organism merely relies on the existing functions of the undamaged brain area. If the injury renders the organisms less effective by altering their biochemistry or anatomy, then the behaviors used will be more or less effective, depending upon the "impact" of the injury.

An important question to ask here is whether all subjects within a given strain or species fall back upon the same response–substitution systems. After visual cortex lesions, for example, would all rats use the olfactory system to solve a maze problem, or might some use olfaction, whereas others depend upon vestibular, tactile, proprioceptive, or even auditory (echolocation) cues? What factors predispose the organism to "select" one pattern of compensation over the other? This issue has not been addressed systematically until recently, and there is only some preliminary evidence to show that animals do *not* always use the same pattern of compensation following similar types of lesions. Recently, one of us (DGS) used a radioactive tracer (C^{14}-2-DG) to analyze recovery from bilateral lesions of the frontal cortex. Following frontal surgery, rats were trained continuously until they performed a delayed-spatial alternation task as well as intact animals. We reasoned that if the brain-damaged animals could learn the task in the absence of frontal cortex, they would do so by depending upon the integrative functions of remaining, intact brain structures. C^{14}-2-DG is taken up by neurons that are functionally active, and since it cannot be metabolized, it remains in those cells and can serve as a marker of functional activity. Armed with this technique, both brain-damaged and intact rats were injected with C^{14}-2-DG just prior to being tested for spatial alternation ability. After 45 minutes, the rats were decapitated and their brains prepared for autoradiography. In brief, the analyses of the autoradiographs revealed that the intact rats showed a remarkably consistent pattern of 2-DG uptake, most of which could be seen in dorsomedial nuclei of the thalamus, superior colliculus, caudate nucleus, and medial frontal cortex. The brain-damaged rats showed similar patterns, but there was also much unexpected variability. For example, some brain-damaged rats showed uptake in the geniculate region, while others had more in the reticular region of the brain stem. Such variability in uptake of 2-DG can be attributed to many factors such as differences in vascularity, patterns of neural degeneration, lesion size, stress, and so on. But the main point is that the brain-damaged rats *did* show subtle differences in cerebral uptake of 2-DG which indicates that the response of the brain to injury varies from one subject to another, despite identical performance in the maze. These preliminary data can be interpreted to suggest that the compensatory processes underlying recovery may be different from subject to subject.

The explanatory value of functional substitution theory can best be seen with rats that have to learn mazes with cul-de-sacs in them, such as those used by Karl Lashley (1929) and his contemporaries (see Figure 16.1). Quite some time ago, C. H. Honzik (1936), of the University of California, conducted a series of experiments to determine which of the sensory systems animals use most during maze learning. He came to the conclusion that vision is by far the most important sense, since maze learning is rapid as long as the visual system is intact. When vision is impaired by peripheral blinding or by ablations of the posterior cortex, rats

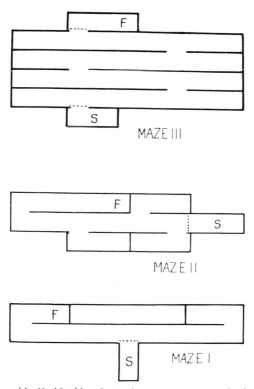

Figure 16.1. *Mazes used by Karl Lashley. S, starting compartment; F, food compartment. Broken lines represent trap doors, which prevent return to the starting box. (Reprinted from* Brain Mechanisms and Intelligence *by K. E. Lashley by permission of the University of Chicago Press © 1929.)*

still manage to learn the mazes, although at a much slower rate. Through various manipulations, Honzik found that the animals who could no longer rely on visual information were now turning predominantly to olfactory cues (odor trails) in navigating the mazes. The simple switching from the dominant sensory system to a "back-up" system, in his opinion, accounted for the apparent recovery (see also Hunter, 1930), that is, the ability to attain the goal. Honzik noted that tactile sensibility can also be important especially with walled mazes where the vibrissae (facial whiskers) can be used. Auditory and kinesthetic cues also have the potential to be called into play to guide maze learning and retention; however, they are not the first choice of the animals. In short, the rats have a hierarchy of cues that they will use, and will fall back on less desirable strategies as their preferred ones are eliminated.

Without recourse to vicariation theory, where structures are thought to assume new and unusual functions, Honzik's work is able to provide a satisfactory explanation for why small cortical lesions have, at most, transient effects on maze learning. Moreover, Karl Lashley's observation (1929, pp. 43–45) that the posterior cortex may be more important for maze learning than the anterior cortex would be expected on the basis of the findings presented by Honzik. This is because the posterior cortical lesions require the subject to switch from the preferred and presumably most efficient system (vision), to one lower on its hierarchy, which may be neither as preferred nor as efficient. In contrast, anterior cortical lesions would leave the dominant, visual system intact. Finally, since large cortical lesions alter the projections of more sensory systems than small cortical lesions, these data may in part explain why Lashley (1929) found a high positive correlation between lesion size and error scores on his mazes. This is shown in Figure 16.2.

The ability of animals to use remaining sensory systems to guide maze learning after localized cortical lesions represents a simple and intuitively obvious way in which response substitution could be effective in obtaining a goal. The changing from a reliance on one sensory system to another, or from one set of efferent fibers to another, can also occur in situations in which it is totally unexpected, the result being that investigators can be completely fooled and misled by the "recovery" that they at first think they are witnessing.

A good example of the use of "tricks" to achieve reinforcement is seen in an experiment that was conducted by Michael Goldberger (1972) on monkeys with lesions of Brodmann area 6 ("supplementary motor area"). After surgery, the monkeys displayed a pathological reflex of forced grasping to light tactile stimulation and an inability to release the grasped object. Goldberger tried to teach his animals to hold and then release a stick to obtain food reward, but he noted that the pathological grasp could not be overcome in the period immediately following surgery. This can be seen in Figure 16.3. A few weeks later the animals showed a definite improvement, which suggested that true recovery

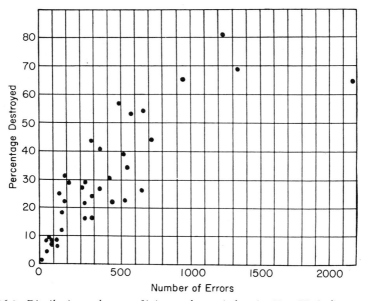

Figure 16.2. *Distribution and extent of injury and errors in learning Maze III. Ordinate represents percentage of neopallium destroyed; abscissa, number of errors made during testing. (Reprinted from* Brain Mechanisms and Intelligence *by K. E. Lashley by permission of the University of Chicago Press © 1929.)*

had taken place. After a number of additional tests and observations, Goldberger rejected the possibility of functional restitution in favor of the hypothesis that the functions lost after area 6 lesions remained lost and that the "restitution" observed was due to different mechanisms. For the monkeys, the process of recovery was identified as being the increased utilization of an opposing, intact reflex called the "tactile evasion" reflex.[1]

Goldberger sees a certain similarity between his work on compensatory acts following lesions of the central nervous system and Roger Sperry's earlier work on "tricks," which give the impression of recovery after lesions of the peripheral nervous system (see Sperry, 1945, 1947). In particular, Goldberger notes that Sperry had observed that seemingly identical movements could be accomplished in different ways by monkeys with surgically "crossed" nerves to antagonistic muscle groups. On closer observation, Sperry was forced to conclude that the monkeys had actually learned to use different and unusual sequences of muscle contractions during the recovery phase.

Roger Sperry recently won the Nobel prize for his work on the split-brain

---

[1] According to Goldberger, tactile evasion responses are normally mediated by the pyramidal system. When evasion is prevented by severing the pyramidal fibers, the pathological grasp reflex reappears (is "unmasked") and there no longer is any recovery.

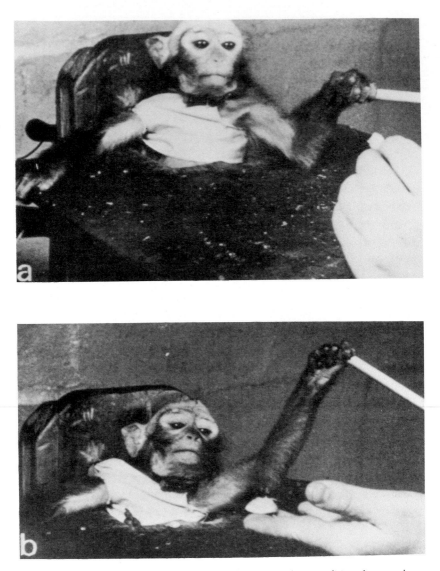

Figure 16.3. *Monkey with bilateral area 6 ablation (9 days) trained in a conditioned grasp-release sequence for food. In (a), the monkey has grasped the stick, but is unable, because of forced grasping, to release it to obtain the food that she is obviously looking at with concentration. The examiner is pulling on the stick making it impossible for the animal to let go, and the tension in the flexor muscles of the animal's left arm can be seen. In (b), the monkey's fifth finger is grasping the stick, pulling opposite to the direction in which the examiner is pulling. This is enough to elicit forced grasping and to recruit the flexors of the digits. (From Goldberger, 1974.)*

preparation—an operation in which the major pathways (corpus callosum, optic chiasm, anterior and hippocampal commissures) connecting the two hemispheres are sectioned (see Sperry, 1952, 1964). This experimental model also provides an excellent example of how a behavioral "trick" can be used to suggest recovery—a trick that has been uncovered only after careful observation and special tests.

After the cerebral hemispheres and optic chiasm are surgically "split," an occluder is placed over one eye (or a special projection device can be used) to restrict vision to only one hemisphere; that which is on the same side as the good eye. Since the major pathway (corticospinal tract) for arm movement crosses in the pyramids, well below the level of the transections, the opposite arm can still exhibit coordinated movements to visual stimuli. For example, the split-brain monkey can still reach for a grape using one eye and the opposite hand. Similarly, because the major somatic pathway (medial lemniscus), crosses deep in the brain stem and escapes the transection, the same hand has no difficulty feeling that which is seen by the contralateral hemisphere.

Michael Gazzaniga, who studied these animals in Sperry's laboratory at the California Institute of Technology, asked an interesting question: Could the monkeys use the hand on the same side as the useful eye to perform coordinated eye–hand actions? That is, could they use their small ipsilateral motor and somatic pathways to retrieve a grape that was shown to them?

Gazzaniga (1964) found that although early deficits were typically noted with the ipsilateral arm in split-brain monkeys with vision restricted to one hemisphere, good eye–hand control often occurred with time and practice (see also Downer, 1959; Myers, McCurdy, and Sperry, 1962; Trevarthen, 1961). Gazzaniga (1964) reasoned that if this were due to direct ipsilateral fibers to and from the "seeing" hemisphere, lesions of the frontal lobe (motor cortex) and part of the parietal lobe (somatic cortex) on the same side of the brain to which the eye projected should affect these behaviors severely. To his surprise, when such lesions were made, the animals *still* learned the visual discriminations and the maneuvers required of their ipsilateral hand, and they did so in about the same amount of time as animals without ablations!

Slow motion pictures were made of the animals and the film analyses showed that the successful behavior was not due to direct projections from the "seeing" hemisphere to the hand on the same side of the body. Instead, it appeared that the opposite, intact hemisphere of the brain was involved; the hemisphere that received *no* information from the useful eye. Gazzaniga (1966) stated:

> Before the animals reached out for the food, they oriented toward the object to be retrieved, starting with eye, head and neck movements. Following this the responding arm rapidly shot out for the object to be retrieved. It was as if the response of the arm was in itself in no way checked or guided by any visual process. It appeared that

the blind hemisphere picked up the information as to where the object was in space via peripheral feedback mechanism available to it following neck and head orientation produced by the visual half-brain. Subsequently, the blind hemisphere, presumably with no further assistance from the other half-brain, followed through with the manual response [p. 294].

Subsequent data presented by Gazzaniga in the same paper confirmed that the integrity of the *contralateral* sensory and motor cortices was needed for these guided movements. He also showed that the "seeing" hemisphere really had very little control over its ipsilateral arm. Through bilaterally innervated somatic structures like the neck muscles, the split-brain monkeys had learned to "cross-cue" the hemisphere that could not see, but which could control the fine arm movements needed to retrieve the grapes in the testing situation. That is, the initial impression that ipsilateral sensory and motor fibers could play an important functional role in these behaviors proved to be illusory. These afferents and efferents never had this ability, and they did not acquire it after split-brain surgery, as may have been thought when the animals were first observed. Instead, the monkeys had learned an extremely subtle behavioral "trick," which only gave the impression that they could do something that was impossible, or at least extremely difficult for them to do, under these experimental conditions.

It would be a mistake to think that these compensatory actions are confined to animals in laboratory studies, and that they do not relate to human beings with brain disease and injury. Geschwind (1974), for instance, recently described a number of cases that were at first very perplexing in terms of the degree of recovery exhibited, but which later were found to be due to similar "tricks" that allowed these subjects to perform well on certain tasks in spite of the losses imposed upon them by brain injuries. One of his examples involved a patient with corpus callosum damage who evolved a maneuver for responding with the left hand to a verbal command that was only understood by the left hemisphere. This patient's strategy closely resembled that displayed by the split-brain monkeys in the study just described.

Consider a patient with a callosal lesion who apparently carried out verbal commands correctly with both the right and left hands. . . . The patient would first carry out the command with his right hand and would only then carry out the movement with the left arm. . . . The patient, or rather the left hemisphere of the patient, had learned that by signalling nonverbally it could get the right hand to imitate the movement. Clearly, no language comprehension by the right hemisphere was necessary for this performance, but one could be easily fooled [p. 501].

Many other cases of response substitution and roundabout solutions can be found in the human clinical literature. In fact, so pervasive is this phenomenon that Kurt Goldstein (1875–1965), the noted German-born neurologist, included it as a basic principle of organismic functioning in his best known treatise, *The*

Organism: A Holistic Approach to Biology Derived from Pathological Data in Man (English Edition, 1939). In his monograph, Goldstein argued that brain-damaged patients tend to avoid catastrophic and dangerous situations and try to maintain conditions with which they can cope by special techniques, such as rigidly ordering their environments. If dangerous situations cannot be avoided, the patients will rely on substitute performances as a last resort to avoid catastrophe. These substitute performances are meaningful and adaptive acts to Goldstein since they enable the patients to come to terms with their environments. To Goldstein, a true recovery of function will occur only as a result of restoring the anatomical substratum, or, under exceedingly limited and rare conditions, by a tedious relearning process which requires the help of the substratum which participated in the original function. He conceived of recovery as a readjustment process, by which patients learn to utilize best their remaining functions and to get along without the functions that have been lost. As stated by Goldstein (1939), ''If lost performances return, this is either possible through restitution of the damage, or through the restitution of performances which are similar only in their effect [p. 475].''

Models based on cue and strategy selection can be applied in a number of ways to instances of good perceptual learning after serial lesions (see Finger, 1978b). For example, if the first of a series of subtotal lesions can be assumed to effect a partial loss of an important capacity, brain-injured subjects may now explore the environment and learn to attend to other relevant cues that might differ from those originally sampled. After additional damage, they may still be able to solve the problem, but this time by relying on new cues, whereas other subjects with one-stage composite lesions may never have learned that these other (sometimes very subtle) cues are available in the testing situation.

In addition, the model may apply to situations in which the same cues can be examined with different receptors than those used previously. In this example, a rat may quickly learn to distinguish among different tactile stimuli by using its vibrissae after the first of a series of lesions of the cortical forepaw projection regions. Such a capacity to shift to different receptors may take considerably longer when the forepaw areas are damaged all at once since the bilateral ablation would not permit a simultaneous comparison of forepaw and vibrissae information, which may be helpful in defining the utility of the vibrissae.

Exposure to highly complex environments may also facilitate behavioral compensation. Here it can be contended that experiencing complex environments may allow a subject to learn many different strategies and hypotheses for dealing with some types of problems. In particular, maze learning represents a task that can be approached in many ways (visually, tactually, proprioceptively), and it seems possible that animals raised in ''enriched'' environments may come into the maze-learning situation with experiences that the ''deprived'' animals may not have. Although these strategy hierarchies and learning sets may be useful and associated with relatively good postoperative performance, it may take time and/or trials to make a successful shift from a preferred strategy and group of receptors to less preferred and possibly less efficient ones after a brain lesion. This might be why enriched animals (with lesions) may still take longer to learn or relearn a maze than control animals without lesions who can still rely on their original, most effective strategies (see Finger, 1978a).

In addition to providing explanations for better recovery after serial lesions than after one-stage lesions, and after environmental enrichment than after rearing in more restricted environments, response and stimulus substitution theories also seem applicable to overtraining and to certain age-related recovery effects (see Finger, Simons, and Posner, 1978). With regard to age-related recovery, it is possible that subjects with brain damage created in infancy may use spared fragments of a damaged system more readily than adult-injured organisms because they do not have to overcome previous learning sets and fixed ways of responding with particular receptors after injury. That is, subjects given surgery as adults may associate certain receptors with established functions, not realizing that they can be used in other ways as well (e.g., they may be less likely to use their faces to feel textures after limb projections are damaged). We might speculate that as a result of more education or a wider range of life experiences, some people may even deteriorate less with age because they may be able to switch from one operational system to another as nerve cells are lost and as brain diseases (e.g., arteriosclerosis) progress to affect preferred structures.

Whether compensatory actions are the sole explanation for recovery after the initial period during which the effects of neural shock may subside is debatable. In fact, different subjects may rely on different substrata and different mechanisms for recovery even after lesions that, for all intents and purposes, appear to be the same. This last point is made especially clear in the studies in which "recovered" animals with one-stage lesions or serial lesions are given drugs or additional lesions. Sometimes the responses to the additional lesions or drugs are different in the two groups (see Chapters 9 and 15). This may also be noted when nonconventional procedures are used to examine the "recovered" animals in the absence of additional lesions or drugs. In one recent experiment, for instance, Gentile, Green, Nieburgs, Schmeltzer, and Stein (1978) subjected rats to single-stage or two-stage lesions of the motor-parietal cortex and examined their ability to negotiate a narrow elevated runway. Both groups eventually appeared to recover this capacity, and a conventional analysis would have left it at that. When the animals' ballistic and temporal movements on the runway were analyzed frame-by-frame with a high-speed camera, it was found that the rats suffering one-stage lesions, who were at first less impaired on this task than their two-stage counterparts, had learned to navigate the runway with postoperative response patterns that were *significantly different* from those used in the preoperative condition. This would be an example of response substitution accounting for the apparent recovery. In contrast, as can be seen in Figure 16.4, after a period of initial impairment, some of the rats with comparable serial lesions returned to a movement pattern which very closely resembled that displayed by the sham-operated animals.

Because behavioral compensation theories are applicable to a wide range of events and circumstances, they have a broad appeal, which is not diminished by the fact that they do not require that "new and unusual events" take place in the mature mammalian central nervous system. Of course, in some circumstances, sprouting may play a role in behavioral substitution (see Goldberger, 1977). Indeed, collateral and anomalous projections can be incorporated into substitutional models in the sense that these projections can be maladaptive, thus forcing the organism to abandon one system in favor of another, or beneficial in that they may facilitate the use of an alternate, existing pathway or system. Whether or not sprouting is incorporated into the model, the key point is simply that the subject learns to use whatever remaining capacity it has to obtain a particular goal after a lesion. When put in this light, the effectiveness of the compensatory response would only depend upon the integrity of the remaining systems, the past experience and learning history of the organism, and perhaps some secondary factors such as motivation to resume a normal life. In this sense, the view outlined here is compatible with much of the thinking of John Hughlings Jackson, who proposed that the nervous system was characterized by hierarchical organization. Jackson's idea was that a general function may be represented more than once in the nervous system, but that at higher levels it is more finely tuned. A center at a lower level may be released from inhibition when a structure at a higher level is damaged. Following a lesion at a high level in the system, the lower level structure would then mediate performance as best it can.

As we stated in the beginning of this chapter, despite their appeal, behavioral compensation theories are not immune to criticism. One glaring problem is that a brain lesion may lead to a change in behavior not because something is lost, but only because of a change in cue or response *preference* on the behalf of the subject. The problem here is that if a subject switches from using tactile cues in the maze to using some other type of cue, it cannot be stated with any certainty that the action is taken to compensate for a system that is disrupted and no longer as effective as it had been. The idea that a change in strategy or a shift in problem-solving behavior may only reflect a change in response preference, rather than a loss of the neuronal substrate that was previously used to mediate performance, has been discussed by one of us on a number of occasions (e.g., Finger, 1978b), but is still rarely considered when substitutional models are applied to data. In particular, when a new solution is less effective than an old one, we may be too willing to concede that the lesion has resulted in a loss of function. However, with a slight change in the testing procedure, we may be surprised to find that the subject can still solve the problem in the original way. This is significant because it

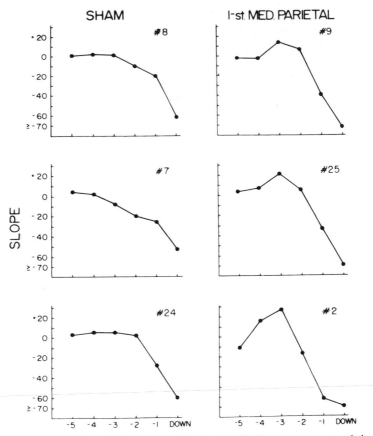

Figure 16.4. *Slope analysis of cinematographic data for hindlimb movements of three sham-operated, three one-stage, and six two-stage medial parietal animals. Data points represent the slope between X, Y coordinates of two successive frames during the terminal phase of the movement, ending with replacement of the paw on the runway (zero on the ordinate scale of each graph). (From Gentile et al., 1978.)*

shows that altered strategies and different behaviors do not *necessarily* signify a loss of original function, as might initially be thought.

If recovery is defined in terms of "goals" rather than "means," the question of deficits versus preferences may not seem terribly important. But this issue must be considered more seriously by those who are interested in how the subject attains the goal and in the implications of such data for recovery of function and how therapy might be applied.

A related issue which deserves some consideration revolves around the fact that substitutional theories can never be "disproved." This is because whenever postoperative behaviors resemble preoperative behaviors, it can be claimed that

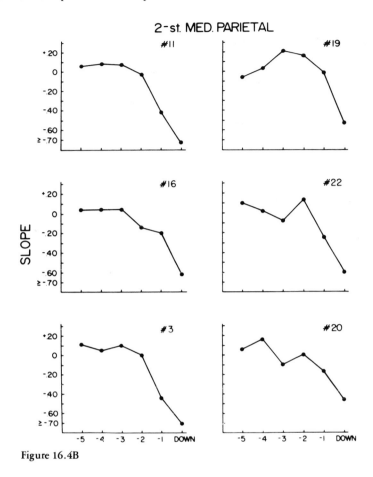

Figure 16.4B

the tests used to evaluate posttraumatic performance are simply insensitive to the nature of the residual impairments. Even when the most careful measurements are made of the receptors being used or the efferents or muscle groups employed to make a response, someone can always argue, a posteriori, that the lesion may have changed the cognitive strategy that is being used, or some ideational process.

We might turn to the field of mathematical problem solving to illustrate this point. Before brain damage, a problem such as 3 × 2 might be solved by rote memory by a person with a few years of education. Although rote memory may fail the patient immediately after the damage, it may again return with the passage of time. If we take the theoretical position that the memory area of the brain for mathematical problem solving was completely destroyed by the lesion, the possibility for recovery might not be taken seriously. Instead, it could be argued that the subject is using some compensatory technique to mask the loss, such as relying on a visual image of columns and rows of numbers to solve these simple multiplication problems. If this could be tested and if it is found not to be the case, another, and still another change in processing could be postulated, rather than accepting the possibility that recovery could indeed have taken place.

Since behavioral change is no guarantee that a function has been lost and since the apparent remission of symptoms cannot be regarded as a proof of true recovery, we find ourselves in a position whereby we cannot help but question the tenets of a recovery model such as this one. At the heart of the dilemma is again the issue of whether we know the functions of the brain and are able to localize them accurately into neat compartments. If one is willing to argue from convergent operations (e.g., combined anatomical, physiological, neurological, and behavioral data) that we know much about the functions of different brain areas, many of the questions that we have raised can be addressed with some satisfaction. If not, deliberations about whether we are witnessing vicariation or compensation can at times seem more and more like theoretical blind alleys.

Although philosophical biases may differ with respect to how much we do or do not know about the organization of the brain, or how testable certain models of recovery may be, we must emphasize that it is also possible to look at the data reported throughout this book in a strictly practical way. In the next chapter we will discuss how the findings of many of the experiments reported here can be used to help brain-damaged people, regardless of one's theoretical bias. In Chapter 18 we will return to the issue of the contribution of brain lesion research to the neural sciences and medicine, where we will reexamine in greater detail some of the questions that brain lesion experiments can and cannot answer directly.

References

Dawson, R. G. Recovery of function: Implications for theories of brain function. *Behavioral Biology,* 1973, *8,* 439–460.

Downer, J. L. de C. Changes in visually guided behavior following midsagittal division of optic chiasm and corpus callosum in monkeys (*Macaca mulatta*). *Brain,* 1959, *82,* 251–259.

Finger, S. Environmental attenuation of brain-lesion symptoms. In S. Finger (Ed.), *Recovery from brain damage: Research and theory.* New York: Plenum, 1978, Pp. 297–329.(a)

Finger, S. Lesion momentum and behavior. In S. Finger (Ed.), *Recovery from brain damage: Research and theory.* New York: Plenum, 1978, Pp. 135–164. (b)

Finger, S., Simons, D., and Posner, R. Anatomical, physiological and behavioral effects of neonatal sensorimotor cortex ablation in the rat. *Experimental Neurology,* 1978, *60,* 347–373.

Gazzaniga, M. S. Cerebral mechanisms involved in ipsilateral eye-hand use in split-brain monkeys. *Experimental Neurology,* 1964, *10,* 148–155.

Gazzaniga, M. S. Visuomotor integration in split-brain monkeys with other cerebral lesions. *Experimental Neurology,* 1966, *16,* 289–298.

Gazzaniga, M. S. Is seeing believing?: Notes on clinical recovery. In S. Finger (Ed.), *Recovery from brain damage: Research and theory.* New York: Plenum 1978, Pp. 409–414.

Gentile, A. M., Green, S., Nieburgs, A., Schmeltzer, W., and Stein, D. G. Disruption and recovery of locomotor and manipulative behavior following cortical lesions in rats. *Behavioral Biology*, 1978, *22*, 417–455.

Geschwind, N. Late changes in the nervous system: An overview. In D. G. Stein, J. J. Rosen, and N. Butters (Eds.), *Plasticity and recovery of function in the central nervous system*. New York: Academic Press, 1974, Pp. 467–508.

Goldberger, M. E. Restitution of function in the CNS: The pathological grasp in *Macaca mulatta*. *Experimental Brain Research*, 1972, *15*, 79–96.

Goldberger, M. E. Recovery of movement after CNS lesions in monkeys. In D. G. Stein, J. J. Rosen, and N. Butters (Eds.), *Plasticity and recovery of function in the central nervous system*. New York: Academic Press, 1974, Pp. 265–337.

Goldberger, M. E. Locomotor recovery after unilateral hindlimb deafferentation in cats. *Brain Research*, 1977, *123*, 59–74.

Goldstein, K. *The organism: A holistic approach to biology derived from pathological data in man*. New York: American Book Company, 1939.

Honzik, C. H. The sensory basis of maze learning in rats. *Comparative Psychology Monographs*, 1936, *13*(64), 1–113.

Hunter, W. S. A consideration of Lashley's theory of equipotentiality of cerebral action. *Journal of General Psychology*, 1930, *31*, 455–468.

Lashley, K. E. *Brain mechanisms and intelligence*. Chicago: University of Chicago Press, 1929.

Laurence, S., and Stein, D. G. Recovery after brain damage and the concept of localization of function. In S. Finger (Eds.), *Recovery from brain damage: Research and theory*. New York: Plenum, 1978, Pp. 369–407.

LeVere, T. E. Neural stability, sparing, and behavioral recovery following brain damage. *Psychological Review*, 1975, *82*, 344–358.

Myers, R. E., McCurdy, N., and Sperry, R. W. Neural mechanisms in visual guidance of limb movements. *Archives of Neurology*, 1962, *7*, 195–202.

Sperry, R. W. The problem of central nervous reorganization after nerve regeneration and muscle transposition. *The Quarterly Review of Biology*, 1945, *20*, 311–369.

Sperry, R. W. Effect of crossing nerves to antagonistic limb muscles in the monkey. *Archives of Neurology and Psychiatry*, 1947, *58*, 452–473.

Sperry, R. W. Neurology and the mind-brain problem. *American Scientist*, 1952, *40*, 291–312.

Sperry, R. W. The great cerebral commissure. *Scientific American*, 1964, *210*, 42–52.

Trevarthen, C. D. *Studies on visual learning in split-brain monkeys*. Unpublished doctoral dissertation, California Institute of Technology, Pasadena, 1961.

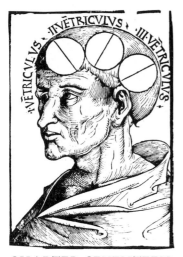

Recovery and the Human Patient

Many a patient has been discouraged by the words of his physician at the very beginning of his disability. A physician may tell a man who has been paralyzed because of a cerebral hemorrhage that he will never walk again. The statement that the paralyzed leg never can regain its functions remains stamped in the patient's mind; he comes to regard his condition as hopeless, and he makes no plans for a future in which he shall be able to walk again [Shepherd Ivory Franz, 1923, p. 35].

CHAPTER SEVENTEEN

Most of our discussions about neuroplasticity have focused on experimental models that have used animals as subjects. With respect to anatomy and in terms of physiological alterations in response to brain damage, this can hardly be avoided. Events such as central synaptogenesis, rerouted projections, and failure of synaptic boutons or dendrites to retract following early brain injury have only recently been discovered and required the kind of detailed and controlled experimentation that so far has only been possible and verifiable in the animal laboratory.

While clinical case studies are not as rigorously controlled as animal experiments, such investigations, although they represent only a small fraction of the work, do show quite clearly that the factors that enhance or retard recovery in rats, cats, and monkeys can play the same role in man.

To take one example, we have seen in previous chapters that age at the time of injury is a critical factor in determining the outcome of brain damage. Even after massive lesions, there is a very good chance of extensive or even complete recovery of certain functions if the injury occurs early in life. The transitory nature of language deficits in children who have suffered prenatal brain damage was first noted by Bernhardt (1885), whereas Freud (1897) was one of the first to observe that *temporary* language difficulties in brain-damaged children could occur after injury to either the left or right hemisphere.

According to Eric Lenneberg (1967), recovery after prenatal lesions is rapid and complete if the damage occurs prior to 2 years of age. If aphasia develops before children are 10 years old, recovery also occurs, but it is more gradual and less dramatic. Between 11 and 14 years, the symptoms are more like those of adults, and whereas some recovery of function is usually seen, it typically is incomplete.

A dramatic case of the extent to which recovery of language as well as other cognitive skills may be possible following early brain damage can be found in a report by Aaron Smith and Oscar Sugar (1975). They followed the progress of a 26-year-old man who had a total left hemispherectomy performed when he was 5 ½-years-old. When he was tested on a comprehensive battery of neuropsychological tests 15 ½ years after surgery, the patient was able to perform normally on all of the measures. This individual worked as an industrial executive and completed a college degree in business administration and sociology. Remarkably, his superior performance, especially in language skills, occurred in the absence of all of the areas thought to be critical for the mediation of language. As Smith and Sugar (1975) stated, ''The initial and long-term studies following excision of the diseased left hemisphere clearly indicate that the loss of the 'classical language zones' in the left hemispere early in life does not preclude the development of superior adult language and verbal reasoning skills [p. 816].'' [1]

Although anecdotal reports have to be considered with a great degree of care, there is now enough literature to suggest that recovery from brain injury in humans is more pervasive than previously thought. Cases where individuals describe their own progress following brain injury or disease are especially enlightening in this regard and often make fascinating reading, especially for those who have not worked with brain-damaged people or imagined how these patients feel after such debilitating, and often life-threatening events as strokes and gunshot wounds of the head (Luria, 1972).

One of the most interesting early case reports was provided by Samuel Johnson, the gifted literary scholar and man of letters (see Critchley, 1962). In June of 1783, Johnson was 73 years old, overweight, and in generally poor health. That night he awoke and realized that he had experienced a stroke. He immediately tried to compose a prayer in Latin to satisfy himself that his mental powers were still intact, and whereas he was moderately successful in doing this, he noted that his voice was gone when he endeavored to speak out loud. His speech was still nonfunctional the next day when he handed his bewildered servant a note to fetch his physician.

On the third day of his affliction, Johnson wrote the following message to Mrs. Thrale in Bath:

> On Monday, the 16, I sat for my picture, and walked a considerable way with little inconvenience. In the afternoon and evening, I felt myself light and easy, and began to plan schemes of life. Thus I went to bed, and in a short time waked and sat up as has long been my custom, when I felt a confusion and indistinctness in my head

[1] Despite the excellent performance of this patient, critics, of course, could always argue that had both hemispheres remained intact, he would have been a remarkable genius. That is, that the lesion rendered him ''merely'' normal. With anecdotal material such as this, it is not possible to accept or reject such arguments as definitive statements of fact. As with other interpretations, however, they must be recognized.

which lasted, I suppose, about half a minute; I was alarmed and prayed God, that however he might afflict my body he would spare my understanding. This prayer, that I might try the integrity of my faculties I made in Latin verse. The lines were not very good, but I know them not to be very good. I made them easily, and concluded myself to be unimpaired in my faculties.

Soon after I perceived that I had suffered a paralytick stroke, and that my Speech was taken from me. I had no pain, and so little dejection in this dreadful state that I wondered at my own apathy, and considered that perhaps death itself when it should come, would excite less horrour than seems now to attend it.

By the fourth day of his illness, Johnson's speech began to return. He described his condition as one in which he tired and faltered easily. During the third week, the impediment continued to subside as evidenced by a letter that he wrote on July 3, 1783, to James Boswell, his noted biographer, who was living in Edinborough:

Dear Sir, Your anxiety about my health is very friendly and very agreeable with your general kindness. I have, indeed, had a very frightful blow. On the 17th of last month, about three in the morning, as near as I can guess, I perceived myself almost totally deprived of speech. I had no pain. My organs were so obstructed, that I could say "no," but scarcely say "yes." I wrote the necessary directions, for it pleased God to spare my hand, and sent for Dr. Heberden and Dr. Brocklesby. Between the time in which I sent for the doctors, I had I believe, in spite of my surprise and solitude, a little sleep, and nature began to renew its operations. They came, and gave the directions which the disease required, and from that time I have been continually improving in articulation. I can now speak, but the nerves are weak, and I cannot continue discourse long; but strength, I hope will return. The Physicians consider me as cured.

By November of the same year, Johnson seemed to have overcome his fatigability:

What a man am I: who have got the better of three diseases, the palsy, the gout and the asthma, and can now enjoy the conversation of my friends, without the interruptions of weakness or pain.

Johnson lived for 18 months after his stroke, but remained a sick man suffering from a variety of ailments, including gout and emphysema. His literary output did not cease during these months, and he continued to spend many evenings translating Greek epigrams into Latin. He also wrote dedications for other literary pieces, translated Horace's ode, *Diffugere nives, redeunt, jam gramina campis* into English, and started, but failed to complete a preface for the collected works of John Scott. Samual Johnson died on December 13, 1784, from cardiorenal failure.

Johnson's aphasia, which proved to be both mild and brief, certainly cannot be considered representative of all cases. In fact, some neurologists have speculated that his lesion was either very small or that he had experienced a passing clot rather than a hemorrhage. Critchley (1962) even raises the idea that he may have had speech somewhat equally represented in the two hemispheres, so that one was able to perform at a high level after the other was damaged. These explanations are speculative, but they are important because they show how resistant we sometimes are to the idea that near total recovery can follow severe initial deficits resulting from brain damage.

Although Johnson's description of his own stroke was written almost 200 years ago, we see how perceptive he was of his own condition. In this context, another excellent self-description, written by Alf Brodal, a widely read and highly respected professor of anatomy at the University of Oslo, merits attention. Brodal, who spent his entire life studying the organization of the mammalian central nervous system, experienced a stroke in 1972, when he was 62 years old. Although he did not lose consciousness, he experienced unusual sensations (parathesiae) on the left side of the head, was dizzy, had double vision, a paralysis of the left arm and leg, and dysarthria (slowed, stammering, and slurred speech).

Brodal states that his left side paralysis was almost complete on the first day, but that it gradually improved so that on the fifth day he was able to flex both his fingers and elbow although extension of the fingers was still impossible. He still could not demonstrate dorsiflexion of the left foot or the toes. In addition, knee and hip flexion were weak in contrast to extension of these parts, which was fairly good.

Brodal surmised that he had suffered an occlusion of the right middle cerebral artery and that his left hemisphere had escaped direct damage. He went on to state that his recovery progressed fairly rapidly and was quite extensive. Two months after the stroke, he was able to handle a fork when eating and could button and unbutton his clothes. After 6 months, he could again walk fairly well and was able to use his left arm and hand for most things, although performance was not perfect. He also reported a gradual improvement in dysarthria and in dizziness and mental capacity.

In his manuscript, Brodal (1973) describes the course of recovery for specific functions such as reading, writing, and remembering series of figures (see Figure 17.1). He also suggests some explanations for why marked improvements were found on some tasks and not on others. As he himself noted, "It is often amazing to see to what degree restitution may take place [p. 689]."

In looking at these reports and considering all of the data discussed in this book, what conclusions can we now draw that would have relevance for brain-damaged patients and those who must attend to and care for these individuals? Are there means of treating such patients that may be more advantageous than those typically used? Are there other things that can be done that might be beneficial? Are we following "rules" that may no longer be sound? And where might we expect major advances in the near future?

The first and perhaps most important point we can make is to emphasize that

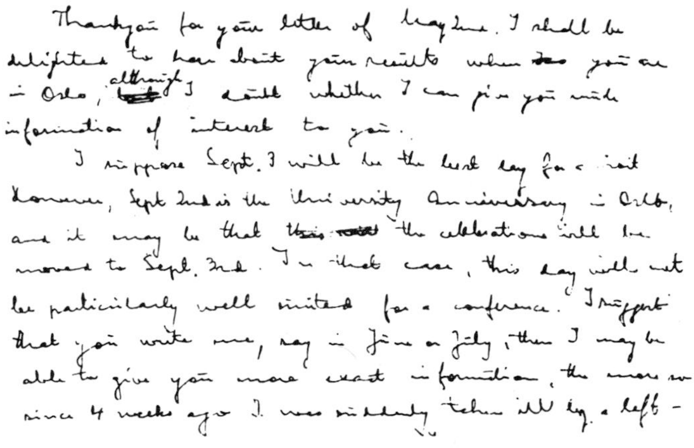
Thankyou for your letter of May 2nd. I shall be delighted to hear about your results when you are in Oslo, although I doubt whether I can give you much information of interest to you.
I suppose Sept. 3 will be the best day for a visit. However, Sept 2nd is the University Anniversary in Oslo, and it may be that the celebrations will be moved to Sept. 3rd. In that case, this day will not be particularly well suited for a conference. I suggest that you write me, say in June or July, then I may be able to give you more exact information, the more so since 4 weeks ago I was suddenly taken ill by a left-

A

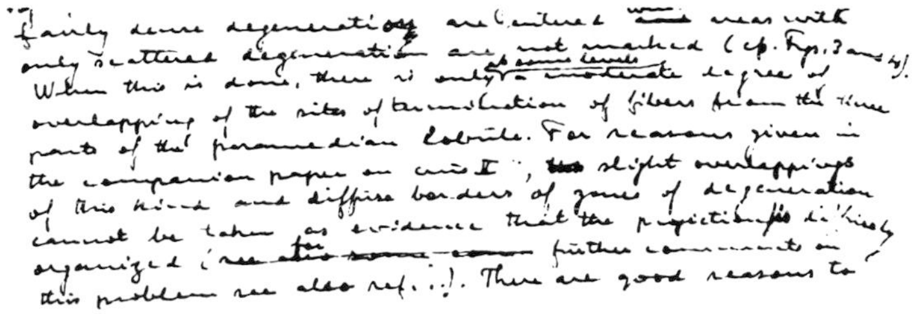
fairly dense degeneration are limited to areas with only scattered degeneration are not marked (cf. Figs. 3 and 4). When this is done, there is only a moderate degree of overlapping of the sites of termination of fibers from the three parts of the paramedian lobule. For reasons given in the companion paper on cat II, slight overlappings of this kind and diffuse borders of zones of degeneration cannot be taken as evidence that the projection is diffusely organized (see further comments on this problem see also ref...). There are good reasons to

B

Figure 17.1. *(A) Part of a letter written on lined paper by Brodal a month after the stroke. (B) part of the first draft of a paper written 6 months before, on plain paper. Note the irregularities of letters, lines, and intervals in ("A"). (From Brodal, 1973.)*

the time course for recovery depends upon many different variables, including the locus of the lesion, the kind of damage inflicted, experiential history, and age at the time of injury. Regarding age, whereas we have just noted that there may be excellent recovery following focal lesions early in life, it is worth repeating that recovery can often also be observed after damage in adolescence or even at maturity. This observation is important because it allows us to ask how recovery can be enhanced or maximized in adults and because it suggests that with appropriate treatments, the outcomes of therapy on mature patients may be more gratifying for both the patient and the therapist.

From the research literature, we know that the degree to which adults can recover from brain damage is often more dramatic than expected. Recently, Paul Glees (1980) described several cases of hemispherectomy performed on young adults between 19 and 20 years of age. In one of the cases, a patient had complete removal of the right hemisphere, and despite this loss, he was able to obtain a university degree. Sensory testing on the left side of this person's body showed normal recognition of shapes and objects and cutaneous localization of pain and touch. He held a responsible administrative job, and according to Glees, "proved convincingly that one hemisphere is sufficient as a substratum for an apparently complete personality [p. 117]."

Even with hemispherectomies performed on much older individuals, dramatic recovery can be seen. A short time ago, Burklund and Smith (1977) examined a patient for 18 months after he had a left hemispherectomy at 41 years of age for removal of a malignant glioma. It should be noted that the hemispherectomy was the third operation for neoplastic removal; subtotal frontal lesions and removal of the entire left frontal operculum preceded the hemispherectomy. In each of the first two operations, initial impairment (inability to speak, paralysis of right arm) occurred and was followed by rapid recovery. Following the last of the operations, verbal performance clearly deteriorated, although the patient could make appropriate nonverbal responses to simple commands. Restitution was slow, and the patient never fully recovered by the time he died 2 years after the surgery. Yet there was, all things considered, dramatic improvement despite the absence of the entire left hemisphere and further glial damage to the remaining right side of the brain.

With time, both verbal and nonverbal abilities became better and more consistent, and the dysarthria that was seen immediately after surgery largely subsided. In repeating phrases (Schnell test of speech), the patient made only one error in 32 items and was able to count and recite the days of the week and perfectly repeat 6 of 8 complete sentences. Within a few months he also showed that he could do fairly well in digit span and on a motor test (Purdue Pegboard). Moreover, the patient made no errors on a test of visual memory (Benton test).

What is noteworthy in this case is certainly not the fact that the patient still had some verbal difficulties. If we assume that the left hemisphere is critical and necessary for the mediation of verbal performance, the surprise is that he had any verbal and cognitive skills *at all* in the absence of a left hemisphere removed at maturity. Thus, the idea that recovery is unlikely after the period of infancy can be seriously challenged, even after extensive injuries in man.

Another concept which should also be reconsidered in the face of new evidence is the idea that if any recovery will occur, it will be essentially confined to the first few weeks after trauma, with little more improvement after that time. We now can say that, in some instances, this conception of recovery may be entirely too pessimistic. In fact, too strong an adherence to this view may even be harmful in the sense that therapeutic interventions could be terminated before they can really be effective. Also, the patient who has no expectation of recovering any further may respond to the world in a way that would inhibit additional restitution or progress which could be within reach.

There is now some new evidence that "delayed" recovery from brain damage need *not* be limited only to cognitive processes, but may also occur after injury to specific sensory systems as well.

For example, patients with lesions of the visual cortex most typically develop "scotomas." This means that when objects are moved across the patient's visual field, there are gaps or "defects" in the ability to see the target. There is literally a hole in the visual field. Until now it was thought that brain injury would produce "permanent" scotomas or "blind spots" even though Poppel, Held, and Bowling (1977) have shown some residual vision in patients who were unaware that they could, in fact, make discriminations within the impaired zone.

In 1981, at a conference on recovery of function held in Rotterdam, The Netherlands, J. Zihl, of the Max Planck Institute of Munich, reported that, with appropriate training techniques, the scotomas of patients with damage to the visual cortex could be made to shrink. To accomplish this, Zihl gave intensive visual discrimination training by requiring his patients to press a key whenever they could "see" a small target (blanks were occasionally presented to make sure the subjects were not making "false positive" responses). The stimuli were presented to specific areas within the scotoma, and as training progressed, Zihl noted that the size of the defect (i.e., the area of blindness) began to shrink. After carefully guided training, some recovery of visual function began to emerge. Visual acuity as well as some color vision also improved, although it seemed that such improvement was limited to the edges of the scotoma, rather than to its center. Zihl also noted that the recovery was still observed 1 year after all training had been terminated, so the changes in visual performance that were induced were not due to temporary changes in arousal or neuronal activity.

At the present time, the specific mechanisms for recovery of vision after cortical lesions have not been determined. Nonetheless, intensive training sometimes seems to be an important factor. Whereas one might be tempted to speculate that the patients were able to use new strategies for "seeing," it is difficult for us to imagine how this might have occurred in Zihl's experiment.

Another good illustration of a delayed recovery effect in man can be seen in a report published by Blakemore and Falconer (1967). These investigators examined 54 patients with left temporal lobectomies and 32 with right temporal lobectomies. Significant decrements in verbal (left side lesion) and nonverbal (right side lesion) performance were found when the patients were tested within 2 months of surgery. These declines proved to be transient, and the patients' scores rebounded to preoperative levels by the end of their first postoperative year. Blakemore and Falconer also reported that the group with left temporal lobectomies displayed marked deficits in paired associate learning and that these impairments showed little improvement during the first 2–3 years. From this point on, performance improved, and by the end of the fifth postoperative year, the patients were performing at preoperative levels.

In addition to these data, the idea that recovery can sometimes take place long after the time of injury can be supported in Hans-Lukas Teuber's (1975) extensive longitudinal work on veterans of the Korean War who had suffered penetrating head wounds. Teuber was able to show considerable recovery (or sparing) on some tests up to 15 years after injury. His data are important because he obtained precise, preinduction intelligence test scores on the men, which could then be compared to their scores obtained in the post-traumatic condition.

In gainful employment, which he considered a "test of life," Teuber found that 68–82% of veterans with different penetrating wounds of the head were fully employed 15 years after first being hospitalized. The higher the initial IQ, the greater the percentage of employment. In comparison to controls, about 20% of the men with brain injury were unable to work. As Teuber himself put it:

> The question of interpretation remains: Should one stress the relative insensitivity of routine psychometrics to the more subtle long-term after-effects of penetrating brain injuries or should one turn the argument around and underline the frequent ultimate recovery of test intelligence after lesions in any but the critical left parietal-temporal zone [p. 165]?

Impressive recovery over time can also be seen in the tables compiled by Walker and Jablon (1961) and Walker and Erculei (1969) on soldiers who sustained head wounds during World War II. These men showed considerable improvement on a number of neurological and psychometric tests when they were examined 5–8 years after injury, although symptom remission was more sporadic and variable over the next 7–10 years. Walker and Jablon, in the initial follow-up study, stated that the chance of a hemiparesis clearing up completely after a penetrating wound of the head was about 25% and that the probability was even higher for a paralysis of just one limb (monoparesis). Earlier, Richie Russel (1951), the noted British neurologist, had reported that motor functions may recover completely in more than half of the patients showing an initial paralysis.

At this point it is important to raise a related possibility—that the recovery witnessed after a brain injury may diminish at a later point in the patient's life. This finding is becoming well known in cases in which lesions are sustained by animals during the period of infancy (see Chapter 8; see also Bogen, 1974; Goldman, 1974; Hicks and D'Amato, 1970; Kennard, 1940, 1942). However, the same declines in behavior have now also been seen after lesions in adult animals (Gruenthal, Finger, Berenbeim, Pollock, and Hart, 1980), and more importantly, it can be observed in certain adult, neurological subjects (Geschwind, 1974). For instance, patients with some types of acute cerebral lesions may assume a posture of flexion like that of spinal animals, many years after the time of injury, and individuals with frontal lobe lesions who may perform normally on a number of psychometric tests soon after insult, often exhibit a decline in performance many years later (Hamlin, 1970).

The bases of these delayed lesion effects are not well understood. Conceivably, they could be due to secondary changes in the nervous system (Schoenfeld and Hamilton, 1977), such as sprouting or transsynaptic and transneuronal degeneration. For example, Yakovlev (1954) found that if 20 or more years have elapsed after a prefrontal lobotomy, the brain of the patient goes from a normal appearance to one showing considerable shrinkage. A comparable effect has been noted in rats by Rosenzweig, Bennett, Morimoto, and Herbert (1978). It is also possible that the limited environmental stimulation that some of these patients are receiving could be contributing to the general deterioration of their behavior (Finger, 1978; Gruenthal et al., 1980). In any case, "late" changes in behavior, whether beneficial or deleterious, are a reality that must be considered when patients are evaluated, when families are counseled, and when goals of therapy are considered. These findings show clearly that the effects of focal brain lesions in man may not be stable after the first few weeks, during which the effects of anoxia, edema, hemorrhage, and trauma are expected to wear off. They also show that some of our conclusions about recovery not taking place, or taking place, may be based on an inadequate period of time for observation. Although there may be practical limits to most therapies and studies, this consideration must always be borne in mind.

Knowing that recovery can occur in mature human subjects, what can be done to maximize it? Part of the answer to this question was provided many years ago in an experiment by Shepherd Ivory Franz and his colleagues (Franz, Scheetz, and Wilson, 1915). These investigators looked at patients ("old cases") who had cerebral accidents many years earlier and who developed paralyses and contractures that seemed permanent in the sense that little improvement was noted long after the time of insult. The arm segment, being the most affected, was chosen for treatment. These patients were then treated with massage and vibration by stroking, shaking, and grasping, passive movements (with emphasis on extentions), and supervised voluntary use of the extensor muscles in simple activities. Franz and his co-workers found a return of function in the paralyzed segment "much beyond the time limit set by some neurologists for possible improvement." On the basis of their observations, they proceeded to argue that not only passive, but active intervention with the environment is essential for maximizing recovery.

The idea that specific, active interactions with the environment can be an important factor in some types of recovery was further explored under better controlled conditions by Franz in his experiments on monkeys. Robert Ogden and Franz (1917) destroyed the motor cortex on one side of a group of animals and then permitted them (a) time for "spontaneous" recovery with no intervention; (b) forced usage of the affected arm resulting from strapping the good arm to the trunk; or (c) general massage of the affected limbs. The experimenters found

that motor recovery after the production of a hemiplegia does not result if the animal is left to its own devices, and this management (or lack of management) it is almost unnecessary to remark is what is given to most human paralytic cases.

... The method of treatment recommended by neurologists, general massage, does produce a slight amount of improvement but not to an extent to enable the animal to use the arm and hand properly for such ordinary operations as feeding and climbing, although these activities may be carried out after such treatment in an awkward manner. When, however, efforts are directed to the special nerves and muscles, and when the sound side of the animal is restrained so that movements of climbing and feeding must be made, if at all, by the use of the paralyzed segments the improvement is rapid and the recovery is practically complete [pp. 44–45].

The importance of active interactions with the environment has been a recurrent theme through almost all of the chapters of this book. We noted that ''serial lesion effects'' might not appear in the absence of active, environmental exploration and eye–limb interactions between multiple surgeries (Dru, Walker, and Walker, 1975). The failure of the developing organism to thrive in the absence of adequate social contact and interactive stimulation has also been discussed (*hospitalism*, Chapter 10), and there now is growing recognition of the finding that following restricted visual input to one eye early in life, forced usage of that eye and extensive training and handling can lead to previously unexpected behavioral recovery (e.g., Chow and Stewart, 1972). With all of these findings in mind, a strong case can be made for the significance of active participation on the behalf of the subject, rather than just passive stimulation, as an essential element in recovery programs, especially those dealing with motor functions and sensorimotor integration. As stated by Josephene Moore (1980) in her chapter examining ''ten cardinal principles of (re)habilitation'':

Active involvement has repeatedly been shown to be superior to passive participation in order for the nervous system to learn, mature and remain viable. . . . In rehabilitation it is necessary at times to use passive treatment techniques in order to prevent contractures, atrophy and general deterioration. However, every effort should be made to get the patient involved in the (re)habilitation process so that the patient learns how to carry out purposeful and sequential movement patterns [p. 72].

Closely related to these ideas is the notion that ''nonspecific'' environmental stimulation can enhance recovery on general learning tasks and intellectual functions (Chapter 10). Here too, we have noted that it is important for the subject to be more than a passive observer if significant brain and behavioral changes are to occur as a result of the enriched experience (Ferchmin, Bennett, and Rosenzweig, 1975). Furthermore, with general maze learning as a measure, there is convincing evidence from animal studies that environmental stimulation can serve as an effective therapy for not only both early and later focal lesions of the brain, but, at least to some extent, for dysfunctions due to more generalized insult, such as those due to early malnutrition. Although the literature on environmental complexity and brain lesions in man is primarily represented by relatively poorly controlled studies and appears to be both anecdotal and speculative, one would be hard pressed to argue that social contact, more attentive staff, and more stimulating hospital rooms (with pictures, television, colored chairs, etc.) would be harmful to the patient. Rather, such conditions would be ineffective at worst, and could very possibly be beneficial to the subjects on a wide variety of tasks as they attempt to cope with an altered world.

Needless to say, hospital settings are becoming more cheerful than they were even 10 or 20 years ago, and one need only to look at old photographs or paintings (see Figure 17.2) to realize how unstimulating they had been at the turn of the century. Although there is a great need for more controlled research on how environmental variables of this nature specifically affect brain-damaged human patients, on the basis of the evidence currently available to us, the trend toward making hospitals brighter and more interesting and stimulating can only be viewed favorably. The importance of this factor should not go unrecognized as new hospitals are built, as old buildings and rooms are improved, and as quarters in private homes are modified for sick or injured family members.

Another principle to emerge from the data reviewed in this monograph is that

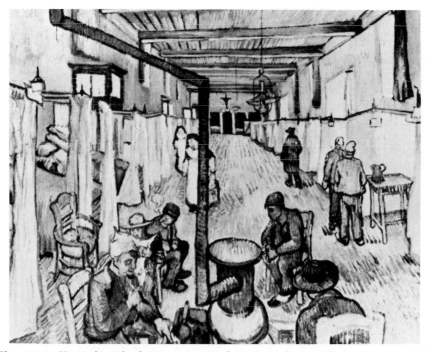

Figure 17.2. *Hospital in Arles, by Vincent Van Gogh (1889). (Collection of O. Reinhart, Winterhur, Switzerland.)*

therapy should be initiated as soon as possible. Although this idea is widely followed and usually stated without qualification, the research literature would suggest that this may be an even more important rule to follow when the brain is damaged while in a stage of rapid growth. In particular, it is now well known that the effects of early malnutrition and sensory restriction, which can be looked upon as physiological "lesions" of the brain, can be relatively permanent if therapy starts after the "critical period" has passed (Layton, Corrick, and Toga, 1978; Winick, 1976).

With adults, Teuber (1975) points out that near the end of the World War II, Wepman assigned some of his aphasic patients to immediate therapy, whereas others had to wait ½–1 year for retraining because of inadequate personnel and facilities. When tested later on, those who had the earlier therapy were performing significantly better than those who were forced to wait for such assistance.

It now seems that recovery is most likely to follow early interventions in the forms of physical therapy, occupational therapy, and the like; although, as we have seen in the reports of Franz, the effects of later-starting therapies can sometimes be substantial. Yet, the exact reasons why it is important to start therapy as soon as possible after injury are not always clear. Quite possibly, many factors are involved. The more disuse atrophy that there is in the muscles, for example, the less effective (or more prolonged) the therapy might have to be. It may also be that therapeutic interventions result in neuronal activity that can block or prevent certain degenerative changes from occurring in the central nervous system. Therapy may also be psychologically important. Patients may feel that attention is being paid to them, and by seeing early progress, they may more easily achieve the motivation and frame of mind needed to "fight back" for an active and normal life.

In this context it should be noted that the whole issue of psychological factors in determining the course of an illness is again being given the recognition that we believe it merits. The role that stress and mental attitude can play in the spread of cancer may be among the best known of these effects, having both anecdotal support in popular books by recovered patients such as Normal Cousins (1980) and some verification in controlled laboratory studies (Wozniak, Finger, Blumenthal, and Poland, 1982).

Some of the same principles that apply to these cases probably play a role in recovery from brain damage. The depressed brain-damaged patient does not interact with his environment in the same way or to the same extent as the patient with the "healthier" mental attitude, and the latter, of course, would also be the better, more cooperative patient in therapy. Help from other patients who have been through the long and tedious process could also be very beneficial; knowing that someone else cares and can share the experience is a valuable adjunct to supportative therapy.

Our belief in the potential for recovery from brain damage is important in this regard. If the family and medical staff believe that partial or complete recovery can take place, this should be emphasized to the patient as it can undoubtably affect mental attitude. If the prevailing view is one of a static nervous system and fixed deficits, at least after the first few weeks, it seems entirely possible that the patient may simply adapt to this pessimistic view and perform in a way that will be consonant with the expectation that there will be no (further) restitution. Such a patient may not strive for additional improvement and may not try to do things that he or she might find could come within reach with additional effort or practice. As noted by Franz (1923) almost 60 years ago:

> Relatives who only bemoan the fate of a man in need of reeducation, who pity him and regard him as a helpless burden, place a real obstacle in the way of his recovery. The family which encourages its patient-member, which makes with him plans for the day when he shall be "recovered," which regards him as a potential asset instead of a burden, and which cooperates with the instructors in charge of the patient, is a potent factor in the eventual recovery [p. 44].

Moreover:

> The production of a sound, normal mental attitude in the patient must have a primary place in all reeducation work. It is an integral part of rehabilitation in all its stages. An attitude of hope and hopefulness must be instilled at the start. A will to get well must be created if it does not exist. . . . The discouraged and helpless patient believes nothing can help him . . . . Each time something is done for him, each time treatment is prescribed, he asks himself, "What good will this do?" And always he answers himself, "This will do me no good." He feels he is helpless, and it may almost be said he has reached a state at which he "doesn't want to get well" [p. 44].

It is particularly easy for a harried hospital or nursing staff to "pathologize" the patient in order to treat the disorder. In some cases pathologizing leads to the conclusion that nothing can or should be done to deal with the individual's attempts to cope and to adjust to his or her altered world. If the staff's attitude is that nothing can be done, the patient may soon conform to the institutional beliefs.

In this context, Thomas LeVere (1980) raised an interesting, new possibility. He argued that a negative response to brain injury may lead to compensatory reactions (alternate strategies, cues, and muscle groups), which if somewhat successful, may even prevent, inhibit, or preclude the course of true recovery from the damage.

Thus, psychological factors such as "set" and expectation and stress and depressive reactions certainly should not be treated lightly. In fact, the importance of these variables cannot be overstated. We should emphasize, however, that we are not advocating that the patient should be deceived. Obviously, there are cases where it is difficult to be optimistic, even with regard to the possibility of using compensatory devices to circumvent lost functions. Nevertheless, one of the themes of this book is that there are many situations and instances in which we have been entirely too pessimistic about the possibility of restitution, and it is not difficult to argue that these attitudes and beliefs can affect how patients actually perform in the period after brain injury.

As we have noted, one of the most basic messages of this book is that each subject must be considered individually. Although group norms may set guidelines and be appropriate for summarizing data in an experimental setting, there is no such thing as an "average" brain injury. Each case is an individual and unique occurrence. One's developmental status, the environmental conditions prior to insult, and the speed of growth of the lesion are just a few of the variables that can influence the course of recovery in a patient. These factors, as well as motivation and the personalities involved, must be considered in planning a treatment program. Since these factors differ from case to case, it should not be expected that a particular treatment will be effective on all patients, nor that "spontaneous" recovery would be seen to the same degree in each case. On the one hand, the individual with a stroke may show more deficits immediately after such an incident than a person with a slow-growing tumor in the same general area. On the other hand, the stroke victim may also have the better prognosis for the remission of symptoms as time passes or as therapy proceeds.

With such an (idiopathic) orientation, one's emphases and goals must be both flexible and case-oriented. Moreover, as we have suggested, individually designed programs of therapy will probably be most effective if they focus upon providing a supportive environment that emphasizes the skills that the patient can employ at the time of therapy.[2]

As we have seen, age at the time of insult would be one of the factors that would be most important to consider at the time of therapy. The ability of the child to recover speech after a lesion of the left hemisphere is obviously better than that of an old individual. However, the older person may still be capable of some restitution, and because of a richer experiential and learning history, we

[2] With regard to what we have just said about the role of psychological factors in recovery from brain damage, we must emphasize that therapy should not be restricted to deficiencies, but should also capitalize on the strengths of the individual. That is, knowing that some tasks may lead to feelings of failure, practitioners should emphasize what the individual still can do well while attempting to improve performance on the affected functions. For example, although the highly distractable patient with a short attention span may do poorly in reading and writing skills, such an individual may excell in another activity, such as using shop tools or drafting equipment. Thus, while efforts should be made to improve deficient skills, it may be important for such a patient to be able to feel that there are things that he can do as well as, if not better than, others can. If nothing else, the idea of capitalizing on strengths may provide an atmosphere that would be conducive for attaining other therapeutic goals.

might even expect compensatory responses, if not recovery per se, to be better in this population.

The observation that delayed lesion effects may appear after some types of brain damage early in life and that some might even be seen after insult at maturity raises an especially interesting possibility. Specifically, in some of these cases it might be possible to work with the patient in anticipation of the appearance of later lesion effects. This can be particularly beneficial in developing alternate strategies for dealing with problems. If a part of the brain soon to be affected is still functioning relatively well, it can serve as a basis of comparison against which new ways of solving problems can be compared. Alternative solutions and methods could be matched against the "standard" until successful methods of coping are found. Later, when the first part of the brain is infiltrated or suffers transneuronal degeneration, the switch can be made to the new system. In contrast, the learning process may take much longer if it begins after the normal neural substrate is lost. In fact, other subtle, but very helpful, cues may never be noticed in the latter case. This possibility need not be restricted to cases of focal lesions early in life (Goldman, 1974; Kennard, 1940, 1942). It could account for some of the serial lesion effects that we discussed in Chapter 9.

With regard to what we now know about fast- versus slow-growing lesions, we can also suggest that where neurosurgery must be performed, the possibility of doing it in stages should be considered. This is not to say that multiple surgical entries should be the rule, as there are many instances where a single operation would not be expected to result in great losses or deficits and as multiple operations could have a greater risk associated with them.[3] However, in some cases the risk–reward ratio might well justify a series of operations rather than a single surgery. Also, anesthetics and surgical trauma may be minimized in some of these cases by techniques such as using implanted electrodes. If electrodes are implanted in the target zone during an operation, current could be passed in a series of stages without the need for additional anesthetics or the risk of complications that might result from exposing the brain on successive occasions. If the research literature is correct, and there is every reason to believe it is, procedures like this one for making lesions more slowly may have fewer symptoms associated with

---

[3] Serial lesions may have different risks for different types of patients. The removal of a malignant tumor, for example, cannot be equated with the removal of a cyst or debris from a missile wound. This is because it is possible that partial removal of the tumor substance could conceivably trigger the rapid spread of remaining tumor cells to other parts of the brain or even to other parts of the body. Similarly, it is possible that with a disease such as epilepsy, small incomplete lesions may result in the development of additional foci and "recovery" of the epilepsy itself. Thus, while multiple small lesions may be associated with fewer behavioral deficits in laboratory studies on previously healthy animals, serious consideration should be given to the possibility that unexpected complications could emerge when these same techniques are applied to people with diseases of the brain.

them—and more rapid recovery from those symptoms that do emerge—than conventional one-operation approaches.

The fact that lesion effects can change over time would also suggest that patients with brain damage be subject to periodic examinations to evaluate both physical and mental status. This would have to be considered basic to cases in which lobotomies, temporal lobectomies, and other types of psychosurgery have been performed. Here in particular, performance 1 month or 1 or 2 years after surgery should not be viewed as a definitive statement about how behavior will look later on. As John Hughlings Jackson (1879) noted more than 100 years ago, the condition of the rest of the brain may have as much to do with the resultant symptomatology as the site of the lesion itself. This concept is by no means trivial when attempting to predict how patients will respond to and recover from brain damage.

Insofar as human subjects are concerned, the future may permit us to be even more optimistic about both the possibility of recovery from brain damage and the chances of successful compensatory responses to make up for serious losses. In the latter case, new prosthetic devices, are receiving considerable attention, especially in cases of motor neuron and limb damage and in visual and hearing impairments.

With pharmacological treatments, we have already seen the success that the Russian workers have been having with drugs in cases where the primary symptoms of head injury seem to result from depressed functioning (Chapter 12). Their use of drugs, such as the potent alkaloid, galanthamine, may well represent a future trend in aiding focal brain injured patients. In fact, in a recent publication, Bruce Peters and Harvey Levin (1977), of the University of Texas Medical Branch in Galveston, reported that injections of physostigmine, a central cholinergic agonist, could enhance memory in amnesic patients. In one of their follow-up studies, Peters and Levin (1979) reported that this drug, when combined with lecithin (another agent that increases acetylcholine), can even improve the memory functions of patients with Alzheimer's disease, the most common cause of progressive dementia. Figure 17.3 shows this finding. Thus, pharmacological agents can sometimes be useful in promoting recovery, not only in cases of focal brain injury, but in instances where there may even be cumulative and perhaps diffuse cell loss.[4]

[4] With a disorder such as Alzheimer's disease, agents that would increase the amount of acetylcholine in the central nervous system would, however, be time-limited in their effectiveness. Since there is progressive cell degeneration, there would be fewer and fewer cholinergic synapses remaining as the disease runs it course. A point will eventually be reached where agents like physostigimine and lecithin would cease to be effective because there would not be enough cholinergic circuitry remaining for them to affect. In this regard, agents (yet to be discovered) that would halt the loss of synapses and perhaps combine with others like physostigmine, which would increase the amount of available transmitter, would be essential to prevent further deterioration and enhance recovery. Increasing the sensitivity of remaining synapses might also prove to be a rewarding strategy in such cases.

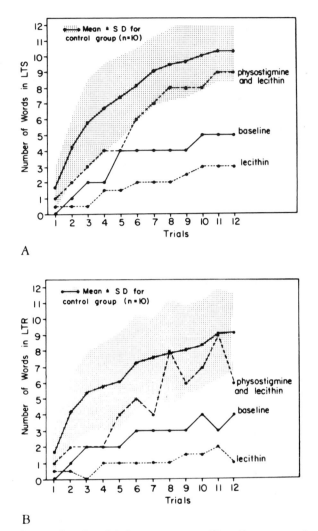

Figure 17.3. *Median number of words in long-term storage (A) and long-term retrieval (B) for three patients under three test conditions, shown with normative data from an age-matched control group (mean age, 71.9 years). (From Peters and Levin, 1979.)*

In conclusion, there appear to be a number of things that can be done to promote recovery from brain damage or at least to increase the probability of seeing
some improvement. Some of these factors are based firmly on experimental
evidence, but others, such as motivation and psychological set and adjustment,
can be just as important in the recovery process, although we are not always certain about the mechanisms mediating their effectiveness. It is our contention that
recovery in man may be more prevalent than we think. Furthermore, the poten-

tial for recovery in adults, even after the first few weeks following injury, is probably not as limited as we have been led to believe. Knowing what we do about the factors that can affect recovery, such as age and environmental stimulation, it should now come as no surprise that patients with lesions in the same general areas do not always show the same symptoms and potential for restitution. With this in mind, a more idiopathic (individual patient) orientation toward therapy is called for—one that would take into account not only features of the lesion, but factors such as motivation, age, experiential history, and the status of the rest of the brain. The variability and differential recovery often witnessed in response to injury and disease begin to make sense only when clinical data are viewed in this way.

References

Bernhardt, M. Ueber die spastiche cerebrale paralyse im Kindersalter nebst einem Excurse uber "aphasie bei Kindern". *Virchows Archives for Anatomie und Physiologie*, 1885, *102*.

Blakemore, C. B., and Falconer, M. A. Long-term effects of anterior temporal lobectomy on certain cognitive functions. *Journal of Neurology, Neurosurgery and Psychiatry*, 1967, *30*, 364–367.

Bogen, J. E. Hemisphrectomy and the placing reaction in cats. M. Kinsbourne and W. L. Smith (Eds.), *Hemisphere disconnection and cerebral function*. Springfield, Ill.: Charles C Thomas, 1974, Pp. 48–94.

Brodal, A. Self-observations and neuro-anatomical considerations after a stroke. *Brain*, 1973, *96*, 675–694.

Burklund, C. W., and Smith, A. Language and the cerebral hemispheres. *Neurology*, 1977, *27*, 627–633.

Chow, K. L., and Stewart, D. L. Reversal of structural and functional effects of long-term visual deprivation in cats. *Experimental Neurology*, 1972, *34*, 409–433.

Cousins, N. *Anatomy of an illness*. Boston: G. K. Hall, 1980.

Critchley, M. Dr. Samual Johnson's aphasia. *Medical History*, 1962, *6*, 27–44.

Dru, D., Walker, J. P., and Walker, J. B. Self-produced locomotion restores visual capacity after striate lesion. *Science*, 1975, *187*, 265–266.

Ferchmin, P. A., Bennett, E. L., and Rosenzweig, M. R. Direct contact with enriched environment is required to alter cerebral weights in rats. *Journal of Comparative and Physiological Psychology*, 1975, *88*, 360–367.

Finger, S. Environmental attenuation of brain lesion symptoms. In S. Finger (Ed.), *Recovery from brain damage: Research and theory*. New York: Plenum, 1978.

Franz, S. I. *Nervous and mental re-education*. New York: Macmillan, 1923.

Franz, S. I., Scheetz, M. E., and Wilson, A. A. The possibility of recovery of motor function in long-standing hemiplegia. *Journal of the American Medical Association*, 1915, *65*, 2150–2154.

Freud, S. Die infantile cerebrallahmung. In *Nothnagel, Specielle pathologie und Therapie IV*, Vienna: Holder, 1897.

Geschwind, N. Late changes in the nervous system: An overview. In D. G. Stein, J. J. Rosen, and N. Butters (Eds.), *Plasticity and recovery of function in the central nervous system*. New York: Academic Press, 1974, Pp. 467–508.

Glees, P. Functional reorganization following hemispherectomy in man and after small experimental lesions in primates. In P. Bach-y-Rita, (Ed.), *Recovery of function: Theoretical considerations for brain injury rehabilitation*. Baltimore, Md.: University Park Press, 1980, 106–126.

Goldman, P. An alternative to developmental plasticity: Heterology of CNS structures in infants and adults. In D. G. Stein, J. J. Rosen, and N. Butters (Eds.), *Plasticity and recovery of function in the central nervous system*. New York: Academic Press, 1974, Pp. 149–174.

Gruenthal, M., Finger, S., Berenbeim, J., Pollock, D., and Hart, T. A. delayed lesion effect following sensorimotor cortex ablation in adult rats. *Experimental Neurology*, 1980, *69*, 4–21.

Hamlin, R. M. Intellectual functions 14 years after frontal lobe surgery. *Cortex*, 1970, *6*, 299–307.

Hicks, S. P., and D'Amato, C. J. Motor-sensory and visual behavior after hemispherectomy in newborn and mature rats. *Experimetal Neurology*, 1970, *29*, 416–438.

Jackson, J. H. On affections of speech from disease of the brain. *Brain*, 1879, *2*, 323–356.

Kennard, M. A. Relation of age to motor impairment in man and sub-human primates. *Archives of Neurology and Psychiatry*, 1940, *44*, 377–397.

Kennard, M. A. Cortical reorganization of motor function: Studies on a series of monkeys of various ages from infancy to maturity. *Archives of Neurology and Psychiatry*, 1942, *48*, 227–240.

Layton, B. S., Corrick, G. E., and Toga, A. W. Sensory restriction and recovery of function. In S. Finger (Ed.), *Recovery from brain damage: Research and theory*. New York: Plenum, 1978, Pp. 331–366.

Lenneberg, E. H. *Biological foundations of language*. New York: Wiley, 1967.

LeVere, T. Recovery of function after brain damage. A theory of the behavioral deficit. *Physiological Psychology*, 1980, *8*, 297–308.

Luria, A. R. *The man with a shattered world*. New York: Basic Books, 1972.

Moore, J. Neuroanatomical considerations relating to recovery of function following brain injury. In P. Bach-y-Rita (Ed.), *Recovery of function: Theoretical considerations for brain injury rehabilitation*. Baltimore, Md.: University Park Press, 1980, Pp. 9–90.

Ogden, R., and Franz, S. I. On cerebral motor control: The recovery from experimentally produced hemiplegia. *Psychobiology*, 1917, *1*, 33–49.

Peters, B. H., and Levin, H. S. Memory enhancement after physostigmine treatment in the amnesic syndrome. *Archives of Neurology*, 1977, *34*, 215–219.

Peters, B. H., and Levin, H. S. Effects of physostigmine and lecithin on memory in Alzheimer disease. *Annals of Neurology*, 1979, *6*, 219–221.

Poppel, E., Held, R. and Bowling, J. E. Neuronal mechanisms in visual perception. *Neuroscience Research Program Bulletin*, 1977, *15*, 323–375.

Rosenzweig, M. R., Bennett, E. L., Morimoto, H., and Hebert, M. Lesions in occipital cortex of rat lead to secondary loss of cells in other cortical regions. *Society for Neuroscience Abstracts*, 1978, *4*, 478.

Russell, W. R., Disability caused by brain wounds: Review of 1,166 cases. *Journal of Neurology, Neurosurgery and Psychiatry*, 1951, *14*, 35–39.

Schoenfeld, T. A., and Hamilton, L. W. Secondary brain changes following lesions: A new paradigm for lesion experimentation. *Physiology and Behavior*, 1977, *18*, 951–967.

Smith, A., and Sugar, O. Development of above normal language and intelligence 21 years after left hemispherectomy. *Neurology*, 1975, *25*, 813–818.

Teuber, H. L. Recovery of function after brain injury in man. In *Outcome of severe damage to the central nervous system* (Ciba Foundation Symposium #34, new series), Elsevier, North Holland, 1975, 159–190.

Walker, A. E., and Erculei, F. *Head-injured men fifteen years later*. Springfield, Ill.: Charles C Thomas, 1969.

Walker, A. E., and Jablon, S. *A followup study of head wounds in World War II*. Washington, D.C.: VA Medical Monograph, U.S. Government Printing Office, 1961.

Winick, M. *Malnutrition and brain development*. New York: Oxford University Press, 1976.

Wozniak, D., Finger, S., Blumenthal, H., and Poland, R. Brain damage, stress and lifespan: An experimental study. *Journal of Gerontology*, 1982, *37*, 161–168.

Yakovlev, P. I. Paraplegia in flexion of cerebral origin. *Journal of Neuropathology and Experimental Neurology*, 1954, *13*, 267–295.

Zihl, J. *Shrinkage of visual field defects associated with specific training after brain damage.* Paper presented at the European Brain and Behavior Society Workshop, "Recovery from Brain Damage," Rotterdam, April 1981. In M. W. van Hof and G. Mohn (Eds.), *Functional Recovery from Brain Damage.* Amsterdam: Elsevier, 1981, Pp. 189–202.

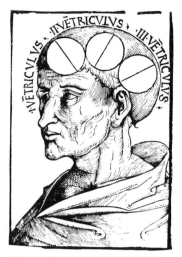

Recovery, Plasticity, and Brain Theory

It seems that if we try to discover the ways in which any part of the brain functions, it is only logical to try and find out in what way it acts within the brain as a whole. There is evidence that whatever the frontal lobes do must in some way affect the reticular formation, hypothalamus, limbic system and a number of other structures about which we do not know very much. I think the point should be made that no part of the brain functions on its own, but only through other parts of the brain with which it is concerned [Nauta, 1964, p. 125].

CHAPTER EIGHTEEN

Throughout the earlier chapters of this book we have examined the response to brain injury from three different perspectives—anatomy, physiology, and behavior. In each of these cases we have tried to look very carefully at the paradigm that has guided the research, and have, at times, questioned some of the basic assumptions underlying the interpretation of the results.

In this, our final chapter, we will attempt to tie some of these divergent findings and ideas together by doing five things. First, we will examine the issue of how central nervous system *function* can be defined. Second, we will ask whether the lesion paradigm is really shedding any light on understanding structure–function relationships in the brain. Third, we will stress why it is important to look not just at the anatomy of the lesion, but also at the condition of the remaining brain and the adaptive nature of behavior following central nervous system injury. Fourth, we will present another paradigm for conducting and interpreting brain lesion studies, an alternative that we favor and believe can be at least as important as using brain lesion techniques to localize behavioral functions into smaller and smaller parcels of tissue. And fifth, we will make three suggestions that can lead to a better understanding of brain lesion effects and recovery of function, regardless of one's theoretical orientation.

Let us first consider the issue of brain lesions and the concept of *function*. As we have emphasized throughout this book, the diversity of the data and the complexity of the problems involved in the interpretation of studies employing lesion techniques must be considered in the context of the unresolved issue of determining how structure–function relationships are to be defined in normal and brain-damaged subjects (see Laurence and Stein, 1978). Our contention is that it is not appropriate to assume that a given part of the nervous system *must* have a given function because a certain type of damage usually results in specific symptoms.

In most papers appearing in the area of contemporary neuropsychology, the word *function* is rarely defined (see Ruckmich, 1913, and Dallenbach, 1915, for early definitions of the word *function*). For the most part, *function* is usually operationally defined in terms of the experimental variables manipulated or performances examined. Typically, in the biological sciences the *function of a given area* is defined as its ability to generate action potentials in response to a specific stimulus or in terms of its capacity to release certain neurotransmitters when electrically excited. Especially, in neurology and the behavioral sciences, areas of the central nervous system differentiated by classical anatomical or morphological criteria have also been assigned functions as global as the mediation of problem solving, aggression, sexual activity, and anxiety. One often encounters discussions of the functions of the four major lobes of the brain as if the lobes were more than convenient anatomical entities.

Therefore, as Luria and his colleagues have pointed out (Luria, Maydin, Tsvetkova, and Vinarskaya, 1969), *function* can be understood to mean two different things. In the first place, *function* can refer to the work performed by a specific organ or tissue, as when we talk about the secretory function of the salivary or pituitary gland. In the second place, *function* may refer to the complex, adaptive activity of individuals who are responding to their environments with such things as written signs for the exchange of ideas, or speech for communication.

Luria contends that this second example of function *cannot* be regarded as a "fixed function" of one particular organ or tissue. As a rule, the accomplishment of these cognitive or psychological functions may be based on a whole system of variable methods that may be performed in different ways. For example, locomotion is not performed by a fixed series of innervations, but always involves a complex and changing "functional system," the links of which are constantly varying as the course of the movement evolves. All that remains constant is either the aim or the purpose of the movement . . . some "plan" or "scheme" that guides the individual to obtain a goal (see also Miller, Pribram, and Gallanter, 1960).

As we noted earlier, the difficult problem of defining a function precisely is often avoided by the logical fallacy of assuming that those changes *caused* by brain damage directly indicate the unified, local functions of the injured area. Sir David Ferrier, in particular, often fell victim to this error. It is a comforting and convenient error because it makes it easy to side-step the problem of explaining instances of recovery or sparing after injury. One simply argues that any definition of function, and hence any restitution of that function, would depend upon the sensitivity of the tests used to measure performance. When recovery is observed, one claim is that the true functions of the areas were never measured because of insensitive or inappropriate tests. Even when a battery of tests is administered, it can still be asserted that the "critical" one was not applied.

The sensitivity of the tests used in the behavioral testing situation is unquestionably important. As we have seen, there are cases that indicate that subtle and sophisticated examination of brain-damaged patients can reveal deficits and impediments of which even the patient is unaware. Nevertheless, the argument that recovery of function is always due to insensitive or inappropriate tests certainly must lose some of its impact in the light of many of the experiments summarized throughout this book. This is because the subjects with lesions in these studies are not simply compared to an unoperated control group, but to other subjects with generally similar lesions who, because of some manipulation, such as a drug or experience, fail to show the same symptoms. For example, as we have seen in Chapter 9, bilateral one-stage lesions may cause severe, long-lasting deficits in performance, whereas the same extent of damage inflicted more slowly may have little or no apparent effects on the same measures (the "serial lesion effect"). Here, it cannot simply be stated that the test is insensitive because deficits are detected when the lesions are made in one stage. Rather, in ways which are not yet clear, the neural response to injury probably differs between the treatment groups in some of these cases, and these differences are reflected in the organism's performance—good in one case and poor in the other.

If nothing else, the materials we have reviewed strongly suggest that lesion sequelae do not necessarily signify the functions of a brain structure. To assume that symptoms represent localized functions in the specific area damaged is like saying that resistors are used in a radio to prevent howling since the removal of some resistors would result in unpleasant noises (Gregory, 1964; see also Zangwill, 1963). John Hughlings Jackson was aware of this logical fallacy at the turn of the last century when he argued that localization of symptoms following central nervous system activity is *not* the same as localization of function in normal, healthy brains. The point he made was that the symptoms of brain damage do not necessarily reveal the functions of the damaged tissue, but more accurately reflect what the remaining areas of the brain can do following injury to a part. Furthermore, it is important to remember that it is the organism that is performing, not its hippocampus or visual cortex, and certainly not a single, isolated cell! If the guiding principle in examining the effects of different kinds of brain lesions is one of studying symptoms and not of localizing "psychological functions," recovery phenomena, in fact, pose little threat to the theory of localization as currently conceived.

The basic distinction between symptoms and functions seems to have been forgotten by many contemporary neuroscientists. It is interesting that Morton Prince, who had been a President of the American Neurological Association, tried to warn his colleagues about using cases of brain damage to make statements about localization of function in the brain. In 1910, Prince wrote, "The present doctrine of cerebral localization regarded as a mapping of the brain into areas within which lesions give rise to particular groups of symptoms is one of the triumphs of neurology which cannot be valued too highly." But then he added, "Regarded as a localization of the psychophysiological functions represented by these symptoms within narrowly circumscribed areas, it is in large part naive to a degree which will excite the smiles of future neurologists [p. 340].

Some of the errors resulting from the assumption that the presence (or absence) of symptoms is a direct reflection of the functions of the disrupted circuitry have already been examined in a number of places in this book. Ferrier (1878) himself once even remarked that the loosening of a pin in a chronometer will damage the whole timekeeping mechanism; but that we should not therefore attribute timekeeping functions to that one part exclusively.

On an empirical level, we now know that if symptoms do appear after a given lesion, they could well reflect not only the direct loss of specific neurons, typically shown by photographs, tracings, or drawings of the lesion site, but could also be due to distal effects, for example, changes in neurotransmitters, degenerating axons, and altered blood supplies in other parts of the brain, to name just a few of the many factors involved (Schoenfeld and Hamilton, 1977). Whether the lesion effect is due to the primary site of damage, to these "secondary" changes and effects, or to an interaction of both factors may be next to impossible to determine with any certainty. Franz Gall (1835), who opposed Flourens' use of the lesion method, seemed well aware of the interpretive difficulties involved in studying such material when he wrote, "How can we remove a part without affecting those that are contiguous to it? How can we remove the cerebellum, especially in the mammalia, without injuring the medulla oblongata and all the parts with which it communicates [p. 244]?" Although the experiments that Gall criticized were certainly not sophisticated by modern standards, his basic idea should still have meaning for contemporary experimenters using the lesion method to localize functions.

In the same way, it is important to realize that a comparable error can be made by assuming that the absence of a lesion effect must mean that the damaged area is in no way concerned with the function in question. If a neuronal system is both diffuse and redundant, an incomplete lesion may not have any obvious effects, even though, prior to injury, the area damaged could conceivably play a significant role in mediating the behavior being evaluated. Although some brain scientists tend to shy away from the notion, at least as applied to the mature mammalian brain, another possibility is that some other area has "taken over" the function normally mediated by the damaged region (i.e., vicariation). Thus, the paradigm that accepts the creation of brain lesions as a means of localizing functions in specific brain areas is not foolproof: *Neither the presence nor the absence of symptoms after a given lesion need necessarily show convincingly what a certain part of the brain is doing prior to injury or over the course of a lifetime.*

Does this mean that the lesion method is of no value in defining structure–function relationships in the nervous system? We do not believe so. Nor do we mean to imply that brain lesion research cannot contribute to a better understanding of how the nervous system works. In fact, in simple systems with few neurons (e.g., sea slugs) it may be possible to come to a fairly good understanding of the functions of specific parts by observing the changes that follow damage to the few elements that make up the animal's nervous system. Similarly, we have been able to learn much about the peripheral nervous system by examining the effects of injury to individual spinal nerves, for instance in determining how sensitivity changes in different parts of the skin following nerve damage. However, when we turn to the central nervous system of mammals, the ability of the lesion method to stand on its own as a way of defining "the functions" of various parts, such as the frontal lobes or the hippocampus, seems to break down in direct proportion to the complex interrelationships that those parts have with other parts of the brain and spinal cord.

Nevertheless, the behavioral data taken from brain-damaged subjects need not be viewed in isolation, and when combined with unit recordings, anatomical records, developmental profiles, and the like, more reasonable inferences can be made. In these cases, we only wish to point out that we are still dealing with *inferences* and not necessarily with proofs or iron-clad associations between structures and functions, although these inferences are sometimes treated as if they really are points of fact. It should be realized that each commonly used technique for determining structure–function relationships in the brain has its own limitations. Thus, when evaluating and integrating the results of a variety of different types of experiments ("convergent operations") it should not be forgotten that:

1. Electrical stimulation does not tell you what the stimulated region does normally; it tells you how the system as a whole responds to abnormal conditions at that point.
2. Infusion of a putative neurotransmitter at a particular locus does not tell you about the responsiveness of that region; it tells you how the whole system reacts to an unusual amount of substance at that point.
3. A single-unit recording tells you, not about the properties of that unit, but about the entire system to which it is connected (Glassman, 1978, p. 8).

In short, with regard to determining structure–function relationships in the brain, the lesion techniques may be less informative than often is believed. Even when combined with other procedures, the distinction between fact and theory should not be overlooked or treated trivially, especially when experiments dealing with recovery of function are evaluated. Recovery may not seem so "anomalous" (Chapter 1) or perplexing if greater recognition could be given to the idea that these phenomena may not be running contrary to fact, but rather contrary to theory.

There are a number of problems that are closely related to the logical and philosophical points that we have raised so far. One of the most fundamental issues that must be faced deals with the concept of *centers*, which was quite popular at the turn of the century and which remains with us even today (see Chapter 3 for more details). In brief, on the basis of the experiments that we have examined throughout this book, we no longer think that it is appropriate to view parts of the central nervous system as isolated, individual controlling centers. As O. L. Zangwill (1963), a respected British neuropsychologist has written

> There can be no doubt that a variety of behaviour patterns may be evoked by stimulation, or lost after ablation, of limited parts of the brain. But I do no think we should therefore postulate special "centres," that is to say, assemblies of neurones whose function it is to generate the behaviour in question. As Sherrington (1906) clearly saw, behaviour does not spring ready-made from the brain, like Athene from the head of Zeus. Rather it must be regarded as an integration of a large number of component activities. . . . No one level, not even the highest, can properly be regarded as the exclusive seat of a behaviour pattern [pp. 338–339].

Walle Nauta, of the Massachusetts Institute of Technology, also realized this at the time that he wrote the words that we cited at the beginning of this chapter. Rather than postulating isolated controlling centers, individuals like Nauta and Zangwill contended that all brain areas are acting as components of dynamic systems in which each part is under the influence of many other parts. But even this concept is often based upon the assumption that we know exactly what the parts are and what they do. Yet, the continually expanding study of neuro-anatomy shows that we are far from this "complete understanding" of neuronal circuitry. Each new technique seems to provide new and sometimes different information about the interconnections between brain parts. Often, the defining characteristics of the regions change as new discoveries are made.

With this consideration in mind, we should stress that despite the anatomical boundaries between parts of the brain, there is no a priori reason to assume that the contribution of any one part remains static over the course of a lifetime or even over shorter periods of time (see Stein and Firl, 1976). In fact, we think it is quite likely that the activity of the central nervous system is constantly in flux, with cells dying, new synapses being formed, and other changes continuously taking place. Thus, many internal and external events will interact to determine the effects of a brain lesion. That is, the genetic endowment of the organism, its past experiences, motivation to learn new responses, and structural changes in various parts of the brain before and after lesions all can contribute to the behavioral pattern that is observed at any given moment in time.

Insofar as behavior is concerned, the status of the rest of the brain can be just as important in determining symptomatology as the specific site of injury being examined. This realization can go far toward explaining why recovery from early brain damage is neither a principle, as Kennard (1938, 1940) had first thought, nor an artifact, as implied in the writings of other individuals.

The importance of the condition of the brain at the time of injury is not only something that pertains to cases of injury early in life. John Hughlings Jackson realized this over 100 years ago. In many of his papers (e.g., Jackson, 1879) he spoke of "negative" symptoms, which reflected the destruction of specific brain areas, and "positive" symptoms (e.g., exaggerated responses), which reflected the condition of the rest of the brain. In 1898, Jackson was most succinct about this when he stated, "One advantage of considering numerous maladies as dissolutions[1] is, that in doing so we are obliged in each case to deal with the diseased part as a flaw in the whole nervous system; we thus have to take into account the undamaged remainder and the evolution still going on in it [p. 422]."

Ralph Reitan, who is best known for a widely used test battery that is employed to localize the site of brain damage and to define the deficits involved, has also emphasized the status of the rest of the brain in cases of central nervous system injury. In 1966, Reitan wrote, "In terms of recovery of functions or deteriorative changes over time following a cerebral lesion, the adequacy of function of the supposedly non-involved areas of the cerebrum may well turn out to be the critical criterion [p. 135]."

Henry Head (1926) once argued that following brain damage, the remaining nervous system should be perceived as a new whole in itself. To this we might add that the response to brain injury must also be understood in the light of the organism's attempt to cope with the environment. That is, symptoms should not be perceived simply as a remnant of normal behavior, but as Kurt Goldstein (1939) would have emphasized, as *a totally new type* of behavior that reflects the adaptive capacity of the organism as it attempts to survive in its radically altered world. This position demands that we not only look at the lesion and the condition of the surrounding brain (the doughnut and the hole analogy), but at how the organism itself responds to interal and external environmental demands. Symptomatology would take on added meaning if interpreted in the context of adaptation, rather than only considering the descriptive nature of the deficits.

Is there another way to view and interpret the data collected in brain lesion experiments? As we have already indicated, we feel that when used alone, the lesion method is of questionable value if one's objective is to define the functions of particular brain areas. We have also pointed out that even when combined with other methods, all of which also have their drawbacks, its contribution toward defining structure–function relationships in the central nervous system is *still* more limited than is frequently assumed.

[1] Opposite of evolution.

Even though the lesion method may be found less than ideal for localizing functions, it can stil have important practical significance. That is, the study of brain lesions can be particularly valuable when it comes to determining the specific conditions under which brain damage would be more or less likely to produce symptoms. This orientation would specifically benefit neurologists, neuropsychologists, and others involved in patient care and rehabilitation (Chapter 17), since their main goal is the treatment and elimination of symptoms. In addition, since symptoms and not functions would be examined, hypotheses and theories about observable events (symptoms themselves) could be generated, which would be directly testable in laboratory and controlled clinical studies.

In previous chapters we have examined in considerable detail some of the factors (other than lesion locus) that may determine the outcome of brain injuries. One such variable is the age of the organism at the time damage is inflicted. Another relates to nonspecific environmental conditions (enrichment, restriction) both before and after brain damage. The role of early undernutrition is also worthy of our attention. The idea that recovery may be less likely after damage to the previously undernourished brain is only now beginning to be investigated, and initial results are suggesting that some differences seen in neurological patients can be accounted for by early nutritional history (Mangold, Bell, Gruenthal, and Finger, 1981).

In addition to these variables, the speed of growth of the lesion should receive more attention. With slow growing lesions, it it sometimes possible to damage even supposedly "critical" brain areas without overt symptoms appearing. As we noted earlier, the functional status of the rest of the brain may be just as important in determining behavior as the zone of destruction itself. In the clinic we may have to pay more attention to whether the lesion is due to stroke, tumor, injury, or disease, and examine in greater detail the patient's complete neurological history.

Some factors that may relate to this new "contextual" approach seem to have hardly been studied. One might be the role of specific skills in the patient's past history, and the issue of overtraining or overlearning prior to brain damage (Gabriel, Freer, and Finger, 1979; Weese, Neimand, and Finger, 1973). Another might be the genetic inheritance of the individual. With regard to the latter factor, not all brains show the exact same patterns of gyri and fissures, and chances are that specific areas differ both in size and physiological characteristics from patient to patient. More than 30 years ago, Clifford T. Morgan (1951) wrote

We find it natural to say that people are different in the measurements of personality, intelligence, or some other aspect of behavior, but we often seem to assume that brains are standard products turned out on an assembly line so that they look as much alike as new cars. The fact is that brains vary a lot in their size and shape. Lashley (1947) has been going into the matter lately, and he assures us that there are individual differences in brain anatomy. If that be true, why are there not individual differences in which areas of the brain get involved in different functions [p. 52]?

How far might we be from asking how this could relate to deficits and recovery? Could there be intrinsic differences in the capacities of different brains to recover? As Robert Glassman (1978) has theorized

> Conceivably, organisms . . . have some range of options as to which sets of neural structures to use in performing tasks. The initial tendency of one subject to use one or the other option might be determined by past experience or by very slight innate differences, say, in the number of cells in a nucleus. Repeated use of particular options would exaggerate individual differences, through learning [p. 24].

If Glassman is correct, genetic differences may help to explain the ease with which individuals may change strategies and, in turn, the high degree of variability that is typically encountered in brain lesion studies.

As we mentioned earlier in this chapter, data showing that the brain is in a constant state of change (cells dying each day, new synapses being formed, perhaps intense competition for vacated synaptic spaces) would be consistent with, and would be an integral part of, the position that we are now taking. Events such as sprouting and factors that would affect these reactions (Loy and Milner, 1980) would permit us to make more sense out of the individual differences that we see in behavior and may eventually allow us to anticipate individual behavior patterns in response to injury or disease. As we have stressed, it is only when the brain is viewed as a dynamic entity that is constantly undergoing change that individual variability in response to disease can be understood. It is only when the brain lesion is viewed in this context that we begin to get some indication of why subjects with lesions that look the same often respond so differently or show differential capabilities for recovery.

If we consider research on recovery from brain damage in this way, its contribution to the theory of localization of function may become ancillary to attempts to determine and manipulate those conditions that offer the most hope for functional improvements to the victims of central nervous system injury. If this is the case, researchers who use the lesion technique should stop confining themselves only to questions such as, "What are the functions of a given area?," and instead also devote themselves to more testable and clinically relevant questions, such as "How can we minimize the symptoms that often follow brain damage?," and "What are the individual limits to such adaptability?"

Despite our inability to determine precisely where functions are localized, an understanding of the conditions that can affect the appearance of symptoms after brain injury seems well within our grasp. As noted, dealing with observable symptoms will also have practical advantages (e.g., patient care) associated with it that are now beginning to be recognized. And in addition, such an orientation may again force us to look at the whole brain and organism with an understanding that seems to have been lost as technology and theoretical predispositions have pulled us further and further away from all but the locus of the damage itself.

As we have seen, the organism's entire response to brain injury is an important area for study and one in which considerably more work needs to be done. Yet, we will be the first to acknowledge that brain lesion studies with behavioral measures have often been confusing and difficult to interpret. We have argued that much of the confusion has come from attending to just the lesion site itself. When this happens, we tend to overlook small, but important differences in the environment, experiential backgrounds, and the like that could very much influence what kind of response the organism will make to its changed perceptual and behavioral status. Still, this may not account for all of the inconsistencies that have appeared in the literature. For this reason alone, it is important to ask whether there are ways in which lesion experiments and reports can be improved, regardless of whether one is doing lesion research with the hope of making inferences about the functions of particular parts of the brain or, as we have advocated, to study symptoms, recovery, and individual differences in response to neural damage.

We believe that lesion studies can take on added meaning with additional efforts in three directions. The first would be to determine if the course of events after damage follows an orderly progression or set of rules. As pointed out by Jay Braun (1978), attempting to describe the phases of recovery can have several advantages. It could provide a comprehensive basis for comparing different cases having damage in the same brain areas. In addition, knowledge of the phases and transitional states of recovery would allow us to assess rehabilitation techniques and patient or subject progress better than we do now.

Perhaps the best known example of this approach to recovery of function has been provided by Phillip Teitelbaum and his co-workers. These investigators examined the effects of lesions in the lateral hypothalamus. Rats with large, bilateral lesions in this region stop eating and would ordinarily die from starvation, even if food were present in their cages. Typically, these animals also refuse to drink. Teitelbaum and Stellar (1954) found that these rats could often be kept alive when special conditions were provided and that their recovery progressed through four stages in the orderly way that is shown in Figure 18.1.[2]

An analysis of the sequence of changes involved in recovery can be applied to human patients. One example of this involves concussions due to blast injuries where there is an initial unresponsiveness to auditory stimulation (see data of Ger-

---

[2] It is of considerable interest to note that the same four stages were found to be involved in recovery from lesions of the anterolateral neocortex, although, in this case, the rats progressed through the recovery cycle in only 7 days. In an experiment conducted by Braun in 1975, cortically damaged rats at first were aphagic and adipsic, then only ate highly palatable wet foods in inadequate amounts (anorexia and adipsia), and next took wet foods and nibbled on dry foods while refusing water (adipsia). This was followed by drinking (water) and an ability to regulate body weight on dry food alone, although the rats still were very finicky and somewhat different from normal animals in other ways.

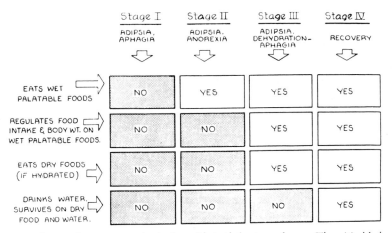

	Stage I	Stage II	Stage III	Stage IV
	ADIPSIA, APHAGIA	ADIPSIA, ANOREXIA	ADIPSIA, DEHYDRATION- APHAGIA	RECOVERY
EATS WET PALATABLE FOODS	NO	YES	YES	YES
REGULATES FOOD INTAKE & BODY WT. ON WET PALATABLE FOODS.	NO	NO	YES	YES
EATS DRY FOODS (IF HYDRATED)	NO	NO	YES	YES
DRINKS WATER. SURVIVES ON DRY FOOD AND WATER.	NO	NO	NO	YES

Figure 18.1. *Stages of recovery seen in the lateral hypothalamic syndrome. (The critical behavioral events that define the stages are listed on the left.) (From Teitelbaum, P., and Epstein, A. N. The lateral hypothalamic syndrome: Recovery of feeding and drinking after lateral hypothalamic lesions.* Psychological Review, 69, 74-90. *Copyright 1962 by the American Psychological Association. Reprinted by permission.)*

shuni, cited by Luria *et al.*, 1969, and also mentioned by Braun, 1978, pp. 191-192). These patients eventually leave this phase to enter another in which intense stimuli are necessary for eliciting physiological responses to sound (e.g., the cochleopupillary reflex—a dilation of the pupil to a sudden intense sound). In this phase there is no auditory perception; patients do not report hearing the intense sounds that they are capable of responding to physiologically. In Phase III the threshold for eliciting the physiological reflex diminishes, and the patients begin to hear loud sounds. Finally, they enter the last phase in which the threshold for auditory perception continues to come down to the point where hearing can occur with stimuli that are not intense enough to elicit the cochleopupillary reflex. This, of course, is more characteristic of normal auditory perception.

Lesion experiments would also be improved if researchers would distinguish more clearly between recovery as defined by means to a goal, and recovery as defined by accomplishing that goal (Laurence and Stein, 1978). Here it must be realized that a description of whether a brain-damaged organism can achieve a goal is *not* sufficient to explain the mechanisms that lead to the improved behavior. If an understanding of the process(es) for recovery is desirable, then the *means* or strategies by which organisms adapt to their environmental demands must also be examined very carefully. As Kurt Goldstein (1939) aptly stressed, we need to think in terms of how the organism solves problems, and this is true even in cases where "goals" are defined arbitrarily by an experimenter working in an artificial testing situation. Furthermore, as noted by Laurence and Stein (1978), it should be recognized that there are no rigid or necessary relationships between means and ends. A particular goal may be accomplished by any of a number of means, and identical means may, in different contexts, accomplish entirely different ends.

Our third suggestion relates to the use of group statistics such as t tests, analyses of variance, and measures of covariance. The point is not whether these procedures are appropriate or not for this type of work. Rather, the question is whether we are truly presenting an accurate picture of the response to brain injury when *only* normative data are presented and discussed.

The fact of the matter is that even in the laboratory where damage and behavioral testing can take place under highly controlled conditions, the behavioral outcome is rarely uniform. Yet, sometimes we seem so entranced by the behavior displayed by some subjects that show deficits that we fail to acknowledge that there may be other subjects who perform more normally or who possibly do not show any lesion effects at all. When this happens, we should first see whether there are differences between the brains of the subjects that do not show the deficit. If there are, the variability can be explained relatively easily. If not, the fact that there are exceptions should still be emphasized since the failure to do so may only lead to more ''principles'' and ''rules'' that in reality must only be recognized as probabilistic statements, at least until more can be learned about them.

Although group statistics have their places, individual differences in response to brain injury should not be overlooked. In terms of relevance for people with brain damage, it may be the latter cases (absence of deficits) that prove most interesting and informative. Indeed, these are the cases that might best teach us how recovery can be enhanced or how performance can be protected from oncoming brain disease.

In conclusion, we can only reemphasize that in the last few years much progress has been made with regard to achieving a better understanding of neuroplasticity and, on a behavioral level, recovery of function. New discoveries are now being made with such rapidity that it is difficult to think that many of the questions that are being asked by anatomists, physiologists, and behavioral scientists today would have seemed out of line even a generation ago.

One of our purposes in writing this book was to present some of the new findings in neurobiology and to associate them with phenomena we think we understand. Another was to probe into the logic that guides most brain lesion research in order to see if appropriate questions are being asked. We also wanted to present another way of looking at brain lesion data—one that would suggest new strategies for rehabilitation and therapy.

We will feel gratified about our efforts if this book is able to stimulate further thinking about such issues as localization in the brain, recovery from brain damage, the meaning of plasticity, and the ability of the nervous system to adapt as a unified whole to trauma and disease. These issues are contemporary and yet, they represent questions that may be with us for many years to come. We think it can be said with some certainty that the more we learn about these issues, the greater will be the benefit to patients suffering neurological damage and to scientists in their endeavor to comprehend the nature of the relationship between brain and behavior in both health and disease. Although the goals are not new, we are still in the early stages of comprehension. And, as we have tried to show, efforts to reach these goals, when based on the "pursuit of anomalies," cannot be considered, in Kuhn's terminology (Chapter 1), "trivial" undertakings.

References

Braun, J. J. Neocortex and feeding behavior in the rat. *Journal of Comparative and Physiological Psychology*, 1975, *89*, 507–522.

Braun, J. J. Time and recovery from brain damage. In S. Finger (Ed.), *Recovery from brain damage: Research and theory*. New York: Plenum, 1978, Pp. 165–197.

Dallenbach, K. M. The history and derivation of the word *function* as a systematic term in psychology. *American Journal of Psychology*, 1915, *26*, 473–484.

Ferrier, D. *The localisation of cerebral disease*. London: Smith, Elder, 1878.

Gabriel, S., Freer, B., and Finger, S. Brain damage and the overlearning reversal effect. *Physiological Psychology*, 1979, *7*, 327–332.

Gall, F. [*On the functions of the brain and each of its parts: With observations on determining the instincts, propensities, and talents, or the moral and intellectual dispositions of men and animals, by the configuration of the brain and head* (Vol. 3.)] (W. Lewis, Jr., trans.). Boston: Marsh, Capen and Lyon, 1835.

Glassman, R. B. The logic of the lesion experiment and its role in the neural sciences. In S. Finger (Ed.), *Recovery from brain damage: Research and theory*. New York: Plenum, 1978, Pp. 3–31.

Goldstein, K. *The organism*. New York: American Book Company, 1939.

Gregory, R. L. The brain as an engineering problem. In R. Thorpe and O. Zangwill (Eds.), *Current problems in animal behavior*. Cambridge, Mass.: Cambridge University Press, 1964, Pp. 307–330.

Head, H. *Aphasia and kindred disorders of speech*. Cambridge, Mass.: Cambridge University Press, 1926.

Jackson, J. H. On affections of speech from disease of the brain. *Brain*, 1879, *2*, 323–356.

Jackson, J. H. Relations of different divisions of the central nervous system to one another and to parts of the body. *Lancet*, 1898. (Reprinted in J. Taylor, Ed., *Selected writings of John Hughlings Jackson*. New York: Basic Books, 1958, Pp. 422–443.)

Kennard, M. A. Reorganization of motor function in the cerebral cortex of monkeys deprived of motor and premotor areas in infancy. *Journal of Neurophysiology*, 1938, *1*, 477–496.

Kennard, M. A. Relation of age to motor impairment in man and sub-human primates. *Archives of Neurology and Psychiatry*, 1940, *44*, 377–397.

Lashley, K. S. Structural variation in the nervous system in relation to behavior. *Psychological Review*, 1947, *54*, 325–334.

Laurence, S., and Stein, D. G. Recovery after brain damage and the concept of localization of function. In S. Finger (Ed.), *Recovery from brain damage: Research and theory*. New York: Plenum, 1978, Pp. 369–407.

Loy, R., and Milner, T. A. Sexual dimorphism in extent of axonal sprouting in rat hippocampus. *Science*, 1980, *208*, 1282–1284.

Luria, A. R., Maydin, V. L., Tsvetkova, L. S., and Vinarskaya, E. N. Restoration of higher cortical function following local brain damage. In F. J. Vinkin and G. G. Bruyn (Eds.), *Handbook of clinical neurology* (Vol. 3). North Holland Publishing, 1969, 368–433.

Mangold, R. F., Bell, J., Gruenthal, M., and Finger, S. Undernutrition and recovery from brain damage. *Brain Research*, 1981, *230*, 406–411.

Miller, G., Pribram, K., and Gallanter, E. *Plans and the organization of behavior*. New York: Holt, 1960.

Morgan, C. T. Some structural factors in perception. In R. R. Blake and G. V. Ramsey (Eds.), *Perception: An approach to personality*. New York: Ronald Press, 1951.

Nauta, W. H. J. M. Cited in discussion of: Stamm, J. S., Retardation and facilitation in learning by stimulation of frontal cortex in monkeys. In J. M. Warren and K. Akert (Eds.), *The frontal granular cortex and behavior*. New York: McGraw-Hill, 1964, P. 125.

Prince, M. Cerebral localization from the point of view of function and symptoms. *Journal of Nervous and Mental Diseases*, 1910, *37*, 337–354.

Reitan, R. Problems and prospects in studying the psychological correlates of brain lesions. *Cortex*, 1966, *2*, 127–153.

Ruckmich, C. A. The use of the term "function" in English textbooks of psychology. *American Journal of Psychology*, 1913, *24*, 99–123.

Schoenfeld, T. A., and Hamilton, L. W. Secondary brain changes following lesions: A new paradigm for lesion experimentation. *Physiology and Behavior*, 1977, *18*, 951–967.

Sherrington, C. S. *The integrative action of the nervous system*. New Haven, Conn.: Yale University Press, 1906.

Stein, D. G., and Firl, A. C. Brain damage and reorganization of function in old age. *Experimental Neurology*, 1976, *52*, 157–167.

Teitelbaum, P., and Epstein, A. N. The lateral hypothalamic syndrome: Recovery of feeding and drinking after lateral hypothalamic lesions. *Psychological Review*, 1962, *69*, 74–90.

Teitelbaum, P., and Stellar, E. Recovery from the failure to eat produced by hypothalamic lesions. *Science*, 1954, *120*, 894–895.

Weese, G. D., Neimand, D., and Finger, S. Cortical lesions and somesthesis in rats: Effects of training and overtraining prior to surgery. *Experimental Brain Research*, 1973, *16*, 542–550.

Zangwill, O. L. The cerebral localisation of psychological function. *Advancement of Science*, 1963, *20*, 335–344.

Author Index

Subject Index